Birth-Throes of the Israeli Homeland

The book brings forth various perspectives on the Israeli "homeland" (*moledet*) from various known Israeli intellectuals such as Boaz Evron, Menachem Brinker, Jacqueline Kahanoff and more. Binding together various academic fields to deal with the question of the essence of the Israeli homeland: from the examination of the status of the Israeli homeland by such known sociologist as Michael Feige, to the historical analysis of Robert Wistrich of the place Israel occupies in history in relation to historical antisemitism.

The study also examines various movements that bear significant importance on the development of the notion of the Israeli homeland in Israeli society: Such movement as "The New Hebrews" and Hebrewism are examined both historically in relation to their place in Zionist history and ideologically in comparison with other prominent movements. Drawing on the work of Jacqueline Kahanoff to provide a unique Mediterranean model for the Israeli homeland, the volume examines prominent models among the Religious Zionist sector of Israeli society regarding the relation of the biblical homeland to the actual homeland of our times.

Discussing the various interpretations of the concept of the nation and its land in the discourse of Hebrew and Israeli identity, the book is a key resource for scholars interested in nationalism, philosophy, modern Jewish history and Israeli Studies.

David Ohana studies modern European and Israel Studies. His affiliations have included the Hebrew University of Jerusalem, the Sorbonne, Harvard University, the University of California, Berkeley, and École des Hautes Études en Sciences Sociales, Paris and life member at Clare Hall College, Cambridge. He is a full professor of History at Ben-Gurion University of the Negev, Israel.

Routledge Jewish Studies Series

Series Editor: Oliver Leaman, *University of Kentucky*

Jewish Studies, which are interpreted to cover the disciplines of history, sociology, anthropology, culture, politics, philosophy, theology, religion, as they relate to Jewish affairs. The remit includes texts which have as their primary focus issues, ideas, personalities and events of relevance to Jews, Jewish life and the concepts which have characterized Jewish culture both in the past and today. The series is interested in receiving appropriate scripts or proposals.

The Making of Modern Jewish Identity
Ideological Change and Religious Conversion
Motti Inbari

Charity in Rabbinic Judaism
Atonement, Rewards, and Righteousness
Alyssa M. Gray

Deconstructing the Talmud
The Absolute Book
Federico Dal Bo

The Divine in Modern Hebrew Literature
Neta Stahl

The Holocaust in Thessaloniki
Reactions to the Anti-Jewish Persecution, 1942–1943
Leon Saltiel

Birth-Throes of the Israeli Homeland
The Concept of Moledet
David Ohana

For more information about this series, please visit:
www.routledge.com/middleeaststudies/series/JEWISH

Birth-Throes of the Israeli Homeland

The Concept of Moledet

David Ohana

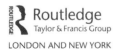

LONDON AND NEW YORK

First published 2020
by Routledge
2 Park Square, Milton Park, Abingdon, Oxon OX14 4RN

and by Routledge
52 Vanderbilt Avenue, New York, NY 10017

Routledge is an imprint of the Taylor & Francis Group, an informa business

British Library Cataloguing-in-Publication Data
A catalogue record for this book is available from the British Library

Library of Congress Cataloging-in-Publication Data
Names: Ohana, David, author.
Title: Birth-throes of the Israeli homeland : the concept of moledet /
David Ohana.
Description: Milton Park, Abingdon, Oxon ; New York, NY : Routledge,
2020. |
Series: Routledge Jewish studies series | Includes bibliographical
references and index.
Identifiers: LCCN 2020001102 (print) | LCCN 2020001103 (ebook) |
ISBN 9780367898694 (hardback) | ISBN 9781003021599 (ebook) |
ISBN 9781000067422 (adobe pdf) | ISBN 9781000067484 (epub) |
ISBN 9781000067453 (mobi)
Subjects: LCSH: Zionism–History. | Israel–History.
Classification: LCC DS149 .O437 2020 (print) | LCC DS149 (ebook) |
DDC 320.54095694–dc23
LC record available at https://lccn.loc.gov/2020001102
LC ebook record available at https://lccn.loc.gov/2020001103

ISBN: 978-0-367-89869-4 (hbk)
ISBN: 978-0-367-49272-4 (pbk)
ISBN: 978-1-003-02159-9 (ebk)

Typeset in Times New Roman
by Wearset Ltd, Boldon, Tyne and Wear

Contents

Introduction
Whence and whither the homeland

The homeland is the original, primordial foundation of our lives, and it is the object of our deepest feelings, our hopes, fears, consolations. It is the source of life, but it sometimes leads one into a dark hole. The questions it poses are the fundamental questions of the great religions: the lust for life and the mystery of what is after, sacrifice and purification, self-denial and consolation, where we come from, where we are going. The homeland transforms "I" into "us," experience into memory, a territory into a land, and both into a nation. It is not surprising if modern nationalism, which made a transposition of many of the concepts of religion, sees the homeland as the cradle, the very beginning of the national collective.

The birth-throes of the homeland are not merely a matter of territory or soil, but of lands with an ancient historical association, the source of a deep-rooted national identity. But the birth-throes of the homeland can also be metaphorical. There are some for whom the birth-throes of the homeland are not enough and who long to be connected with a country together with the rest of their people, half of whom do not yet live in the homeland. There are some for whom the birth-throes of the homeland are unlimited and they long to be connected to the global village. There are some who believe that the time has come to settle their dispute with their neighbors by dividing up the homeland. There are some for whom the birth-throes of the homeland are moral, a "light unto the nations" or chosen people. There are some for whom the birth-throes of the homeland are theological, for "the earth is the Lord's and the fullness thereof," and there are yet other dreamers of dreams for whom the birth-throes of the homeland have a great variety of meanings.

The birth-throes of the homeland are like an umbilical cord. The homeland is the mother who gives birth to the nation in its land. The homeland imprints on its children a seal that can never be removed. The Uganda project failed because it sought to remove the umbilical cord and the seal, an act which meant the erasure of any affinity between the birth-throes of the homeland and the nation longing to return to its bosom. But in many cases the birth-throes of the homeland are tied to the birth-throes of the Messiah. Sometimes a long expectation of the fulfillment of the birth-throes of a country creates a national frustration that gives birth to messianic longings. Where there are birth-throes of the homeland detached from nation-states and there is a demand to restore them or a demand for ownership, it does not result in neutrality. The existence of neighboring states makes these states into bitter enemies, for one is speaking of a dispute concerning mother earth, the homeland, the nation-state umbilically tied to its progeny – the birth-throes of the land. That is how the national controversies and messianic movements in the Sudetenland, among the Basques, in the Balkans and in Alsace came into being. The demand to liberate the ties to the homeland leads to the formation of messianic expectations.

Birth-throes

Moledet in the Bible has a different meaning from more recent terms such as Vaterland (the father-land in medieval Germany), and patria (the land of the forefathers in Latin). The scholar of nationalism Anthony Smith thought that modern man cannot exist without a homeland which has two characteristics that are really one: a homeland requires a national soil and a social body which constitutes a sovereign political entity. Does this modern description of a homeland correspond to the biblical idea of a moledet? In the modern age, said Smith, the activities of the centralized and reflective state are of two main kinds: population censuses and mapping.[1] Clearly, these concepts of a homeland bound up with modern population management and technical development are foreign to the spirit of the Bible. Shalom Rosenberg suggested seeing the biblical idea of the land and Jerusalem as a "mother" as an alternative interpretation to the modern concept of a homeland.[2] In his opinion, the dominant activity characterizing the biblical concept, unlike the activity governing the modern one, is giving birth. Yehuda Elitzur also thought that the biblical meaning of moledet is connected to birth – the progeny, the tribe, the family, the paternal home. The idea of the Land of Israel as a homeland that gives historical rights to an ethnic group is not consistent, in his opinion, with biblical thought. Hence the affinity that I propose between the birth-throes of the homeland and labor pains: the land is the mother, man is what she gives birth to. Man is connected to his homeland by an umbilical cord. This idea of a homeland was given many meanings from the Second Temple period onward. I will now suggest five distinctions to explain the different meanings of this concept.

The first distinction is that between the affinity of the individual and the affinity of the generality. Does the distinction between the individual's affinity to his country and his affinity to his country through his mother – i.e. the collective – have any meaning for the homeland? The concept "homeland" indicates a connection between an individual and a territory, but also one between a people – as a general representation of individuals – and a territory. Philo claimed that the Jews overseas saw the places in which they settled as their homeland. In addition to their loyalty to their various "homelands" they had a loyalty to the Holy City and the Holy Land (Jerusalem and the land of Israel) – the metropolis. By the term "metropolis," Philo meant a place outside the homeland which was the focus of the allegiance of the individual born in the homeland. The innovation represented by the concept "metropolis" created the dual possibility of seeing an individual as born in Egypt, for instance, but at the same time of seeing his people as native to the land of Israel. This possibility indicated a change from the "Jewish homeland" to "the homeland of the Jewish people" which also exists in modern thought. Nathan Rotenstreich, for example, said that "the return to the land" can be understood in two ways: as the immigration of a population and its settlement in a country in a way that does not depend on the rights of the people settling there (the Jewish one), or as the return of a people which claims historical rights – "our rebirth as a return to its historical homeland."[3] It is this form of return that in the last 100 years has created the tragic conflict between two peoples who claim the same homeland.

The second distinction is that between a human love and a divinely ordained duty. If it is a matter of love, the affinity of a people to its land is a natural one; moreover, the question of sovereignty and justification is something separate from that of the affinity and connection of a people to its land. But if it is a question of theology, the connection between the people and its land is a divine commandment, and thus the question of sovereignty has also to be regarded as a theological matter.

In his book *A Land of Two Peoples*, Martin Buber proposed a special approach to the affinity of the Jewish people to the land of Israel.[4] It was not a mass-revelation as Judah Halevy believed, nor ideas like monotheism, nor historical experiences special to the Jewish people, but the special nature of the connection of the Jewish people to the land of Israel. The Jews are the only people that connected the land and people through a divine promise which made it a mission and a duty. Hence, Buber's denial of a "natural," external justification of a connection between the people and land of Israel. The historical right to the land of Israel is "external" to the existence of the Jewish people, and it bestows a legitimacy similar to the right of every people to its country, the universal right given to all peoples through the love and attraction of every man to the "real" place of his birth. But the affinity of the people of Israel to its land is a special one. In this case, the people and land are not two different entities brought together by chance or the laws of logic, but there is an essential connection between the people and its land. The Jewish national movement has a theological significance: the word "Zion" indicates not only a connection between the people and its land given retroactively by chance or by right of birth, but is a connection reflecting a divine and human choice compelling the people of Israel and its God with regard to the fate of the land of Israel.

As against Buber, another connection is made between the people and its homeland through a phenomenological theory that focuses on a relationship of love.[5] Because love is a relationship of passive attention yet requires a subject and an object, this relationship permits the subject to be exposed to the significance of the object of its love. The people of Israel is a people like any other in the sense that its affinity to the land of Israel is an affinity of love. The land of Israel is the place where the soul of the people of Israel seeks to develop its cultural activities, the horizons of meaning opened up by its love. This primordial relationship of love cannot easily be translated into terms of political philosophy such as "rule" and "sovereignty." The love-relationship is an essential condition in that it establishes the affinity between the people and land, but it is not enough in itself to create sovereignty. Sovereignty must be viewed in relation to the practical requirements necessitated by concrete situations. For instance, does sovereignty in the land of Israel today help the people of Israel to develop its culture or does it prevent it from realizing its love? Such questions are really extraneous to the discussion of love and involve considerations of practicality and political philosophy.

The third distinction is that between the Promethean passion (the "pioneering passion" as Boaz Neumann called it[6]) and a historicistic approach to the homeland which by its very nature is passive. The Promethean nature of the modern Jews who sought to return to their country and to history was expressed in their desire to mold the country with their own hands. This voluntary act derived from the modern self-awareness of the individual who creates himself, his world and his country by himself. According to Neumann, the pioneering passion of the Second and Third Aliyahs contained within it an ecstatic element which blurred boundaries, and at the same time a disciplined element which established them. This was not a chronological relationship or a causal, circumstantial or spatial one. The relationship between the elements was simultaneous. The sweat dropping to the earth from the body of the pioneer was a flow that blurred the boundaries between the pioneer and the land of Israel, and thus the pioneer became part of the homeland. At the same time, that same sweat created frontiers, made the soil of the homeland Jewish and established the boundary between Jewish and Arab lands. The ecstatic, boundary-blurring element in the pioneers' relationship to the homeland was expressed in an affinity to the soil, the landscape and the region. On the other hand, the disciplined element secured the homeland through the construction of wells, roads, and settlements. This was representative of a number of historicistic approaches, beginning with Moses Mendelssohn and the Haskalah and ending with a variety of nativistic approaches. The common factor of all these was that they related to the homeland in a passive, natural way, whether the homeland was foreign or whether it was autarchic, a restorative return to the past. To this may be added that the biblical approach also regarded the Jews as exilic: that is to say, a group which had to accept a temporary situation as a moral duty wherever they lived, and even in the land of Israel.

The fourth distinction is that between the land of Israel and exile. If the distinction between the Promethean passion and the historicistic view is one of approach, that between Israel and the exile is one of content. The content of the land of Israel is varied, but it is always a central axis for those committed to it, whether it seen as a spiritual center as envisaged by Ahad Ha-Am, or the country is seen as the Holy Land, or it is a messianic belief that in the future all the Jews of the Diaspora will be gathered into the land. As against this, there is the exilic view with its many gradations. Jean Améry, for example, "a European man, a Jewish man, a man uprooted from his country, who had been in the concentration camps, a man who put an end to his life," saw Austria as his only homeland, and after the Nazis cruelly took it away from him, he never found another. He described in a concise and passionate manner what his lost homeland meant to him:

> Well, one day it happened that the German living below our hiding place felt disturbed in his afternoon rest by our talk and our doings. He climbed the stairs, pounded on the door, and stepped noisily across the threshold: an SS man [...] Every one of us was pale with deadly fear, [...] The man, however, in his unbuttoned uniform jacket, with dishevelled hair, staring at us with sleep-drugged eyes, did not have any intentions appropriate to his trade as a hunting dog. Bellowing, he demanded only peace for himself and his comrade, who was tired from night duty. He made his demand-and for me this was the truly frightening part of the episode in the dialect of my more immediate native region. [...] for the fellow, who at this moment, to be sure, was not exactly after my life, but whose joyfully fulfilled task it was to take people like me in as large numbers as possible to a death camp, appeared to me suddenly as a potential friend. Was it not enough to address him in his, my language in order to then celebrate our regional patriotism and our reconciliation over a glass of wine?[7]

For Améry, his homeland meant first and foremost security: "At most, it can be objected that exile is perhaps not an incurable disease, since one can make a home of foreign countries by a long life in them and with them; that is called finding a new home."[8] But, in fact, he believed that the homeland is an established fact and not something acquired. It is a fixed, unchanging component of one's personality: "Just as one learns one's mother tongue without knowing its grammar, one experiences one's native surroundings." The homeland is the world in which we grow up. It must have political sovereignty and an independent social body, and, as Améry said: "Whoever has no fatherland-that is to say, no shelter in an autonomous social body representing an independent governmental entity-has, so I believe, no homeland either."[9] For some major Jewish thinkers, exile is their true homeland. Unlike those that see "exile" as a text, as alienation, as estrangement, as the spread of universal and avant-garde ideas, in the various formulations of Hermann Cohen, Franz Rosenzweig, Hannah Arendt, Bernard Lazare, Edmond Jabès, George Steiner and the brothers Daniel and Jonathan Boyarin, there are many Jews like Jean Améry for whom "exile" is a real place, not an abstract place like a text or a universal Jewish mission but a concrete homeland that lies outside the borders of the land of Israel.

The fifth distinction is that between Canaanite assertion and crusader opposition. The homeland, according to the Canaanite idea which is based on the French model, is a fusion of place and language. Hebrew nationhood is a territorial, nativistic nationhood born in the Canaanite space, and the homeland exists only in that physical space. The cultural construction of language and place makes the immigrant into a native. Being truly or metaphorically born in the space is what constitutes the people of the homeland. The Canaanite view is that the Israelis are only from here. As against this, the Crusader opposition sees the Hebrew "sons of the homeland" as inauthentic colonialist westerners who have occupied a foreign land and subjugated the locally born natives.[10] According to this view, the Jewish colonialist project is alien to the homeland. The Israelis are not from here.

The Zionists, as we know, returned to the homeland and not to the formative areas of the homeland. Hebron or Shechem were far from the reach or ambitions of the pioneers, the members of the first waves of immigration. The "new Hebrew" took his distance from sacred history and concentrated on building up the new country. When it settled in the land of the Philistines, secular Zionism did not attempt to find a substitute for the places of sacred history found in the biblical narrative. The inability to reach those parts of the country only a short distance away increased the value of what was withheld, the longing for those places, like Moses gazing at the promised land from Mount Nebo. In this way, Zionism preserved a longing for the land of the Bible not in its grasp. In far-away America, the founding of the town of Jericho in the United States created a connection between that town and the biblical Jericho, but it also reflected a discrepancy with the text which was the source of the name Jericho.[11] And the existence of Jericho in a place near to yet inaccessible to secular Zionist settlement only increased the "missing presence" as Martin Heidegger called it.[12] The Jews of the exile related to the Holy Places through language and prayer, and in this way mitigated their lack of immediate presence. The use of the name "Jerusalem" for other towns as in "the Jerusalem of Lithuania" or the name "Hebron" for yeshivas was an indirect form of sanctification. Parallel with this, secular Zionism had unsatisfied longings for places within its reach, longings that came into the open with the conquest of those places in the Six-Day War. Much has been said about the euphoria after that war, but insufficient attention has been paid to the spiritual make-up of secular Zionism which longed to return to the ancient water-holes.

The sanctification of the primeval space is connected with the sanctification of time. In the collective consciousness, the legacies of the past in the historical land are both static and dynamic. They are static in the sense that our imagination is formed by historiography, songs, epics, legends, that create narratives of a continuous connection between areas of the land in ancient myth – in our case, the Holy Bible – and modern individuals living here and now. But these legacies are also dynamic in the sense that their image changes in the course of time. The kingdom of David and Solomon has grown larger or smaller in accordance with the winds prevailing in the historiographical or archaeological intellectual climate. The wish to revive it has also changed in accordance with political circumstances. For instance, David Ben-Gurion, who repeatedly used the expression "weeping for generations" to express his regret at the consequences of not having insisted on conquering the West Bank in the War of Independence, after the Six-Day War recognized the limitations of power and the force of necessity.

The father of the homeland

David Ben-Gurion was a son of the Second Aliyah in which the ideal of halutz-iut (pioneering), which was a central value of the Zionist ethos, grew up and developed. This ideal derived from the European socialist tradition of a van-guard, a special restricted group which went before the camp with a correct vision of the course the future should take. The Nietzschean philosophy of the Übermensch and the centrality of the will and Frederick Turner's thesis about the American frontier and the forming of the individualistic pioneer were very important in the consciousness of the pioneers and in the writings about them.[13] The classic pioneering principles were contentment with little, engagement in manual labor, a preference for agricultural work, a readiness to participate in major national enterprises, an all-round ability rather than limited professional expertise, and cultural and intellectual creativity. The halutz (pioneer) was an individualist but at the same time harnessed himself to national objectives.[14] With the founding of the state, there was a considerable lessening of the importance of the pioneering ethos, and Ben-Gurion's decision to join a kibbutz in the Negev was connected with this development and his attempt to change the situation.

The idea of going to the Negev and continuing with pioneering proposed by Ben-Gurion did not attract the youth or the general public. If in the 1950s there was a strong feeling that the time of pioneering had passed, this was infinitely more true in Ben-Gurion's final years. After the Six-Day War, which shifted the attention of the public to other areas, settlement in the Negev lost the little attraction it had before. A famous song was written in a pioneering spirit by Naomi Shemer praising the settlement of Nahal (the pre-military cadet corps) in Sinai. At the time of Ben-Gurion's death, the public's attention was focused on what was happening on the frontiers of the state, and the vision of pioneering in the Negev was further away than ever. In the years after his death, the debate about settlement was concerned with the settlements of Gush Emunim (The Bloc of the Faithful),[15] and the Negev was even further away.

Ben-Gurion's choice to be buried in the desert, just as he chose to live in the desert, had a dual significance. On the one hand, according to the pioneering ethos, the desert was a virginal place devoid of history, a place in which the future would be written. On the other hand, it was connected with the ancient history of the people and its formative moments, with ancient myths which were a principal component of the Israeli ethos. According to the biblical nar-rative, the people of Israel passed on their way to the land of Israel through Nahal Zin. It is not certain that the wadi called by that name was really the place the children of Israel passed through, not to speak of the fact that archae-ologists today are doubtful of the truth of the historical account of the exodus. The choice of the name "Nahal Zin" was an arbitrary decision of the naming committee for the Negev set up by Ben-Gurion himself in 1949, immediately after the end of the battles of the War of Independence.[16] It can also be said that even if the name was correct, it would have shown that the Negev, and certainly the site of the grave, lay outside the land of Israel, on the way to the country which in the Bible would become the moledet.[17] At the same time, it seems that Ben-Gurion's intention was to connect with the ancient myth which he was eager to cultivate when he identified with the Bible, especially where the exodus from Egypt was concerned. From the mythical point of view, the founding father of Hebrew independence looked from the cliff at the place where the children of Israel passed on their way to the country. In other words, the choice of the place was not motivated by family, community, or political considerations: it was a connection with the founding myth of the nation. As he attempted to do in his life, Ben-Gurion depicted himself symbolically as part of the monumental history of the Jewish people in his own interpretation, while ignoring the questions bound up with the social, political and even physical reality of his time.

Shabtai Teveth noted this in an article titled "King of the Desert," in which he wrote: "Ben-Gurion was not only buried in the land of his ancestors but also in a place that reflected and recalled the Bible. The child of our Bible was gathered to his fathers Abraham, Isaac and Jacob."[18] And Michael Ben-Zohar asked at the end of his biography of Ben-Gurion:

> What did he see when he stood on the cliff face and embraced the endless space with his eyes? The land of Israel which he loved with such a strong, total love? Thus stood Moses on another summit, in a different time, and savored with his eyes the land he had promised to his people. Thus Joshua saw the land he had conquered with the sword. Thus he too had looked towards the land when he came to its coasts as a youth, moved and thrilled, and did not know he had come to inherit it.[19]

A less grandiloquent explanation of his move to Sde Boker was given by Tom Segev in a new biography he wrote of Ben-Gurion:

> It was not only because the place was isolated and had an atmosphere of pioneering […], not only because he dreamed of a new beginning […], but because "the first cowboys' village", as Davar called it, was no longer considered a kibbutz.

On the attraction of this individualistic leader to individualists like himself, Segev added dryly:

> A tour in the desert left him with a deep depression. The vast spaces of the desert – "You don't know what they were created for", he wrote. "Several times the question arises with me in these journeys whether I didn't make a mistake in my position on the conquest of the Negev".[20]

In the Israeli collective memory, Ben-Gurion, the first prime minister, is regarded as the father of the renewed homeland, the founder of the state who even proclaimed its founding, but his image has lost the intensity and the controversial character it possessed in the past. For most of Israeli society, he can be described as a commonplace, inoffensive icon which does not arouse controversy and does not demand action.[21] He has become a picture on the wall, a background like a flag flapping in the wind, or a state symbol which every political camp can and is allowed to adopt for its purposes. The banalization of his memory allows different political camps and opposing public positions to connect to the dead leader, even if in his lifetime he related to many of those who connected to his memory and celebrated his name after his death with hostility and contempt. Moreover, his outlook was opposed to major directions taken by Israeli society. The father of the nation, who was perceived as the main bearer of the values of pioneering and mamlachtiyut (statism), has now become a figure of subversive potential. The contrast between the pioneering outlook and the vast process of privatization in the state of Israel is very marked, and his statist outlook is also opposed to the ever-increasing sectorialization of Israeli society.

As statist and impressive as the ceremonies in his memory may be, there are also ceremonies in memory of his rivals. Here we do not mean consensual statist figures like Herzl or Weizmann but the figure of the Baba Sali, for example, and the huge hillula (festivity) in his memory that takes place every year next to his grave, and to a certain extent the person contemptuously called the "secular Baba Sali," the prime minister Yitzhak Rabin, and the ceremonies and events in his memory. While the figure of Ben-Gurion is said to be uniting and encompassing, its competitors attract particular social groups and repel most of the others.[22] The figure of Ben-Gurion can be seen. despite all the confrontations and disputes in which he was involved in his life, as an inclusive symbol in the face of strong centrifugal tendencies. The lip-service paid at his ceremony by the leaders of Israel, including those who played a large part in promoting the processes of fragmentation and sectorialization overtaking society, reflects the subversive potential of a figure like Ben-Gurion, a potential which is not realized.

Yeshiyahu Leibowitz used to say that the State of Israel (he was referring chiefly to the prime minister, Ben-Gurion) had succeeded in destroying the subversive potential of religion by exercising control over it.[23] Similarly, one may say that the State of Israel attempts, apparently successfully, to destroy the subversive potential of the mythical figure of Ben-Gurion by exercising control over it, and the annual ceremonies that take place by his graveside are the chief means of achieving this. These ceremonies not only exploit Ben-Gurion but to a great extent also erase and blot out the subversive elements in his image. If one examines them, one sees how the centrality and marginality of Ben-Gurion, which go together, appear in them again and again, and give him a preeminent position as the father of the reborn homeland, a homeland which he already might not recognize. The national leadership uses the ceremonies in order to express its values and draw the public to them.[24] These ceremonies, recurring every year, are part of the symbolic aspect of nationhood. Together with the flag, the national anthem, coins and stamps, they constitute the Israeli civil religion.[25] Banknotes, coins and stamps, which change in the course of time, allow an elasticity between the symbol and what is symbolized. The ceremonies have an even greater elasticity. The ceremony is based on a performance recreated each time, and thus it undergoes a process of change in accordance with the changes in the performance.

One of the greatest influences on Ben-Gurion was Micha Yosef Berdichevsky, who formed the young leader to an even greater extent than Ahad Ha-Am. Ben-Gurion needed this Nietzschean thinker to help him liberate himself from the shackles of Jewish tradition, from the excessive Jewish spirituality, from the oppressiveness of Jewish history. He was a thinker who called for a change of values, for a preference for life over study and memory. Living people cannot exist without forgetting, just as they cannot live without memory, but an excess of memory paralyzes the power of action and decision. And this is how Menahem Brinker formulated the main question concerning the culture of the national rebirth: did the Jewish people at the turn of the century have the capacity of renewal to make a new beginning? For, without a renewal, there was no chance that the Jewish people would survive in the modern age. In Berdichevsky, the analysis of the individual in Nietzsche underwent a transformation into national terms. He thought that Jewish culture had become old and feeble and needed energies which would restore its youth. The metaphor of Hebrew rebirth was much used by Ahad Ha-Am, but it was also common in Berdichevsky, who proposed grafting Nietzsche onto Herder. In Nietzsche's opinion, the idea of the equality of human values as applied to the historical consciousness led to mediocrity, suppressed originality and created a feeling of decadence in individuals. This feeling of decadence was applied to the nation by Berdichevsky, who perceived the crisis of a whole national culture which had a deadening effect on its members. Brinker explained the difference between Nietzsche and Berdichevsky. In Nietzsche, an excessive historical consciousness aroused a feeling of decadence, and in Berdichevsky it was a cure for the Jewish nation. Berdichevsky thought that because the Jewish people, having lived outside history, lacked a historical sense, it needed revolutionary values which would give it new life forces. His series of articles that appeared after the one entitled "Old Age and Youth" marked a turning-point in his outlook, a turning-point that the representatives of the Haskalah considered revolutionary and touching the roots of his dispute with Ahad Ha-Am.[26]

Yavne or Canaan

Exile, according to Brinker's reading of Berdichevsky, was the product of an ancient sickness called "Yavne": the "Yavne" that embodied a rejection of political independence and promoted the values of piety and the study of halacha. The emphasis on an inner religious life came at the expense of the existence of vital and material values. The exile was in Berdichevsky's opinion the result of this change of values and not its cause. But most of the thinkers of his time did not accept this idea and thought that "Yavnc" was a historical necessity which permitted the Jews to survive in the absence of sovereignty. In the modern age, the life of the Jews was impoverished because they were cut off from world culture and confined to the exegetic ghetto of talmudic halacha. A "change of values" was required, which in the case of the modern Jews meant a preference for "life" over the "book." Berdichevsky, who sought to "brush history against the grain," was the only thinker who went so far as to perceive an historical change of values, a change that preceded the exile and was the cause of it. As a philosopher of Jewish history, he came to the conclusion that the Jewish leadership had chosen wrong values. Joseph Brenner criticized Berdichevsky's position which he considered idealistic, a position that disregarded social and economic factors and favored an unjustified escape from values.[27]

The critic Baruch Kurzweil is remembered for linking Berdichevsky and the culture of the Hebrew revival with the "Canaanites," who in his opinion did not express an original point of view but were an Israeli breed of a Jewish anti-religious phenomenon that existed in the European exile.[28] From another direction, the critic and essayist Boaz Evron declared that the "Canaanites" who wished to renew the "ancient land" wanted to discard all the later Jewish "accumulations" (his expression) on the ancient Hebrew culture, beginning with the arrival in the country of Ezra and Nehemiah, and leave only the archaic Hebrew substructure common to the whole region, from Ugarit in the north to Moab in the east.[29] Ephron shared the "Canaanite" conviction that at an introverted ghetto-like country within a small area could not exist, but he did not believe that a "renaissance of Hebrew culture" in the sense given by Yonatan Ratosh was possible because not many remnants of archaic Hebrew culture existed apart from the Bible. The poor spiritual coinage of ancient Israelism showed that it represented the myth of a common culture rather than an actual culture. Evron rejected another "Canaanite" idea: to ignore the national consciousness of the Arabs of the area and see them as former Hebrews who had to be brought back to their Hebrew origins. He dismissed Ratosh's idea of divesting the Hebrews in the country of their Judaism and liberating the Arabs and other peoples of the area of the burden of their "Arabism," actions that were supposed to lay the foundations of a great Hebrew nation.

This was the bone of contention between Ratosh and Evron. Evron thought that the past could not be erased. Even if a Jewish immigrant eventually became a Hebrew, he would retain sediments of Judaism and it would be foolish to ignore them. Hebrew culture was strongly connected with the development of Judaism, very little remains of the archaic Hebrew culture, and anyone who adopts the Hebrew language necessarily adopts its linguistic and literary tradition which is mainly Jewish. The reality in the country was enough to make an immigrant into a Hebrew without a Hebrew revolution. Evron did not see any contradiction between the Hebrew language and his Judaism because he had always regarded Hebrew as the "holy tongue." The relationship of the Israeli to the Jew did not resemble the relationship of the Italian-American to his ancestors but rather the affinity of the American to his Anglo-Saxon heritage.

Placing the Hebrew culture solely on its archaic foundations would require a book-burning and an erasure of cultural treasures, and, similarly, one cannot deny the culture and national consciousness of the Arabs, their particular sensibility, their language and tradition.[30]

There is no ancient culture in the country, continued Evron, either Hebrew or Jewish. The Israeli is a tabula rasa and does not wish to live in accordance with the ancient Hebrew culture. The Jewish culture was dying and the recent literature was already breaking away from its Jewish roots. "Only our language remains, and we have to begin from the beginning, from aleph. From the point of view of an autarchic spiritual culture we are barbarians." The new Hebrew nation born in the country was truly new, and any attempt to tie it to an archaic peg would fail. And, in any case, the very concept of an "early archaic culture" was dubious: it did not depict specific values and resembled the "Nordic myth." The culture of the future would definitely be modern and technological. For the same reason, Evron was not happy with the term "Semitic" in the name of his circle ("Semitic Action"), although "Semitism," in his opinion, was milder and less demanding than "Hebraism," and was not a utopian revolt against reality.

The "Canaanites" argued that originally the region was an open space, not a ghetto. It was a mainly Hebrew-speaking area from the Mediterranean Sea to Aram Naharaim. The intellectual climate of early Hebrew culture was cosmopolitan because there were pluralistic cultural currents there. In a small society there was likely to be a situation of closed collective tribes, but in a large society which came in contact with the world there could be social pluralism and a variety of values and spiritual objectives. Decadence set in when a national culture was closed and clerical. There was isolation in a ghetto, but things developed when a living organism was in contact with the great world outside it.[31]

Evron said that Zionism claimed that the Jews were a nation and not a religion. Religion, he thought, was only one of the aspects of Jewish nationhood, although the conditions of exile emphasized the religious factor as the one that defined Judaism. The absence of other elements of nationhood in "exile" such as territory or language led to the Zionist view that Jewish existence in the diaspora was incomplete. The conclusion was that only in the homeland could the defective Jew become a full one through his national existence. According to this view, religion served as a framework which held the Jewish people together until it returned to its homeland, and then it could detach itself from its religion which was only an outward garment of its nationhood. This view made possible the identification of the leaders of the state with the Messiah. The association of contemporary realities with values that were obviously religious, a sort of fusion of dissimilarities, eliminated the distinction between sacred and profane. Evron thought that the Zionist view was essentially flawed because it saw Jewish existence in dispersion as an abnormal one. He asked if a Tel Aviv playboy was really a more complete Jew than Einstein or the Vilna Gaon.

Because Zionism sees Israel as the sole homeland of all Jews, its interests are seen as the interests of the Jewish people as a whole. The difference between the

Zionist view and the Hebraist view is that Zionism sees religion as an axiom and the state as its expression while the Hebraist view sees Hebrew nationhood and the state as the axiom. The connection of the Hebrew-speaker to his country takes first place in his social consciousness:

> He was born or grew up here. He works, loves, fights, and dies here. He is here and nowhere else and does not have any other place. The Israeli has no other place because no other place can be Israeli.[32]

Territory and assimilation

Evron and the historian Robert Wistrich had the same opinion concerning the primacy of the homeland, but with this common starting point they ended with two completely different philosophies of history. While Evron shook off the burden of the exile and the necessity of showing that the Jews living outside the country needed to be protected, Wistrich still saw the Jewish people inside the country and outside it as a single entity. The subject which preoccupied him obsessively was thus the existence and growth of antisemitism, whether directed against the Jewish state or the Jews overseas.

Already in his initial researches on Zionism, Wistrich attempted to connect the history of the Jews in modern times, in Israel as well, with the European historical background. It was impossible, in his opinion, to distinguish between Jewish history and general history.[33] Only in this way, he thought, could phenomena like nationalism and universalism, assimilation and adaptation, Zionism and antisemitism, colonialism and pioneering, be understood in depth. The pioneers of the Second Aliyah brought social-revolutionary ideas developed in the Russian environment to a region of the dying Ottoman empire, a region in which there was no industrial basis, politically organized class or bourgeois capitalism. Everything had to be built up from the start: the country, the people and the new society. Their opposition to the patronizing philosophy of the settlements, which were administered by the agents of the Baron Rothschild, was seen by the latter as clear proof of the social-revolutionary ethos of these early Zionists. They understood that the colonialist social norms, which had begun to take root in the Old Yishuv, would undermine the national ideal of renewal. The ideology of early Zionism never completely rejected the old world. Berl Katznelson, one of the most representative figures of the Jewish labor movement in Palestine, said that Zionism was "a revolt against servility within the revolution." Wistrich thought that the importance of the Zionist revolution did not lie in the birth of a new people as the result of Jewish resoluteness in the War of Independence, but in its attempt to normalize the historical "Jew." For a time it seemed that the split between the Israelis and the Jews would be so great that there would be no basis for a common identity. If that happened, Zionism would have produced a nation of "Hebrew-speaking gentiles," a country in which Israelism as a form of general assimilation would undermine Jewish tradition. Wistrich was of course hinting here at the possibility of the Hebraization or Canaanization of the Jewish State, but he was also pointing to a further danger.

From the very beginning, the Zionist movement saw assimilation as one of its chief enemies, a humiliating position for any self-respecting Jew. Like other national movements, said Wistrich, Zionism saw assimilation as an expression of weakness of character instead of regarding it as an internal logic dictated by the historical situation. The Zionists very readily made a tale of "spiritual servitude" out of the condition of the assimilated. They created a mythical picture of Western Jews who disparaged Jewish existence. The "assimilated" found themselves branded as self-hating Jews or as traitors to their people because they no longer wished to be religious or because of their weak connection to Jewish tradition. The fact that they continued to define themselves in a Jewish context was not understood in liberal societies in nineteenth-century Europe. The Zionist critics of assimilation did not take into account that without the emancipation and exposure to the values of European culture, the Jewish national rebirth would not have come into existence.[34]

Solomon Schechter, President of the Jewish Theological Seminary in the United States and one of the founders of the Conservative Movement, declared in a letter in 1906 that in his opinion, Zionism was one of the main obstacles to assimilation. Assimilation represented for him, as for most Jews, a loss of identity, a process of self-annihilation. The struggle against assimilation, said Wistrich, was a central myth in Zionism, and it continued to be one of its main axes. In Rome and Jerusalem, a work by a German Communist who had once held the ideas of Marx concerning Jews and Judaism, the pattern was already clear: self-rejection was not only in bad taste from the moral point of view, but it was also ineffective. The writer, Moses Hess, wrote that "every Jew, whether he wishes or not, is tied with an unbreakable bond to the entire people." Peretz Smolenskin, a nationalist Russian Jew and one of the leaders of the "Hibbat Zion" movement, believed that the uniqueness of the Jewish people lay in its culture and its past, not in its land. Nathan Birnbaum, one of the founders, in his youth, of Zionism in the Austro-Hungarian Empire, described the "mania for assimilation" as "national suicide." In Wistrich's opinion, none of these early Zionists distinguished between adaptation – the adoption of the external norms of the majority such as language, costume, manners, and so forth – and assimilation, the adoption of the collective identity of the national majority. They regarded assimilation as a vain attempt to bring Jewish history to an end. The assimilated were thought to betray a major value, the duty of national survival. Zionism, as A.D. Gordon said, was the ultimate answer to assimilation: only in the Hebrew homeland could one rid oneself of the contradictions of the exile. The strength of the Jewish nation could only be renewed through connection with the land and physical labor, a creative connection that would enable the new Jews to enter the stage of history. All the major thinkers of Zionism strongly opposed assimilation, just as they rejected the exile. They saw the rejuvenation of the homeland as a renaissance of Jewish nationhood, a process of self-emancipation and a revolutionary move against acceptance of the Jewish fate.

Zionism has not only been received with inner hostility by the movement for assimilation, but also with outward hostility, with the slander that the Jewish national movement is "racist" – a modern version of original sin. The Jewish settlers, according to this view, were European colonialists who brutally expelled the Palestinian natives, and their self-justification reflected a Western racist outlook.[35] Israel's claim to be a "Jewish" state was seen as racist because the Jewish minority was regarded as a religious group rather than a national movement. In practical terms, the Law of Return was attacked as especially racist because it granted exilic Jews an Israeli citizenship Jews denied to exiled Palestinians. But Wistrich asserted that in reality, in stark contrast to the common myth, Zionism was indifferent to the matter of race as a formative element in Israeli society. Unlike in the white colonialist societies in South Africa, Australia and the United States, color was never regarded as important in Israel or as a factor affecting social status. Unlike the whites in South Africa, Rwanda or Algeria, since 1948 the Israelis have been a majority in their country. From Herzl to Jabotinsky, from Weizmann to Ben-Gurion and Berl Katznelson, there was never any hint of racial superiority or of a desire to rule other peoples or enslave them.

A biological-mythical interpretation of the society or the culture was absent from the Zionist philosophy of history. Zionism, which was one of the last of the national-liberation movements which sprang up in Europe in the nineteenth century, combined universalist patriotism as in the French Revolution with the Jewish tradition which stressed a return to Zion.

Unlike most of the national movements, Zionism was characterized from the beginning by a search for territory. It solved the problem of the homeless Jews, a minority without a territory which had lost its sovereignty over Palestine about 1,900 years before. The desperate flight of the Jews of Russia and Eastern Europe – a population that had experienced pogroms and discrimination – in the last quarter of the nineteenth century, created a "Jewish problem" which demanded a political solution. The State of Israel, which absorbed Jews from the Arab countries, the Soviet Union, Eastern Europe and other countries, succeeded in achieving at least one of the objectives for which it had been created. This was made possible by the Law of Return, and, most definitely, if and when the Palestinians will demand a Law of Return of their own, added Wistrich, no one will accuse them of racism because they give preference to Palestinian Arabs. The Israeli Law of Return provided the Jewish victims of Nazi persecution and other forms of oppression with a safe refuge. The Jew who returns to his homeland and obtains citizenship is exercising a natural human right.

Although Wistrich appreciated the historical change of direction effected by early Zionism in the face of the approaching catastrophe, he was critical of the aims of Zionism. Thus, even the early Zionists did not grasp the full significance of antisemitism. Wistrich's Zionism was not intended to cure antisemitism or solve the problem of Jewish existence, but simply to "manage the situation" in the face of antisemitism.

In his final article, Wistrich expressed his credo in connection with his struggle against the new antisemitism and his belief that Israel is the ultimate homeland of the Jewish people. He claimed that the rising tide of contemporary antisemitism was one of the most urgent and disturbing matters for the Jewish communities of the world. He spoke at the conference of the fifth Global Forum for Combating Antisemitism held in Jerusalem shortly before his death, and stressed the need to liberate the Israelis from myths whose time had passed. Even today, he said, Jews in Israel and the diaspora are entrenched in their belief in the danger of a traditional antisemitism from the extreme right, whether the racial, religious or national right. Neo-fascism has not left the scene, but Wistrich thought that it was a secondary threat in most cases. In his opinion, there was an illusory belief that education on the Holocaust and attempts to memorialize it and even the existence of a Jewish homeland would be an effective inoculation against contemporary antisemitism. This way of thinking, he believed, held by many governments and many non-Jewish liberals, is largely unfounded. Rather, the opposite is true. Today, the "reversal of the meaning of the Holocaust" (the perverted transformation of the Jews into Nazis and the Muslims into Jewish victims) is often a weapon to strike at Israel and besmirch the character of the Jewish people.

The Israeli historian quoted in his favor Alexis de Tocqueville, who said that the French Revolution had two stages: the abrogation of all that had existed in the past, and an attempt to reconnect with the past the French had cut themselves off from.[36] Zionism not only wished to destroy the old socioeconomic order and achieve political independence: its main purpose was to rebel against a historical fate, or, as Ben-Gurion put it, "against the unique fate of a unique and special people." Zionism wanted to make the Jews masters of their fate and put an end to their material, moral, cultural and political dependence on others. The success of the Zionist revolution lay in changing the course of Jewish history, giving birth to the new Israeli people and the creation of a renewed homeland.

The homeland as a plurality of places

To the skepticism of Robert Wistrich concerning the capacity of the Jewish homeland to solve the problem of antisemitism, and the skepticism of Jacqueline Kahanoff concerning the hope that a Jewish homeland would solve the problem of identity, Menachem Brinker added his skepticism concerning the validity of the Zionist movement after the Jewish homeland arose. He thought that the existence of the Zionist movement side-by-side with the State of Israel could be unnecessary and even harmful, as it gave rise to the mistaken notion that the state needed the Zionist movement to strengthen it. In reality, the relationship between the two was the other way round. It was the Zionist movement that needed the state to give it a raison d'être as long as large sections of the Jewish people lived outside Israel. The claim that Israel is the home of all the world's Jews is an untruth and a platitude. Israel is not the state of all Jews, but only the state of the Jews (and non-Jews) who live there. Israelis tend to think that all Israel's difficult problems of existence can be solved through "Zionist solutions." The activists of Gush Emunim sought Zionist legitimation for their actions in their demand to realize the right of the Jews to sovereignty in the whole of the land of Israel, a demand that appeared to be a Zionist objective. The activists of "Peace Now" claimed that Israel was gradually becoming a bi-national state, a situation that was not in accordance with the original aims of Zionism. Dragging Zionism into the dispute between the supporters of the Greater Land of Israel and its opponents does not help to solve the dilemma. Brinker wrote: "In Zionism, as in the words of the Sages, one can find almost anything. Zionism, like money, cannot solve everything."[37] A Zionist state could be a national state in which one people rules over another, or it could be a humanist state. Zionism has only one meaning. It is a means to realize a human objective in which concerns only one group of people (a group which includes Brinker): that is to say, it is a means to bring about the State of Israel, which is itself a means to ensure the existence of the Jewish people in history.

Brinker's article "After Post-Zionism" was written in 2007, a quarter of a century after the appearance of his article "After Zionism."[38] When the first article appeared, Brinker said that there was no reason to fear any confusion that might be caused by the title of his lecture/article. But, at the beginning of the twenty-first century, the accepted meaning of post-Zionism (after Zionism) is the subversion of the Zionist ideology, or of Zionist historiography, or of the Zionist enterprise itself, or of all of these. Post-Zionism is seen as a euphemism for anti-Zionism, but Brinker was thinking of Ben-Gurion's surprise, for example, in the early days of the state, at the continued existence of the Zionist Federation and its institutions after the vision of the founders had been realized.[39]

The conquest of the territories in the Six-Day War was a watershed, a difficult "complication" which changed the significance of many Zionist values. Brinker admitted that he was one of those who strongly rejected the post-Zionist description of Zionism as a colonialist movement from the beginning. In his opinion, previous to 1967, Zionism had no colonialist characteristics. There was no armed conquest to exploit conquered lands and their inhabitants, or to obtain raw materials or manpower cheaply or without payment, or for the use of the conqueror who lived mainly abroad. He thought the description of the growth of modern Jewish nationalism, of which Zionism was the political expression, in neo-Marxist terms as a "superstructure" of colonialist imperialism, was particularly distorted. It was a description given by historians who had no conception of the conditions governing the growth of modern Jewish nationalism, but the conquest of the territories made this distorted description of Zionism in its early days a fairly accurate description of Israeli policies in the occupied territories, which are colonialist in all respects.

Brinker said that, in a lecture he gave at the beginning of the 1990s, he reflected on the line in the national anthem, "we have not yet lost our hope," which was still being sung many years after the founding of the state. It did not seem to him that the equality of all Israeli citizens was part of the Zionist vision, but it was clear to him that most of the Zionist thinkers (at least, the secular ones) thought that the "Jewish state" was a "state of all its citizens," even if most of the citizens were Jews, but purely on demographic grounds and not in terms of legislation. They spoke of a modern nation-state like France and Britain. A nation-state is not the "state of a people," for the state of a people belongs exclusively to a historical collective characterized by a common origin. With a change of direction in the development of a historical movement there is a change in the formulas with which it is accompanied, and they sometimes acquire a significance quite opposite to their original meaning. This happened to the word "socialism" in the communist movement. Brinker wrote: "Nothing will remain of the initial bloom of Zionist terminology if the State of Israel becomes a means of protecting the Jewish diaspora beyond its borders."[40] Although most Israeli citizens have an affinity to the Jewish people at large, this should not head their order of preferences. Ben-Gurion, called by Brinker "the last Zionist politician," who claimed that with the founding of the state the task of the Zionist movement was over, was a case in point.

Birth-throes of the homeland, birth-throes of the Messiah

The affinity claimed by the settlers between the Bible and the Land of the Bible – the realms of memory of Judea and Samaria – is the most important feature in their political theology. The link with the Bible is a seismograph for viewing the relationship of Zionism in general and the settlers in particular to their ideological and political outlook. To where in the Bible are the settlers returning? Is it a return to the land of Canaan, to the land of the Patriarchs, or is it perhaps to the Davidic kingdom? And what is the significance of this return? Underlying this question is not only the land but the relationship of the land of Israel to the people of Israel. This "credo" is basic to the settlers' conception. While the founders of the Zionist movement and the members of the Second Aliyah turned to the Bible in order to anchor their affinity to the land but were unwilling to base their right to the land on the divine promise,[41] religious Zionism fused the divine promise with the Zionist ideology, which is essentially secular. But only after the Six-Day War did the settlement project of the believers in the biblical promise to the land become a messianic promise and the sole basis of legitimacy: a basis both political and theological. Gush Emunim, which brought this project to fruition, represented the most forceful and systematic political theology in the State of Israel's seventy years of existence.

One should remember that the secular Zionist settlement did not take place in the land of the Patriarchs but in the land of the Philistines, not in Judea and Samaria but mainly in the coastal plain. The names it chose for the settlements in the country (many of which were foreign to the place or names that represented wishes, such as Petah Tikva – Gateway to Hope, or Rishon le Zion – First in Zion) did not express a deep theological affinity to the ancestral land but a modern, secular, national vision. Thus, there was a dual distance, geographical and linguistic. Unlike the secular Zionism, the Zionism of the settlers, returning to the wellsprings of the Bible, reflected a theological rationale both with regard to the land and with regard to the ancient biblical language, although many of the people of the Greater Land of Israel were secular. The return to the Philistine areas was due to historical reasons: while the hill regions were populated, the swamps and desert regions were desolate. The pioneers turned this obstacle into the secular ideal of redeeming the soil by making the desert bloom and draining the swamps. The settlers, for their part, expressed their Zionism not by returning to the desert but to abandoned and ruined historical sites. While the secular ideal of making the desert bloom represented hope for the future within a desolation, the project of the settlers sought a restoration of ruined sites which it wished to bring back to life.

After 1967, the land of Israel became close and accessible. While secular Zionism returned to David, Saul and Samson in a weakened interpretation which modified the literal sense – an interpretation whose purpose was to strengthen the ideology – the settlers' return to the origins enabled them to pass from this weakened interpretation of the Bible to one that was direct and messianic. The homeland became the "ground" for them, a basis of interpretation which anchored a mystical messianism.[42] The accessibility of the ancient biblical sites brought ancient history closer and made the land of the Bible within reach of the Israelis. The stories of the Bible underwent a concretization. The settlers succeeded in replacing the political-security discourse on the territories with a theological discourse. Stretches of land that only yesterday were in the possession of the enemy became Holy Places. After 1967, many Israelis flocked to Rachel's tomb in Bethlehem and the Tombs of the Patriarchs in Hebron.

Secular Zionism, whose origin was in European nationalism, in many cases falsified place names.[43] The preservation of the affinity to the place and the name bought the settlers closer in this respect to the Arabs than to the secular Zionists who came from Christian Europe. Does the Canaanite-nativist common denominator of the Palestinians and the settlers overrule the national, foreign, European crusading element? Did the "crusaders" who settled in the land become "Canaanites"?[44] Secular Zionism returned to the land of Israel and restored names of the biblical homeland, but it did so in a way that many regard as Canaanite and not religious. Ashkelon and Hazor are not places sanctified in Judaism and are not significant from the religious point of view, but names that belong to a biblical narrative unconnected with religious motifs.

Rabbi Zvi Israel Thau and Rabbi Yitzhak Ginsburgh represent, each in his way, theological views of the homeland. Their differing interpretations of the Davidic kingdom have a significant effect on the attitude of their followers to the State of Israel. In the Thau model, the State of Israel is perfectly in keeping with the messianic project of the settlers, but the dialectical logic of Ginsburgh demands the destruction of the secular foundations of the state, which are regarded as defiled.

This study, which discusses the opinions of various thinkers and scholars on the character of the homeland, omits the views of many of the citizens of the State of Israel. Missing from the text are the interpretations of Arab intellectuals like Emile Habibi, whose inscription on his grave, "I stayed in Haifa," is a declaration about himself and his feelings as a son of the homeland. Also missing is the ultra-Orthodox interpretation of the concept "homeland," the physical place, which the ultra-Orthodox discourse dismisses completely in favor of the metaphysical Place, the Holy One, Blessed Be He. The discourse in this study concerns the character of the homeland, its essence, its directions, the controversy about the birth-throes of the homeland, the birth-throes of redemption at the beginning of the twentieth century and the birth-throes of the Messiah at the beginning of the twenty-first. Here there are a number of different and even conflicting interpretations, by statesmen and thinkers, a literary scholar, a historian, a woman author, a sociologist, pioneers and settlers, of where the homeland comes from and where it is going.

Everyone has his own image of the homeland, but it is precisely the multiplicity of images and interpretations and their existence next to each other that enables the citizens of the homeland to live together in a society that is not one-dimensional. An exclusive interpretation, a one-and-only homeland, necessarily prevents many communities from having other narratives. The potentialities of the homeland are examined here in a broad hermeneutical perspective and reveal a variety of ideas expressed in ideological and philosophical views of history and utopian visions. Each to his own homeland.

Notes

1 Anthony Smith, *Ethno-symbolism and Nationalism: A Cultural Approach*, Routledge, Abingdon 2009.
2 Shalom Rosenberg, "The Affinity to Eretz Israel in Jewish Thought – A Struggle of Outlooks," *Katedra*, 4 (1977): 148–166 (in Hebrew).
3 Nathan Rotenstreich, "Being Zionist in 1976 – An Interview with Yeshayahu Ben Porat," *The Yearbook of Journalists*, Tel Aviv 1975 (in Hebrew).
4 Martin Buber, *Between a Nation and its Country*, Tel Aviv 1944 (in Hebrew); Paul Mendes-Flohr, "Chapter 9: Professor and Political Activist," *Martin Buber: A Life of Faith and Dissent*, Yale University Press, New Haven 2019.
5 Avi Sagi, "Between Love and Politics of Sovereignty," *Against Others: The Ethics of Inner Regression*, Tel Aviv 2012, 107–137 (in Hebrew).
6 Boaz Neumann, *Land and Desire in Early Zionism*, Brandies University Press, Waltham, MA 2011.
7 Jean Améry, *At The Mind's Limits: Contemplations by a Survivor on Auschwitz and its Realities*, Indiana University Press, Bloomington 1980, 49.
8 Ibid., 47.
9 Ibid., 54.
10 David Ohana, *The Origins of Israeli Mythology: Neither Canaanites Nor Crusaders*, Cambridge University Press, Cambridge 2012.
11 Yehoshua Arieli, *Individualism and Nationalism in American Ideology*, Harvard University Press, Cambridge MA 1964.
12 Following Martin Heidegger, many post-modern theologians discuss God's presence through its absence. See: Louis Marie Chauvet, *Symbol and Sacrament: A Sacramental Reinterpretation of Christian Existence*, Liturgical Press, Collegeville MN 1995, 62; David Ohana, *Nietzsche and Jewish Political Theology*, London 2018, 20–23.
13 On Nietzsche and pioneers, see: David Ohana, "Zarathustra in Jerusalem: Nietzsche and the 'New Hebrews'," *The Shaping of Israeli Identity*, eds., Robert Wistrich and

David Ohana, Frank Cass, London 1995, 38–61; On Turner's thesis, see: Frederick Jackson Turner, *The Frontier in American History*, Toronto 1920.

14 On the pioneer's ethos, see: Shmuel N. Eisenstadt, *Israeli Society*, CRC Press, New York 1967; Henry Nir, "Like all the Gentiles? The Zionist Pioneers in Inter-cultural Context," eds., Anita Shapira, Yehuda Reinhertz and Jacob Harris, *The Age of Zionism*, Jerusalem 2000, 109–126 (in Hebrew); Boaz Neumann, op. cit.; On the development of the ethos and its decline, see: Luis Roniger and Michael Feige, "From Pioneer to Freier: The Changing Models of Generalized Exchange in Israel," *Archives Europeennes De Sociologie*, 33 (1992): 280–307.

15 For a further discussion on the subject: Michael Feige, *Settling in the Hearts: Jewish Fundamentalism in the Occupied*, Wayne State University Press, Detroit 2009.

16 Meron Benvenisti, *Sacred Landscape*, University of California Press, Berkeley 2000.

17 Yael Zerubavel, *Desert in the Promised Land*, Stanford 2018.

18 Shabtai Teveth, "King of the Desert," *Haaretz*, 5/12/1973 (in Hebrew).

19 Michael Bar-Zohar, *Ben-Gurion*, Vol. 3, Tel Aviv 1987, 1604–1605 (in Hebrew).

20 Tom Segev, *A State at Any Cost: The Life of David Ben-Gurion*, Farrar, Strauss and Giroux, New York 2019.

21 On the concept of banal nationality, see: Michael Billing, *Banal Nationalism*, SAGE Publications, London 1995.

22 On the Baba Sali see: Yoram Bilu and Eyal Ben-Ari, "Modernity and Charisma in Contemporary Israel: The Case of Baba Sali and Baba Baruch," *The Shaping of Israeli Identity*, 224–237; On the commemoration of Rabin, see: Vered Vinitzky-Seroussi, *Forget-Me-Not: Yitzhak Rabin's Assassination and the Dilemmas of Commemoration*, SUNY Press, Albany 2009.

23 See especially: Aviezer Ravitsky, *Yeshayahu Leibowitz: Between Conservatism and Radicalism- Reflections on his Philosophy*, Jerusalem 1995, 219–284 (in Hebrew).

24 On national rituals, see: Eric Hobsbaum and Terrance Ranger (eds.), *The Invention of Tradition*, Cambridge University Press, Cambridge 1983; Don Handelman, *Models and Mirrors: Towards an Anthropology of Public Events*, Berghahn Books, Cambridge 1990; Gabriella Elgenius, *Symbols of Nations and Nationalism: Celebrating Nationhood*, Palgrave Macmillan, Basingstoke, UK 2011.

25 Charles S. Liebman and Eliezer Don-Yehia, *Civil Religion in Israel*, Berkeley 1983.

26 Avner Holzman, *Towards the Tear in the Heart: Micha Josef Berdichevsky – The Formative Years (1886–1902)*, Jerusalem 1995 (in Hebrew).

27 Menachem Brinker, *Narrative Art and Social Thought in Y. H. Brenner's Work*, Tel Aviv 1990, 165–176 (in Hebrew).

28 Baruch Kurzweil, "Essence and Origins of the 'Young Hebrews' Movement ('Canaanites')," *Our New Literature – Continuity or Revolution?* Tel Aviv 1964 (in Hebrew).

29 Boaz Evron, "Clarifications for our Time – or: Perceived Difference and Real Difference," *Etgar*, 93, 1/10/1964 (in Hebrew).

30 Ibid., "The Dimond Hardness of his Thought," *Haaretz*, 4/4/2001 (in Hebrew).

31 Ehud Ben-Ezer, *Unease in Zion*, ed., Robert Alter, New York 1974.

32 Ohana, " 'Civil Cannanism' in the philosophy of Boaz Evron," in: Israel Segal, *Civil Israelism*, Jerusalem 2018, 157–194 (in Hebrew).

33 Robert Wistrich, "Zionism: Rebellion against History," *Tfuzot Hagola*, 83–84 (1978): 98–105 (in Hebrew).

34 Wistrich, "Zionism and Myths of Assimilation," *Midstream* (Aug–Sept 1990), 3–8.

35 Wistrich, "Zionism, Colonialism and the Third World," *The Jewish Chronicles*, 7.1.1976.

36 David Ohana, "From Rousseau to Tocqueville," *The Intellectual Origins of Modernity*, Routledge, London 2019.

37 Brinker, "After Zionism," *Israeli Thoughts*, Jerusalem 2007, 31 (in Hebrew).

38 Ibid., 35–37.

39 For a contemporary perspective on what the Zionist project has achieved until now, see: S. Ilan Troen and Rachel Fish, *Essential Israel: Essays for the 21st Century (Perspectives on Israel Studies)*, Indiana University Press, Indianapolis 2017.
40 Ibid., 37.
41 Anita Shapira, *The Bible and Israeli Identity*, Cambridge University Press, Cambridge MA 2004.
42 Ground, or Grund is the principle of interpretation in Heideggerian terminology.
43 David Ohana, "Michael Feige's Realms of Memory," in: Michael Feige, *Al Da'at Ha'makom: Israeli Realms of Memory*, Kiryat Sde Boker 2017, 9–47 (in Hebrew).
44 David Ohana, *The Origins of Israeli Mythology: Neither Canaanites nor Crusaders*, Cambridge University Press, Cambridge MA 2012; ibid., *Nationalizing Judaism: Zionism as a Theological Ideology*, Lanham 2017.

1 Pilgrimage to the backside of the desert

"One of the splendid things about Ben-Gurion's decision to be buried at Sde Boker," said a perspicacious woman-journalist, "was that it forced every offici-ating prime minister to go down to the Negev once a year. I feel that I am not exaggerating if I say that this was Ben-Gurion's original intention."[1] David Ben-Gurion, founder of the nation and Israel's first prime minister, passed away on December 1, 1973, and his annual commemoration takes place at his grave-side at the Midreshet Ben-Gurion. Many political, administrative and military leaders are present, and usually the prime minister, the president, members of the government and official representatives of the state institutions. Once a year there is a solemn moment when the Israeli nation comes face to face with the figure and outlook of its founder and leader, David Ben-Gurion. The ceremony is a confrontation of the real Israel with Ben-Gurion's vision, the potentialities it sought to realize and the problematic nature of the place where the ceremony is held. The metamorphoses the ceremony has undergone bear witness both to the changing face of the country and the relationship of its society to the image of its founder.

The impressive state ceremony is a meeting between the Israeli elite and the nation's founding ethos, but its importance should not be exaggerated, espe-cially if one considers the public's view of it. The day of commemoration for Ben-Gurion, known as Ben-Gurion Day, is a relatively marginal event com-pared to some other days of remembrance in the Israeli calendar. Holocaust Remembrance Day, Remembrance Day for the Fallen, and Independence Day are events that take up a whole day. They include many activities and arouse strong feelings. The commemoration of Prime Minister Yitzhak Rabin lasts for about a week and is filled with ceremonies and events. The ceremony that takes place at Ben-Gurion's graveside is generally the only significant event of Ben-Gurion Day, and it is hardly felt outside Midreshet Ben-Gurion. At the same time, the annual state ceremonies in his memory fulfill an essential role: they represent the continuity of the state and symbolize the Israeli nation above and beyond day-to-day politics.

Even if the ceremony is marginal both from a geopolitical point of view and from the point of view of the attention it receives, it would be wrong to say that the figure of Ben-Gurion, the founder of the state is forgotten. Israelis, both young and old, remember him and to a greater or lesser degree are familiar with his image.[2] This chapter focuses on a certain element of special importance in the commemoration of Ben-Gurion, in which one may perhaps discern the changes in the image of that leader. There is a great distance between the historical Ben-Gurion – a demanding, energetic leader with clear positions and supporting and opposing camps – and his image in the Israeli collective memory, and the distance only increases with the passage of time.

The canonical element and the self-referential element

In the first commemorative ceremony for Ben-Gurion, which took place in December 1974, the form of the ceremony was fixed, and it did not change in the course of time.[3] A member of the family said "Kaddish," a cantor sang "El malei rahamin," the president and the prime minister made speeches, and if the latter was not there, he was replaced by a senior member of the government. State representatives, the diplomatic corps and the family laid wreaths on the grave. The participants in the ceremony were invited in accordance with the rules of diplomacy. The laying of wreaths by the public and family was organized in accordance with protocol, and the subsequent changes were slight and insignificant. The religious element changed almost from year to year, and here a certain amount of freedom was given to the chief body organizing the ceremony: the information center in the Prime Minister's Office. From the first ceremony in 1974 until 2004, the emphasis was generally on a subject chosen each year by the Ministry of Education, and very often it was a passage that was read from Ben-Gurion's writings. Sometimes a poem was included in the ceremony, and sometimes Ben-Gurion's voice was heard over the loudspeakers.[4] Despite the slight changes in the religious content, the ceremonies had a monotonous, conservative character, expressing the continuity of the state like other official ceremonies.

While this fixed structure is the basic element in the ceremony, symbolizing the eternity of the people and state and the unchanging relationship of the nation to the figure of its founder, the changes in the ceremony every year reflect social changes. Here the distinction made by the anthropologist Roy Rappaport between the canonical element in ceremonies and the self-referential element is instructive.[5] The canonical element is the liturgy, the ceremonial element recurring year after year, for in the opinion of the organizers of the ceremony changes in its structure and order of appearance would harm its effectiveness. In a broad historical perspective, we can discern the changes that take place in ceremonies that on the face of it seem eternal (the service for the eve of the Day of Atonement, for example, or the Seder night) and see how adaptations are made in accordance with the period. But where the participants themselves are concerned, the ceremony seems fixed for all eternity, and this continuity provides it with its sanctity.

But, side-by-side with the canonical element of the text, there is another, self-referential element which changes from one ceremony to the next, and which is expressed in routine matters dictated by its purpose. It can take the form of the names of couples getting married or a child entering adolescence on his Bar-Mitzva. Weddings and Bar-Mitzvas are canonical ceremonies, but the specific content of the ceremony which takes place in honor of particular people is an individual and changing factor. This factor represents a limited measure of freedom of choice within the accepted forms of the ceremony: for instance, in the decision whether to participate in the ceremony, how one should behave, how one should dress, or what it is permissible to say on the platform. The canonical element, on the other hand, cannot be changed, because the success of the ceremony is measured by its exact execution in the proper order, as prescribed.

The importance of the ceremony derives from its canonical element. It provides a sense of stability among the changes of life and reminds the participants that that there are eternal, transcendental values beyond their daily lives, whether they are religious, national, or some other kind. The canonical element gives the self-referential element its validity: the ceremony is moving and significant because it connects the life of the individual to the eternity beyond it.

The canonical element in the Ben-Gurion memorial ceremony is based on a more sacred ritual. In fact, it represents a hybridization of two ceremonies which make it "right" and even self-evident. The gathering by the graveside, the saying of "kaddish," the singing of "El malei rahamin," the speeches of the president and prime minister, the placing of wreaths on the grave by senior public officials: none of this is unique to Ben-Gurion Day and no special tradition has developed for that ceremony.[6] The Ben-Gurion memorial ceremony imitates other ceremonies, and its canonical character could be described as second-hand. If it has any freshness, it is owing to the landscape which surrounds it and the special location of the grave facing the desert, which make it completely different from other state ceremonies.

The evolution of the self-referential element, which changes from year to year, is the focus of this chapter. Those who take the trouble to come to the ceremony, the messages delivered by the speeches of the president and prime minister and the kind of people brought to the ceremony: these things illustrate the dynamic of the Israelis' relationship to their country, and stand out against the static background of the canonical element.

The death of the leader. Why Sde Boker?

The subject of this study is not the death or funeral of Ben-Gurion: This research has been conducted elsewhere.[7] The annual memorial ceremonies reflect the evolution of Ben-Gution's image and his status with the Israeli public. However, the fixed canonical element and the dynamic of the commemorations are by-products of an original decision by Ben-Gurion himself a number of years before his death. The place of burial reflects a consistent set of values, and he was buried on his orders in a place he had carefully chosen. In his writings and in his diaries, he did not give the reasons why he chose to be buried on the cliff overlooking Nahal Zin, but from his biography and from the accounts of people who were with him one can learn the motives for this choice. Is it possible that he wanted a ceremony that would force the head of state to make a pilgrimage to Sde Boker once a year? Perhaps that was one of his considerations, but there is no indication of it in his speech or in his writings.

Ben-Gurion's place of burial was the direct result of the decision he made at the beginning of the 1950s to go and live in the Negev. The move to the Negev derived from his commitment to pioneering values, and when he made his home in Sde Boker he called on the Israelis to join him. But this step did not bring about a revival of the pioneering movement, and few chose to follow his lead. In the 1970s, towards his death, Ben-Gurion's failure to persuade the masses to move to the Negev was clear. Pioneering had lost the power of attraction it possessed in the early days of the state, but by choosing to be buried in the Negev, Ben-Gurion showed consistency and demonstrated his commitment to the idea of making the desert bloom.

His decision to act according to the pioneering ethos to some extent contradicted another value associated with Ben-Gurion: *mamlachtiyut* (statism).[8] The place of burial of a prime minister was supposed to be Mount Herzl in Jerusalem, next to the great national figures and the slain of the armed forces, and opposite Yad Va-Shem, a place that he himself had nurtured as a symbol of the revival of the nation.[9] His decision to be buried elsewhere resembled the decisions of some other prime ministers: Moshe Sharett, who was buried in the Trumpeldor cemetery in his city, Tel Aviv, and Menahem Begin, who chose the ancient Jewish cemetery on the Mount of Olives. Ben-Gurion's place of burial testifies to his choice between pioneering values and *mamlachtiyut*, and in this case its location was different. He chose not to be buried in the cemetery of Sde Boker but in a burial plot devoted solely to him and his wife. No one else is buried there.

Ben-Gurion ended his tenure as prime minister and minister of defense in 1963 and returned to his home in Sde Boker in 1963, when he was seventy-seven years old. He finally left politics in 1970, when he was eighty-four.[10] He made his decision about his place of burial on the death of his wife, Paula Ben-Gurion, on January 29, 1968. The decision on where she would be buried was also a decision about his own place of burial. A reporter of Haaretz described the happening in Ben-Gurion's household when the message about the death of Pola Ben-Gurion arrived.[11]

His choice to be buried in the desert, like his choice to live in the desert, expressed both the emptiness and the special significance of the desert.[12] On the one hand, in the pioneering view, the desert was a virginal place devoid of history, a place on which the future would be written. On the other hand, the desert was connected to the ancient history of the people and its time of origin, to the ancient myths which were a central feature in the making of the Israeli ethos. Ben-Gurion's biographer Michael Bar-Zohar reflected on the mythological significance of the choice of this particular spot:

> What did he see when he stood on the cliff face and embraced the endless space with his eyes? The land of Israel, which he loved with such a strong,

total love? Thus stood Moses on another summit, in a different time, and savored with his eyes the land he had promised to his people: "And Moses went up from the plains of Moab to Mount Nebo, to the top of Pisgah, which is opposite Jericho. And the Lord showed him all the land, Gilead as far as Dan" (Deuteronomy 34:1). Thus Joshua saw the land he had conquered with the sword: "So Joshua took all that land, the hill country and all the land of Goshen and the lowland and the Aravah and the hill country of Israel and its lowland" (Jushua 11:16). Thus he too had looked towards the land when he came to its coasts as a youth, moved and thrilled, and did not know that he had come to inherit it.[13]

Ben-Gurion passed away on December 1, 1973. His funeral was an event of great symbolic significance: the nation's farewell to its founding father and a moment of collective orphanhood, which was all the more significant because of the shock of the Yom Kippur War which had ended a few weeks earlier.[14] The funeral ceremony began in Jerusalem. The coffin was placed in the Knesset enclosure and from there was taken by helicopter to Sde Boker. Ben-Gurion did not want any eulogies, and so the military presence and the religious ceremonies stood out, and there was a limited number of participants. The specifications in Ben-Gurion's will imposed silence on those present. When the commemorative ceremonies began, there were speeches from the leaders of the nation and various texts were read, and visitors could enter freely (in contrast to conditions in the funeral ceremony, to which a limited number of people were invited), and the ceremony underwent a process of gradual formation. Ben-Gurion decided on the place where the ceremony would take place; its changing character reflected the development of Israeli society and the status of the father of the nation.

The first years of commemoration: the dead leader in search of an identity

With the passage of time, there were changes in the activities that accompanied the commemorative ceremonies. The first years after Ben-Gurion's death were characterized by intense activity around the official ceremony, and it was almost swamped by it. Institutions were founded, exhibitions were shown, symbolic gestures were made, and there were various attempts at memorializing, most of which had no follow-up. Ben-Gurion Day was an opportunity to inaugurate institutions and enterprises whose establishment had been decided on beforehand. On the first anniversary, the Institute for Desert Research, which already operated within the framework of the University of the Negev (later called the Ben-Gurion University of the Negev), was officially instituted in the Midrasha (later called Midreshet Ben-Gurion). Ben-Gurion's *shrif* (hut) was opened to the public in a state ceremony at the kibbutz of Sde Boker, Ben-Gurion's house in Tel Aviv was opened to the public, and there was a ceremony in which Keren Kayemet Boulevard in Tel Aviv was renamed Ben-Gurion Boulevard.[15]

There were also some one-time symbolic activities. Thus, for example, the inhabitants of the Jezreel Valley brought twenty-one date-palms to the Midrasha, corresponding to the number of members in the council; there were exhibitions of pictures and documents illustrating Ben-Gurion's life in Tel Aviv; there was a congress of the Bible Research Society devoted to Ben-Gurion; there were large commemorative gatherings in London, New York and Paris; various products were issued such as a poster, a stamp, a picture-album, volumes of Ben-Gurion's letters and even a record containing his speeches in English – some of them financed by the government and some paid for by the public.

In the first memorial ceremony, a struggle began over control of the ceremony and the character of the commemoration. For instance, a political rivalry between the Prime Minister Yitzhak Rabin and the minister of defense Shimon Peres was shown in their contest over which of them was to give the main speech. Due to his position, Rabin gave the main speech in the state ceremony, but Peres preceded him by giving a speech to thousands of members of *Gadna* (the cadet corps) on the eve of the ceremony. Another notable example of the struggle over Ben-Gurion's memory was the role of the Histadrut (the Federation of Labor) in the ceremony. The coordinating committee of the Histadrut held a special meeting in memory of Ben-Gurion, its founder and first secretary, in which the secretary-general of the Histadrut Yoram Meshel represented him as the first leader to oppose the polarity in Israeli society and to work for social justice: "We can gain much strength from his party doctrine." Meshel himself was not invited to certain official ceremonies, something that the party newspaper Davar noted as an insult, and represented in a way the growing marginalization of the Histadrut in the Israeli society.[16] He presented him in this way despite the fact that Ben-Gurion was already seen at that time as a national-statist figure rather than a figure of the labor movement or the Histadrut.

A further motif which first appeared in the first memorial ceremony and became central in the succeeding ceremonies was the prime minister's assertion of continuity and his commitment to the legacy of the father of the nation. Prime Minister Yitzhak Rabin declared: "We knew that he was conscious of the great mission that as leader of the nation had been laid upon him."[17]

At the time of the second memorial ceremony in November 1975, there were likewise many events demonstrating the important place occupied by Ben-Gurion in the Israeli consciousness. There was Ben-Gurion Day in the schools, there were exhibitions in Jerusalem, Haifa and Tel Aviv, and institutions were founded that were to be influential in the future. Keren Ha-Negev (The Negev Fund), which looked after the legacy and commemoration of the leader, changed its name to "Yad David Ben-Gurion" and undertook to help in developing the Midrasha, the Ben-Gurion Heritage Institute and the Institute for Desert Research, and also to be responsible for the publication of his books and for exhibitions and to take care of his house in Tel Aviv and his *shrif* in Sde Boker. Shimon Peres (a future prime minister) was elected president of the Fund, and Yitzhak Navon (a future president) was made chairman of the council. The government decided henceforth to officially mark the day of Ben-Gurion's death.[18]

Yet, nevertheless, some of the elements of the first ceremony began to be questioned, and especially the necessity for a government presence at the event. In the ceremony on the second anniversary, the absences were already more noticeable than those present. The journalist Yishiyahu Ben-Porat noted those who came to honor Ben-Gurion's memory, including the president, the chief of staff and a group of followers, but above all he gave an account of those who failed to come. Premier Rabin did not come, nor did he appear at the next anniversary, the last in his first term as prime minister. The Ben-Gurion Law was passed in the course of the year and institutionalized the ceremony as an event in the national calendar, but its status was still uncertain. The memory of Ben-Gurion as a stormy and divisive leader was still too strong. One may recall here that Ben-Gurion himself did not go to the funeral of Levi Eshkol, the prime minister who succeeded him, in 1969, and one therefore may not be surprised that many of Eshkol's supporters in his struggle against Ben-Gurion did not trouble to attend the latter's memorial ceremonies.

Because of Ben-Gurion's special status as the founder of the state, there was also some surprise at the importance of the ceremony among the days of commemoration. In those years, many people said that Ben-Gurion's true memorial was the state he founded, and ceremonies were less important than the people's memory of him. On the third anniversary, an editorial in the *Haaretz* newspaper expressed this sentiment:

> Ben-Gurion's memory has no need to be commemorated, not in the calendar and not in stone. The State of Israel is his monument, and as long as Jews live in this country his name will be engraved in their hearts.[19]

In those years, the ceremony tried to find a form of commemoration that would steer a path between celebration of the greatness of the leader, which was beyond the ceremony and anything said about him, and the old hatreds and rivalries which were not forgotten. Ironically, it was Ben-Gurion's great rival Menahem Begin who gave the ceremony its state character and nobility and placed it above the bitter political struggles in which the leader was involved throughout his political career.

Menahem begin and the nationalizing of Ben-Gurion

When David Magen, a member of the Likud party, became mayor of Kiryat Gat in 1976, he threw the portrait of the founder of the state out of his office and placed it in the municipal storerooms. His provocative act anticipated the first great test of the Ben-Gurion commemorative enterprise. In the "turn-around" of 1977, the party Ben-Gurion founded and which he had headed for so long ceased to be the ruling party for the first time in forty years. Moreover, the elected prime minister Menahem Begin had been Ben-Gurion's political rival for many years and their relationship was accompanied by bitter personal grudges. Ben-Gurion's role in the "Altalena" affair, one of the great myths of the right in Israel, caused great resentment. As long as he was prime minister,

Ben-Gurion refused to allow the transference to Israel of the bones of Vladimir Jabotinsky, the hero of Begin and his movement, who had a central place in the evolving symbolic order of the Likud government. Even if in his final years Ben-Gurion's attitude to his main political rival softened, among other things because of the warm relationship of Ben-Gurion's wife Paula to Menahem Begin, Ben-Gurion was still seen as the mythological rival of the Israeli right and of Menahem Begin in particular.

At the time of the fourth Ben-Gurion Day, the first under the Likud government, there was another event which gave the ceremony a deep historical significance. The president of Egypt, Anwar-e-Sadat, was about to come to Israel and speak in the Knesset. In the Knesset session before the ceremony, prime minister Begin said that he asked for the debate on Sadat's visit to take place on Ben-Gurion Day because he was the first person to turn to the Arab rulers and declare his readiness to meet them at any time and place to talk about peace. The chairman of the Knesset, Yitzhak Shamir, said that Ben-Gurion had united the nation and forged a national unity for a war against the enemy before the state was founded, at the time of its birth and when it made its first steps. He opposed the weaknesses of the exile, irritability and small-mindedness, molded the army, the educational system and the administration, and superintended the mass-immigration to the country.[20]

The words of Begin and Shamir embodied two significant motifs. One was the exploitation of Ben-Gurion's image, despite historical resentments. The Likud used his image to give legitimacy to its new position as the ruling party. The other motif was the emphasis on the theme of national unity in Ben-Gurion's teachings, and thus his legacy was regarded as "the possession of the whole house of Israel," as Shamir put it. Myths and exemplary figures serve various political purposes, and each period makes use of them in accordance with its interests. Begin and his party used the figure of Ben-Gurion with a stress on the elements that suited them and less emphasis on other elements. Jewish national unity was a recurring theme in the ideology of the Likud and its predecessor, Herut, and it enlisted for that purpose the figure of a leader, one of whose celebrated sayings was "Without Herut and Maki!"

Begin wished to separate Ben-Gurion from his party, and the Labor Party reacted by holding events of its own, including a memorial session preceding the official ceremony. The minister of education in the previous government, Aharon Yadlin, who had played a central role in creating the Ben-Gurion Law, tried to extricate the leader of his party from the embrace of Begin and the Likud, which he did by recalling the fact that Ben-Gurion had supported the Peel Commission's program of partitioning Palestine even though it did not include the Negev, to which he was devoted.[21] The difference between the speeches of the leaders of the Likud and those of the leaders of the Labor Party was that the Likud stressed the unity of the nation and the land as Ben-Gurion's primary objective, and the Labor Party stressed the difficult decisions he made, including those that created divisions, especially with respect to the maximalist approach of the Revisionists and their leader Begin.

Menahem Begin and the new ruling party tried, through a selective choice from Ben-Gurion's legacy, to prove that in many respects they were the true successors of the founder of the state, but this was a two-way process. For Ben-Gurion to give authorization to Begin as his political successor, one had to strengthen his status as the founder of the nation.[22] By their very participation in the ceremonies, the leaders of the Likud expressed their loyalty to the ethos of *mamlachtiyut* (statism) and their acceptance of Ben-Gurion's elevated status. The recognition of the lofty status of Ben-Gurion was all the more remarkable in view of the new government's revision of various events in history such as the new positive attitude to the underground movements and the emphasis on the importance of the Holocaust in the creation of the Israeli ethos.[23] Paradoxically, Menahem Begin contributed more than anyone else to institutionalizing the image of Ben-Gurion as the leader of the whole nation, but at the same time he enjoyed the legitimation which the ceremony bestowed on him as his heir.

When a national unity government succeeded the Likud government, there was a noticeable absence of Likud ministers at the ceremony. The legitimacy of their public status had ceased to be a controversial matter. The Likud representatives were sometimes oriental Jews who had come to the country in the framework of Ben-Gurion's absorption policy, but their encounter with the image of the founder of the nation was different in nature and had a tension of its own. The deputy prime minister David Levy said at the 1981 ceremony:

> The people will remember the man of the people, the man of the earth, the shepherd and leader of the workers who devoted himself constantly to a struggle for Hebrew labor, his untiring work on behalf of the ancient people in its renewed homeland.[24]

In a similar way to Begin, David Levy bestowed the legitimacy of the "second Israel" on Ben-Gurion and thus himself gained legitimacy from the figure of the national leader.

The absence of prime minister Benjamin Netanyahu from the ceremony indicated that a process was taking place in which leaders who did not know Ben-Gurion, had not worked with him and had not vied with him as political rivals had begun to come on the stage. For them, the "old man" was a mythical figure from the past.

In the decades of speeches and events, there was a moment of ambiguity in which a deputy prime minister from the ranks of the Likud used Ben-Gurion's memory to defend a controversial policy. Prime Minister Ariel Sharon was absent on account of his health, and his place was taken by his deputy Ehud Olmert. His speech was the first intimation of the program of withdrawal from Gaza and northern Samaria, seen as a radical change in Sharon's policy and a blow to the settlement enterprise in which he himself had been involved in promoting and supporting. Minister Olmert made the following declaration: "In the near future, our leaders will have to summon all their spiritual strength, all their

Zionist faith, in order to decide on our future […]." He then proceeded to quote Ben-Gurion:

> Let us suppose that by military means we could conquer the whole of the western land of Israel, and I am sure we could do it. What would happen then? We would have a single state, but that state would want to be democratic. There would be general elections and we would be in the minority. When we were faced with the question of the whole country without a Jewish state or a Jewish state without the whole country, we chose the Jewish state.[25]

It is hard to know whether the use of Ben-Gurion to support a dramatic change in government policy influenced the course of events. At the same time, it was the only occasion when the ceremony played a significant self-referential role in which the late Ben-Gurion gave his stamp of approval to a certain policy, and his moral authority bestowed legitimacy on a controversial political act. Two leaders of the Likud, Sharon and Olmert, made use of their great adversary David Ben-Gurion in order to promote a policy that contradicted the ethos and tradition of the Likud, as though Ben-Gurion had been one of the leaders of their party. However, this episode is the exception which proves the rule, which was that the founding leader became increasingly less relevant to Israeli society and was no more than a commonplace memory accepted by all.

The importance of the Negev

On the third anniversary of Ben-Gurion's death, there was a television program titled "The Negev is Still Waiting." In a review of the program, a female journalist wrote, concerning the founder of the nation who went to live in the south of the country, that "he decided to be an example of settlement in the Negev, but nobody followed him. What has happened since then? Occupiers, settlers, but not in the right places."[26]

She wrote this during the Rabin government's first term of office, and the observation was aimed at the beginnings of the "Gush Emunim" settlement. The idea that settlement of the Negev was the central and sometimes even the main or only message of the commemoration of Ben-Gurion became more pronounced with the overthrow of the government and the continued development of the territories conquered in 1967. It was a crucial moment in which the spokesmen of the Labor Party confronted the policies of the Likud government with Ben-Gurion's vision, and thus there was a split between the founder of the nation and the government that presumed to speak in his name. At the same time, the development of the periphery was an idea that the Likud government could not ignore either, although it did little about it. The theme of developing the Negev gave the ceremonies an ironic aspect, for it was a criticism of the leaders in the political and geographical center of the state, a criticism that threw a searchlight on their failure to develop the periphery.

Already in the ceremony in 1978, President Yitzhak Navon spoke about this in the presence of Menahem Begin:

> The birthplace of our nation was the south and the Negev. They are the vulnerable, dangerous areas of our country, but they are also its great hope […] We may be standing on the threshold of a new period of our history. If a peace treaty is signed with Egypt, it will have a special significance with regard to the Negev […].[27]

Shimon Peres, the prime minister of the national unity government, seconded this statement in 1984, hinting strongly at settlement:

> Today we are gathered next to his monument and not only at the foot of his grave […] We still have to settle the Negev, […] also because in the Negev there is no question of relationships with our neighbors.[28]

And on another occasion, he added: "If there were Arabs in the Negev, Gush Emunim would certainly have come here and settled in the Negev."[29]

From the 1980s onward, the inhabitants of the Negev tried to exploit people's bad conscience for their benefit, making use of the rare visits of heads of state to ask for the area to be developed in Ben-Gurion's name. The portrayal of the Negev as a central component of the state in the ceremonies only emphasized the fact that the local leaders who had no status and played no part in the ceremonies were not invited and did not speak there. The dean of the Faculty of Humanities and Social Sciences in Ben-Gurion University, Professor Yehuda Gradus, asked the television authorities every year to photograph the heads of state arriving at the ceremony in a helicopter and taking off in a cloud of dust, as if to show that there had been no progress in the development of the Negev dreamed of by Ben-Gurion.

By 1988, however, the Negev had become the most important, or even the only, matter dealt with in the Ben-Gurion memorial ceremonies, but it was precisely his family that tried to limit the protest and to preserve at least the appearance of a ceremony of mourning. When minister Navon said that Ben-Gurion University was struggling to survive, the members of the university started clapping, which was out of place at an official event, and certainly in a commemoration. The behavior of the university people annoyed the Ben-Gurion family, and they were angry when they passed by the graveside with banners of protest, and they insisted that they should leave the place immediately.[30]

National leaders saw the annual event as a suitable occasion to make declarations about the future of the periphery of the country, and from the point of view of the people who lived there it was an opportunity to meet the leaders of the nation and ask for the resources to develop the Negev.

The vision of developing the Negev was brought up on every day of remembrance, and greater emphasis was placed on it on each occasion. In 1999, prime minister Ehud Barak was made an honorary member of the council of

Ramat Ha-Negev. He made a speech at Revivim, and said, "I have ordered a program to be prepared for the development of the Negev in the spirit of Ben-Gurion's vision and in accordance with the requirements of our time." Among his promises was the building of a casino in the Negev, the construction of a high-tech city in Beersheba and the building of three new Bedouin towns. The emphasis in the ceremonies on making the desert bloom, developing the Negev and the neglect of the periphery gave Ben-Gurion's legacy a critical and moral character in relation to the politicians who came to the ceremony, as an assignment from a former leader who presented them with a vision they were supposed to carry out. In these matters, related to the peripheral location of the ceremonies, Ben-Gurion looked like an angry prophet confronting Israeli society and showing it the path it had to take. On the yearly occasion of the ceremony in which Ben-Gurion's demand for pioneering was repeated again and again, one felt each time the ever-increasing gap between this demand and the Israeli reality.

The emphasis on the Negev and the periphery and the location of the ceremony became its chief motif and obscured the former leader's other demands of the nation and the leaders who succeeded him. His legacy was reduced to this single issue which took the form of a kind of lip-service to the periphery.

The relationship to the periphery as the sole prism reflecting the demands of the founding father reduced the place of Ben-Gurion in the Israeli political experience to a view through a narrow crevice. The motif of the periphery and the Negev can be used to advance various claims – that against settlement in the occupied territories, for instance, or against the provision of funds for other purposes – but there was never a demonstration at the annual memorial ceremonies for anything other than settling the Negev. In all the years of the ceremony's existence, subjects like the settlements in the West Bank, the Palestinian uprisings, the fragmentation of society, and unemployment never penetrated the enclosed area in which Israel contended with the founder of the nation except for some sarcastic remarks and hints from the speakers on the podium.

The focus on the center-periphery relationship on one day in the year gave Ben-Gurion a limited relevancy. This was accompanied by a growing distancing of Israeli society from the image of the founding father, an estrangement even expressed physically, especially after the murder of Yitzhak Rabin.

The distancing from the leader

The memorial ceremony in 1995 took place three weeks after the murder of Prime Minister Yitzhak Rabin, and was overshadowed by it. The unprecedented safety measures resulted in a list of regulations. The restrictive precautions, which distanced the participants from the visitors and created an estrangement, were a direct result of the reaction to the murder, but they also reflected a deeper process, the distancing of the figure of Ben-Gurion and its transformation into a less emotive image. The yearly gathering had been a state ceremony from the time of Ben-Gurion's death, but its formal character grew stronger with the years. This process was mainly due to reasons related to time. People who did not know Ben-Gurion personally began to come to the ceremony, people most of whose lives were passed in the post-Ben-Gurion era. The family and the Sde Boker community, which gave the ceremony a more personal flavor, grew smaller in the course of time, and the state aspect, which was already strong before, grew even more pronounced and emphasized the impersonal character of the ceremony.

Here the location of the ceremony was important. It took place on the edge of an area belonging to a community, in a settlement today called Midreshet Ben-Gurion which was founded in accordance with the vision of the leader and with the assistance of the Ben-Gurion Heritage Foundation. The inhabitants settled there in direct or, generally, indirect response to Ben-Gurion's idea of creating an academic community, a "Yavne or Oxford" in the Negev. The inhabitants, who seem to embody the fulfillment of Ben-Gurion's vision of settling the Negev, are cast aside during the ceremony. They have no special status there, and many of them attend due to curiosity, commitment to the ethos of the place, its relative accessibility, and sometimes the performance of minor tasks in the enactment of the ritual. In effect, the area is taken from the inhabitants for a day and is given to the state for a national ceremony.

The Midreshet Ben-Gurion community would appear to be a "community of memory" founded in memory of the late Ben-Gurion next to the *shrif* (hut) in which he lived, in the area in which he chose to live his life and near to the grave in which he was buried. Unlike many settlements in the country named after major figures (Herzliya, Zichron Ya'akov, Mizkeret Batya, and so on), the Midreshet Ben-Gurion community is directly and consciously connected to the figure of Ben-Gurion, his vision and his legacy. At the same time, the community has liberated itself in the course of the years from the basis of its foundation, and it is sometimes even opposed to the national memory. The event that demonstrates this more than anything else is the community's chief ritual, the Adloyada organized by the high school for environmental studies at Purim. Anyone attending the event would never know that it is taking place in a settlement whose main attraction is that it is a national site commemorating the founder of the state. In the Adloyada, the Midreshet Ben-Gurion community creates an autonomous identity, separate from the image of the founding father, the father of the nation, who was also the father of the community living in the Midrasha. This demonstrates the alien character of the state ceremony all the more.

The memorial ceremony: between Zionism and cynicism

The memorial ceremonies for Ben-Gurion are national state ceremonies, and as such they express the continuity, the importance of the nation, and give a form to political power. In their identification with the figure of the "father of the nation," they embody in themselves the tensions that characterized this figure and demonstrate the dialectical gap between his historical image and the society that moves further and further away from his view of the world. The ceremonies are a blend of grandeur and cynicism, memory and forgetfulness, centrality and total irrelevance. Although the Israeli leaders declare their commitment to continuing the path of the founder, for most of them it is their only visit to the southern periphery of the country in the year. In the state ceremony, the officials and the public express admiration for the figure of the founder of the nation, but outside the ceremony Ben-Gurion is hardly present in the social and political discourse in Israel. His impressive image has become banal and has lost much of its relevance.

With regard to those who are present, the ceremony represents the Israeli power-elite, which is mainly Europocentric and belongs to the Israeli upper class. Oriental Jews, religious Jews, Haredi Jews, Arabs and women are not represented, or certainly not to a degree close to their percentage in the population. The presence of the army is particularly noticeable. The Ben-Gurion Midrasha is a relatively well-established community situated in an environment of development towns and unrecognized Bedouin villages whose inhabitants do not see the ceremony as having anything to do with them. Although taking place in the periphery, it can be seen as one of the mechanisms symbolizing and re-instituting the Israeli power-structure and giving it an aura of sanctity under the patronage of the founder of the nation.

Moreover, the message conveyed by the ceremonies and by Ben-Gurion's legacy contradicts the path taken by the aforementioned elite and confront the promise of the beginnings of the state with the complex realities of today. There is a real expectation that the Israeli leaders coming to the ceremony would feel some shame or at least a certain modesty. Because of Ben-Gurion's decision to be buried in the periphery of the country, the leaders of Israel from the whole political spectrum have to make a pilgrimage to a center of bygone values, "out there," to use Victor Turner's expression,[31] south of the political, cultural, social and economic centers of power.

This pilgrimage-cum-ceremony in which the Israeli political center tears itself away from its surroundings and enters the geographical space of the inhabitants of the Ben-Gurion Midrasha places the founding father in the position of an onlooker and judge who decides if his successors have maintained the high standards required by his legacy. By means of the ceremony, Ben-Gurion has become a great eye that looks down on the nation from above and expects the heads of the state to report on their deeds and failures. The peripheral site stresses the uniqueness of Ben-Gurion and distinguishes him from all previous prime ministers, presidents and office-holders. It also distinguishes between pilgrimage to his grave and pilgrimages (if such exist) to graves which do not have such a strong character of confrontation with a demanding legacy. Deference to the great leader is seen in every ceremony and is sometimes expressed in words. Prime minister Ehud Barak said in the memorial ceremony in 2000: "Ben-Gurion's testimony cannot be evaded. His testimony demands vision and action, and we are committed to it."[32]

But this testimony must not be falsified. Apart from these two hours once a year, Ben-Gurion does not serve as a national conscience except on rare occasions. The ceremony serves to elevate him, and it simultaneously confines him and tames him and permits the Israeli governments to continue on their way (which can also be opposite to his way): tendencies to fragmentation, dismemberment of the welfare state, neglect of the periphery and distancing from the moral ideal of "a light unto the nations" which was dear to the heart of the founding leader. The Ben-Gurion memorial ceremonies are a "successful" national ritual in that they honor Ben-Gurion as the first and greatest of the Zionist leaders, the father of the nation, the founder of the state who gave it its status. They are also "successful" in that they divest his image of the subversive potential it contains. Another reason for their success is that they provide a platform for every new generation of leaders and permit it to connect itself with the figure of the first prime minister of Israel.

There is no doubt that Ben-Gurion's greatest achievement was succeeding in his ceaseless struggle for the revival of the Jewish nation, but even before it was founded, and certainly afterwards, there were plenty of questions about the character the reborn nation would have. Would the homeland have a secular character in which the religious part of affairs of state would be limited, as in the Haskalah slogan: "Be religious at home and an Israeli citizen outside"? Or would the Jewish "added value" determine everything and create an equation between nationality and religion, between the earthly homeland and theological or even messianic conceptions? These debates on the character of the future Moledet were already present in the thinking of Ahad Ha-Am, Berdichevsky, Brenner and many other writers and poets of the culture of the Hebrew revival cannot be ignored. The philosopher, literary critic and intellectual Menahem Brinker has undertaken their up-to-date elucidation.

Notes

1 Bat-Neomi Neumar, "Go to the Desert," *Sheva*, 18.11.1998.
2 On the concept of "National Banality" see: Michael Billing, *Banal Nationalism*, SAGE Publications, London 1995.
3 On national rituals, see: Eric Hobsbaum and Terrance Ranger (eds.), *The Invention of Tradition*, Cambridge University Press, Cambridge 1983; Don Handelman, *Models and Mirrors: Towards an Anthropology of Public Events*, Berghahn Books, Cambridge 1990; Gabriella Elgenius, *Symbols of Nations and Nationalism: Celebrating Nationhood*, Palgrave Macmillan, Basingstoke 2011.
4 See the interview of the writers of this study with Hannah Shtilman, 15.4.2008.
5 Roy Rappaport, "The Obvious Aspects of Ritual," in: ibid., *Ecology, Meaning and Religion*, North Atlantic Books, Berkeley 1979, 173–221; Paul Connerton, *How Societies Remember*, Cambridge University Press, Cambridge 1989.
6 On lament rituals in Judaism see: Nisan Rubin, *New Rituals, Old Societies: Invented Rituals in Contemporary Israel*, Academic Studies Press, Boston 2009. As for national rituals in Israel and Zionist symbols see: Avner Ben-Amos and Ilana Bet-El, "Rituals, Education and History: The Memorial Days of the Holocaust and the National Memorial Day in Israeli Schools," in: Emanuel Atkes and Rivka Paldachi, eds.,

Education and History, Jerusalem 1998, 457–479 (in Hebrew); Maoz Azaryahu, *State Rituals*, Sde Boker 1995 (in Hebrew).

7 Michael Feige and David Ohana, "Funeral at the Edge of a Cliff: Israel Bids Farewell to David Ben-Gurion," *Journal of Israeli History*, 31:2 (2012): 249–281.

8 On the concept of "Mamlachtiyut" see: Eliezer Don-Yechia, "Mamlachtiyut and Judaism in the Dictum of Ben-Gurion," Zionism, 14 (1989): 51–81 (in Hebrew); Nir Keidar, *Mamlachtiyut: The Civil Conception of David Ben-Gurion*, Sde Boker 2009 (in Hebrew); David Ohana, *Modernism and Zionism*, Palgrave Macmillan, New York 2012, 80–122; Maoz Azaryahu, "Mt. Herzl: An Historical Outline of the National Cemetery in Jerusalem," *Ophacim BeGeographia*, 64–65 (2005): 369–383 (in Hebrew).

9 On the last years of Ben-Gurion, see: Avi Shilon, *Ben-Gurion: His Later Years in the Political Wilderness*, Rowman & Littlefield, Lexington 2016.

10 Mordechai Eretzieli, "Pola Ben-Gurion has Died," *Haaretz*, 30.1.1968 (in Hebrew).

11 Maoz Azaryahu, "Mt Herzel."

12 On the Desert in the Zionist conception see: Yael Zerubavel, "The Desert as a mythical landscape and as a memorial site in the Hebrew Culture," in: Moshe Idel and Itamar Greenold, eds., *The Myths in Judaism: History, Thought, Literature*, Jerusalem 2004, 223–236 (in Hebrew).

13 Michael Bar-Zohar, *Ben-Gurion*, New York 1986 (pages 1604–1605 in the Hebrew Edition).

14 For a more elaborate discussion of the funeral and its implications, see: Feige and Ohana, "Funeral."

15 These events were reported in the newspapers: See, Sopher "Davar," "Memorial Events, Science and Culture in the Day of the Year for Ben-Gurion," *Davar*, 7.11.1974 (in Hebrew).

16 Ibid.

17 Sopher "Davar," "Rabin on the Legacy of Ben-Gurion," *Davar*, 21.11.1974 (in Hebrew).

18 "The Memory of Ben-Gurion Will be Present Today at an Official Ritual in Sde Boker," *Davar*, 10.11.1975 (in Hebrew).

19 Board Article, "The Commemoration of the Unforgettable," *Haaretz*, 11.6.1976 (in Hebrew).

20 The Protocol of the Israeli Parliament, 15.11.1997, *Divrei HaKnesset*, 81, 396 (in Hebrew); see also: "The Knesset Remembers Ben-Gurion in the Fourth Year to his Death," *Davar*, 16.11.1977 (in Hebrew).

21 Meshulam Ed, "The Government Gave Last Respect to Ben-Gurion in an Official Ritual in Sde Boker," *Davar*, 17.11.1977 (in Hebrew).

22 Shimon Peres and Yitzhak Navon were significant supporters of Ben-Gurion and occupied important positions under his leadership Peres was the CEO of the Security Office, and Navon his personal secretary. Both of them were members of the Raphi party, quitted the Mapai party and were elected to the parliament.

23 Udi Lebel, *The Road to the Pantheon: Etzel, Lechi and the Limits of the Israeli Memory*, Jerusalem 2007 (in Hebrew).

24 Nissim Taito, "Navon: B.G. warned against the involvement of the IDF not for the sake of defending Israel," *Yediot Aharonot*, 3.12.1981 (in Hebrew).

25 Aluph Ben, "Olmert and Sharon Were Assisted by Ben-Gurion: A Jewish State is Better than the Whole Land," *Haaretz*, 1.12.2003 (in Hebrew).

26 Neomi Gal, "Settling in the Negev: The Perspective of the Radio and Television," *Maariv*, 29.11.1976 (in Hebrew).

27 Shlomo Givon, "Navon: Ben-Gurion Took into Account the Strategic Value of the Negev," *Maariv*, 7.12.1978.

28 Amir Rozenblit, "The Tombstone of Ben-Gurion is Disturbing those who Follow Him: The Negev is Still to be Settled," *Davar*, 3.12.1984 (in Hebrew).

29 Shelly Yachimovich, "Navon: I Feel Shame that we Did Nothing to Settle the Negev," *Al-HaMishmar*, 9.12.1986 (in Hebrew).
30 Rozenblit, "Ben-Gurion Always Claimed that we are Prone to a Sick and Laughable Party Division," *Davar*, 16.11.1988 (in Hebrew).
31 Victor Turner, "The Center Out There: Pilgrim's Goal," *History of Religion*, 12:3 (1973): 191–230.
32 Oded Ben Meir and Gal Levinson, "We must follow his way," *Col HaNegev*, 8.12.2000 (in Hebrew).

2 The Hebrewism that engendered the homeland

Non-mythical Judaism

In the Bat-Zion synagogue in the Romema neighborhood in north Jerusalem founded by Haim Beer's father, there were "some ritualistic Jews whose feet, despite the fact that they had lost their faith in the course of time, continued to lead them to the house of the God of their youth."[1] In the synagogue, there were two cantors who stood in front of the Ark. The second was Shalom Gad Brinker, father of Menahem, "the sound of whose long-departed voice, like a violin, wafted at night over the roofs of Peki'in Street." Beer's mother confessed that "when he sang the Kol Nidrei prayer, even the rusty hinges of the doors of my heart would open before the sweetness of his voice." Eventually, Menahem left in his adolescence for a kibbutz in the north and adopted the socialist creed. In 1989, the two sons of the neighborhood Menahem Brinker and Haim Beer, were in Moscow after attending the "Kol Nidrei" prayer in the Achipova Street synagogue, and were walking by the walls of the Kremlin. Beer asked Brinker, "What's on your mind?," and Brinker answered,

> I'm trying to picture my father standing in front of the open Ark with a thin prayer-shawl draped around his neck like a scarf. He taps his tuning-fork on the sides of the Ark, raises it to his ears, and starts to sing, "Behold, we are like clay in the hand of the potter, who lengthens and shortens it at will. Thus we are in your hands, giver of life and death."[2]

Did such sights, scraps of memory, religious-heretical biographical bits and pieces, constitute a hidden link between Brinker and the subjects he investigated, from the Jewish existentialists Berdichevsky and Brenner to the non-Jewish existentialists Nietzsche and Sartre?

On the lines of Brinker's statement that "unifying Berdichevsky's work is a great problem for scholars,"[3] I would like to delineate the unity of the work of Brinker himself, to analyze and interpret it, and I claim that this could contribute to his status as an intellectual in the public sphere in Israel. Underlying his essays on the literature of the Hebrew revival, his critical studies of secular and post-Zionist Judaism, his philosophical studies like those on Friedrich Nietzsche and Jean-Paul Sartre, his discussions with opponents like Yehoshua Leibowitz, and many other matters that he dealt with, was the comprehensive world-view of a thinker and scholar who surveyed the literary crossroads and theoretical inter-sections in the discourse of the last 100 years, the "century of the Jews." In accordance with this genealogy and parallel with it, there was his position as a politically involved intellectual engaged in many activities: philosophical study, literary editing, publicity and education.

Brinker asserted that Hebrew literature developed on two planes: the vertical and the horizontal.[4] The horizontal plane was the connection with non-Jewish culture and literature, and the vertical plane was the connection of the new Hebrew culture and literature with the literary, linguistic and cultural tradition of the Jewish people. Hebrew literature, which combined these two tendencies, should not, in his opinion, depend only on one of them, a position that would be one-dimensional. It would either mean an introverted and pent-up particularism or a total loss of self-identity. All eight chapters of his last book, *Hebrew Liter-ature as European Literature* (2016) – "The Split-up Unity of the Work of Berdichevsky," "European Romanticism and the New Hebrew Literature." "Nietzsche in the Generation of the Hebrew Revival," "Hebrew Literature and Zionist Historiography," "Time and Form in Saul Tchernikovsky," "Biography in the Shadow of Myth in the Manner of Brenner," and "Revolutions in Poetry" – demonstrate the intersection of the horizontal and the vertical plane. Brinker's theory of intersection raises an interesting question: the significance of a Jewish existence which is non-religious, secular or heretically religious, or is in some way not dependent on religion.

In his final article, Brinker attacked the idea of a "national spirit," a sort of Jewish immanence. That, he believed, was connected to the idea that Jewish thought was the essence of Judaism, replacing the Jewish religion. He proposed replacing the national or religious way of thinking with the idea of the two planes in the new Hebrew literature, "the tradition of the forms and images of the Jewish imagination and thought on the one hand, and what takes place in the surrounding European literature on the other."[5]

Brinker believed that the cure for the situation would draw on both sources: the more distant source, existentialist, non-metaphysical thought which shifts the emphasis from metaphysics to the concrete questions of Jewish existence, and the nearer source, connected to both the existentialist tradition and to literature: the idea that concrete existence is understood most deeply through literature rather than through speculative philosophy. Brinker, like the writers of the Hebrew revival, thought that literature, and especially Hebrew literature, had replaced philosophy and theology because it provided a tool by means of which people could consider their actual Jewish existence.

This view explains Brinker's strong attraction to four figures: Berdichevsky, Brenner, Nietzsche and Sartre, between whom there runs a thread of existen-tialism. Throughout his life, these characters accompanied Brinker, who, like them, was a critic and an existentialist, a commentator, and laid stress on peo-ple's concrete existence rather than on theories and ideologies, and also had a

tremendous sense of responsibility for the people around them. Brenner and
Berdichevsky placed in the center of things the actual existence of people as
Jews, and made the question of affinity to Jewish tradition a question of affin-
ity to the cultural-literary tradition.

Brinker regarded Brenner and Berdichevsky as cultural heroes of Jewish life
because they represented a Judaism that was not mythical but existential.[6] In
Brinker's opinion, Hebrew literature had its own independent character. It was
not an imitation of European literature because the counterbalancing Jewish
element was an integral part of it, nor, on the other hand, was it a return to some
religious or mythical past because of its openness to European literature.
Hebrew literature consequently reflected the rhythm of Jewish existence itself,
suspended between the two forces underlying that existence, the past and the
present. It represented an absolute conformity between literature and life. The
classic question of the relationship of literature to life, which troubled Brenner
and Berdichevsky, was answered by the equilibrium they had in common.
Brinker proposed this equilibrium to us a challenge and as the basis for a possible Jewish existence in our time. This is what he had to say in his article, "The
Special Character of the Secular Jew":

> From his mental and spiritual sources, the secular Jew summons up and
> receives the freedom to decide the elements of light and darkness in the tra-
> dition of his people as in every other tradition, and the lack of a direct, pre-
> ordained, unquestioned identity linking him to a large collective with a
> history longer than the exile is compensated by his readiness to withstand
> all the vicissitudes of private and collective life, guided as he is by his
> thinking periodically renewed like life itself with its challenges, forms and
> fulfillments.[7]

Brinker, who was a professor of Hebrew literature and philosophy in Tel Aviv
University and in the Hebrew University in Jerusalem, also engaged in
editing. In addition to editing *Masa*, the literary supplement of the newspaper
Davar (1969–1970), he also edited the socialist journal *Emda* (1974–1978),
which brought together many intellectuals of the Israeli left. The connection
between the editor of *Emda* and the editor of *Ha-Meorer*, a journal edited by
Brenner in London (1906–1907), is clear when one sees Brenner's appeal to
his readers in the journal: "The purpose of HaMeorer is the manifestation of
our Human-Israeli spirit, its broadening and dedication of our national literary
works, sublation of our Hebrew-Human element."[8]

Berdichevsky: brushing Jewish history against the grain

Berdichevsky, known as the "Hebrew Nietzsche," was in all stages of his life
involved in "heretical religiosity." With regard to the theologian George Lindbeck's
distinction between two approaches to religion, the cultural and experiential models

of faith, David Neumark can be classed in the first category and Buber and Berdichevsky in the second.[9] In his critical article "Jewish Modernity" discussing the four volumes of Berdichevsky's articles which appeared in Warsaw in 1900, Neumark criticized Berdichevsky's quasi-Nietzschean Hebrew revolution which he thought would lead to an historical and theological nihilism.[10] In contrast to the unifying theological approach of Ahad Ha-Am and Neumark, Berdichevsky believed that "in every period there was a different kind of Judaism."[11] In this way, Berdichevsky brushed Jewish history against the grain and sought to include in it not only the conformists and believers but also the heretics who were cast outside the camp, for what was significant for Berdichevsky was mythical time and not historical time.

How does one connect the individual with a revolutionary movement? This was a classic problem for intellectuals who wished to create a "new man." They ended up by congregating in avant-garde belligerent orders or in elite movements which had no contact with the masses. Like the Nietzschean cultural critics at the turn of the century who wanted to make Zarathustra into a political militant, Berdichevsky was faced with the problem of translating the philosophy of the cabbalists into sociological language. Many artists and intellectuals turned their backs on integral nationalism of the kind of Heinrich von Treischke, based on ancient traditions, privileges and social distinctions, and created an existentialist species of nationalism which stressed the individual rather than the community, the present rather than the past, aesthetics rather than ethics.[12]

Brinker devoted half of his book *Hebrew Literature as European Literature* to a discussion of Berdichevsky's work. Why did this Jewish critic and author of the period of the Hebrew revival deserve such attention from the Israeli scholar? In his entry, "Micha Yosef Berdichevsky (Ben-Gurion)" in *New Jewish Time: Jewish Culture in the Secular Age – an Encyclopedic View*, Brinker spoke of Berdichevsky's influence on the Jewish youth and intelligentsia at the turn of the nineteenth and twentieth centuries and described his subversion of accepted norms in the historiography and culture of the Jewish people. Like Ahad Ha-Am, Berdichevsky's starting point was the critical situation of the Jewish people at the turn of the century, but, unlike him, his solution was what he called "the complete Europeanization of Jewish culture."[13] The conformism and introversion of traditional Jewish culture which made the youth and the intellectuals seek out foreign cultures created what he called a "rent in the heart." The meaning of this was their desire to be faithful to their people together with a wish to become "Hebrew Europeans." The cure for this rent was through a spiritual revolution of the modern Jews who would abandon the world of *halacha* and become a sovereign people in their historical land.

Brinker examined Berdichevsky's revolutionary call, a call made in a variety of ways such as novellas, novels, historical research, Bible criticism, the editing of *aggadot*, reviews and publicistic articles. In different periods of his life, the Hebrew writer adopted changing positions on basic matters concerning Jewish identity and culture. Brinker's intention was to find the unity in Berdichevsky among the multiplicity and change. Bar Halafta, a figure of the Haskalah who wandered around in the new movements of literature, may possibly not have been an exact portrait of Berdichevsky, but this imaginary figure tells us something about the many changes and reversals that took place in his outlook."[14] In Reuben Brainin's journal *Mi-Mizrach u-mi-Maarav* (From the East and West), there was an article "Age and Youth" which was the first of a series Berdichevsky wrote on national subjects signed with the pseudonym "Bin-Gorion." Brinker explained that the name-change reflected his change of position from that of a radical representative of the Haskalah to a national point of view.[15] Previous to that turning-point he was first a yeshiva-student from Volozhin and later a religious reformer seeking a compromise between religious tradition and the ideas of the Haskalah. His new national outlook was intended to unite the Jewish people. In the following stage, he became a heretical member of the Haskalah, an enemy of *halacha* and a man with a "rent" in his heart. The rent in his heart brought him to the realization that the influence of the Haskalah on the young was a positive contribution to the Jewish collective, and that the individual who abandoned the traditions of the past was the modern representative of the Jewish nation. In Brinker's opinion, these frequent changes in the space of only eight years took at least eighty years among Jewish intellectuals as a whole.

In Brinker's opinion, Berdichevsky "did not fit any theology, whether liberal or eclectic, whatsoever. He was somewhat pagan, somewhat pantheistic [...] and, at the same time, theistic."[16] A one-dimensional reading which saw Berdichevsky primarily as a thinker and preacher of secularism was rejected. His main criticism in his national-Zionist phase was not of religion as such but of rabbinical Judaism, the school of "Yavne" which ignored nature, the health of the body, beauty, the senses, the instincts and the love of life. Like Tchernikovsky, Berdichevsky subscribed to the romantic view of a unity of experience that was thought to have existed in the pre-monotheistic era, the view that already at "Sinai" and before "Yavne" the original Hebrew unity ceased to be total. There began a division of soul that prohibited sensory pleasure, and conscience and a sense of guilt came into being. The split from the unity of existence began at "Sinai" where spirituality arose, causing an alienation of man from nature, but only at "Yavne" were the spirit and tradition completely victorious over nature. Amos Oz gave a good account of Brinker's Berdichevsky:

> Brinker comes and says to us, Berdichevsky did not begin with, but ended with relationships between the past and the future, with arguments against Yavne and in favor of the Canaanites, with a revolt against the shtetl. There were various phases and even contradictions in Berdichevsky's thought, and in those very same periods there was a discordance and sometimes an opposition between Berdichevsky's essays and his stories. In Berdichevsky's world there is a counterbalancing movement to the force of gravity: the gravitational pull of Nietzsche and Schopenhauer. There is a discordance and even an opposition between his early thinking – vitalistic, optimistic – and the stories he wrote in those very same years. Brinker confronts us with

this contradiction. It was Berdichevsky who told us that there was an opposition in the curse of Yavne which was preceded by the curse of Sinai: the disconnection with nature and the instincts in favor of the book, in favor of parchments. There is an opposition between this way of thinking and what Berdichevsky wrote in his early stories, things steeped in fatality. Not determinism but fatalism in the darkest and gloomiest sense of the word, far from the romanticism of vitalism, of the instincts and senses.

The sources of nature in Berdichevsky are distant, perhaps Rousseau and Nietzsche, but at the same time there was another Berdichevsky, and Brinker makes this clear. To use a formula that was not Berdichevsky's or Menahem's, I would say that his main contention was this: our past belongs to us, but we do not belong to our past. At certain stages, in certain moments, both Berdichevsky, Brenner and Menahem Brinker would perhaps have accepted this formula. If we belong to our past, it is bad and hateful; if the past belongs to us, then things are possible.[17]

Nietzsche – the banality of holiness

A central figure in Brinker's thought and writing was Nietzsche. To give a succinct description of Nietzsche's purpose, it was a punitive celebration of the immanent over the transcendental. This was something very deep and had both an existential and a theological aspect. In its existential aspect, it was an affirmation of life as it is without hope of redemption or an afterlife, and without regrets at one's present existence. And theologically, Nietzsche did not make the death of God dependent on the elimination of religious feeling. He did not deny anything, and he recognized the deep pathos there is in man, a pathos that allows him to transcend himself.

Nietzsche gave the generation of the Hebrew revival and its writers a major gift: the liberation of Jewish life from the concept of holiness. Israel has no Messiah, wrote Brenner, so we have to work. Nietzsche transferred the religious passion to life itself where it became a motivating force: one must not yield to the difficulties of day-to-day existence. This passion knows despair and the temptation of religion but continually directs man to his immanent existence. Brinker saw Nietzsche as the herald of the generation of revival because he provided a profound basis for life in actuality devoid of messianic ecstasies.

In his national-Zionist period, Berdichevsky expounded on the book *The Genealogy of Morals* by Nietzsche, the philosopher who gave an interpretation of the fateful turning-point that had been reached in the history of the Jews and in European culture in general.[18] Brinker pointed out the use Berdichevsky made of the idea of "desecration" (as in "the desecration of natural values"), a use that ascribed sanctity to nature. For Nietzsche, the history of the Jewish people was the history of someone who was rooted in his country, and whose God was a local God and not a universal one. Here, Brinker saw significant differences between Nietzsche and Berdichevsky. He regarded Nietzsche as anti-romantic in his positive attitude both to "Yavne" and to "Sinai," while Berdichevsky was seen as having a romantic approach to nature. But they both shared the view that the real lives of the Israelites of the biblical period were not as depicted in the Bible, for in the Bible divine providence is shown as guiding humanity according to moral criteria. Berdichevsky closely followed Nietzsche in his biblical criticism which claimed that the editors of the Bible had distorted Jewish history.

Brinker pointed to a dialectical paradox: the attempts of the traditional Jewish national culture to absorb European culture gave rise to the Jewish rebirth and the revival of the Hebrew language. The modern language of the younger generation, which used it for purposes of assimilation, at the same time gave rise to a national consciousness among other Jews.

Brinker explained the sociological context. As a result of the tendency to assimilation, the children of those who had left the yeshivas were given a European education and a command of the Russian language, and there was a crisis in the publication of books and journals in Hebrew. Most of the Hebrew newspapers shut down and the number of readers of Hebrew authors such as Mendele, Ahad Ha-Am, Berdichevsky and Tchernikovsky decreased astoundingly. As Amos Oz wrote:

> Hebrew literature had many more readers before the year 1900 and after the year 1920 than in the formative years of Zionism between 1900 and 1920. The main years in the production of Bialik, Tchernikovsky, Brenner, Berdichevsky and Brainin were years with few readers of Hebrew literature.[19]

Fortunately for the Hebrew language, this was also the period of the flowering of Zionism and the beginning of settlement in Palestine, processes which revived the ancient tongue. The first two decades of the twentieth century were a time of searching for a path among the Jewish youth. The process of secularization made conservative views obsolete and caused the old elites to be repudiated. The young people sought inspiration and guidance from the new literary intelligentsia, and Hebrew authors like Smolenskin, Lilienblum, Frishman, Ahad Ha-Am, Berdichevsky and Brainin responded to the call.

Zionism was an exceptional phenomenon in the history of European nationalism, being the only national movement created by writers and intellectuals.[20] It could be said that Hebrew literature at the turn of the century in Russia and Eastern Europe gave birth to Zionism. It is interesting to note that this literary and national rebirth was bound up with the crisis at the turn of the century, with the moral skepticism with which it was accompanied, the stress on aestheticism, radical individualism and decadence. It was precisely the writers, poets and critics who were especially open to Jewish decadence such as Berdichevsky and Brenner that became the guides of the national transvaluation of values. This process involved, among other things, the major influence of Friedrich Nietzsche.

Brinker stressed the major role of Nietzsche in the crisis between the generations and his influence on the writers of the culture of the Jewish revival in the years 1880–1920.[21] This influence began to be seen in the European literature of the last decade of the nineteenth century when the books of Brandes, Shestov and Simmel served as intermediaries between the German philosopher and the Hebrew writers. Although *Thus Spake Zarathustra* was popular among readers in eastern and Western Europe, Brinker thought that this book was not of special importance for Hebrew writers and critics; Berdichevsky, for example, admitted that he did not finish reading it. The essays most read on the right and left were *The Use and Abuse of History*, *The Birth of Tragedy*, *Schopenhauer as an Educator*, and later works such as *The Genealogy of Morals* and *The Antichrist*. Brenner also read *The Twilight of the Gods* and *Ecce Homo*.

Brinker discerned three stages in the encounter of Hebrew literature with Nietzsche. The first was the popularization of war-cries such as "God is dead!," "the *Übermensch*" and the "will to power." The second was the indirect acquaintance with Nietzsche through European literature, which we have mentioned, and the third was the reading of Nietzsche's actual works and immersion in his radical ideas. Brinker came to the conclusion that in all these stages Nietzsche was a more fruitful influence on Hebrew literature than any other nineteenth-century thinker or writer.[22]

In the first decade of the twentieth century, there were two opposing camps: those who rejected Nietzsche and those who supported him, those who advocated a connection with Jewish tradition and those who spoke of a renewal of Hebrew culture with a direct reference to Nietzschean ideas. Brinker saw Berdichevsky as the most outstanding example of a thinker who made an extensive use of the Nietzschean "transvaluation of values." The influence of the German thinker was seen in the five volumes of stories that Berdichevsky published in 1899, to which he added four books of reflections. In *On the Road*, one sees Nietzsche's influence on Berdichevsky in his affirmation of the "positive" values of doubt, extremism, opposition, war and heroism and his condemnation of the "negative" values of authority, certainty, peace and compromise. The call for an alteration of values was made in the context of a call for a comprehensive transvaluation of values in the Jewish national culture. At the head of his article "Age and Youth," he quoted Nietzsche's aphorism, "in order to build a temple one must destroy a temple."[23] A sentence signed with the initials F. N. was printed as a war-cry against conservative opponents.

In the debate about the future of Hebrew culture and the Jewish nation, Nietzsche's name was commandeered by the revolutionary side. In opposition, at the head of the conservative camp, stood Ahad Ha-Am, who supported the unity of Jewish culture and the preservation of its continuity in all generations. This position reflected his adherence to the concept of the "spirit of the people," involving a belief that the Jews had always preferred thought to feeling and ethics to aesthetics. The "national spirit" was seen by Ahad Ha-Am as a permanent feature of Jewish culture. In accordance with this idea, he wrote an article, "The Transvaluation of values" in which he examined Nietzsche as the source of inspiration of the opposing camp. According to Brinker, his knowledge of the German philosopher was very limited as it was chiefly derived from a reading of

Brandes' book. Nietszche's main thesis, according to Ahad Ha-Am, was that human achievements were not to be seen as actions in society but in terms of individual excellence. Ahad Ha-Am said that Jews could agree with this idea on condition that the achievements were judged by the criteria of intelligence (science) and morality (justice) and not by those of aesthetics or heroism. He thought that, according to these criteria, certain figures could be regarded as examples of the *Übermensch*: for instance, prophets who sought justice, in the Jewish tradition. The synthesis of "Judaism" and "Europeanism" and of "Judaism" and "humanism" was the main subject of discussion in the cultural discourse of the period. In this context, Brinker exemplifies Ahad Ha-Am's attitude, for him, Nietzsche was the outstanding example of a non-Jewish thinker of general significance, some of whose ideas could on certain conditions be absorbed into Jewish culture.[24]

Like Ahad Ha-Am, who complained about the "Aryan form" of Nietzsche's thought, his star pupil, Bialik, also had his reservations. Hinting at a lion – the "blond beast," the chief symbol of *Zarathustra* and which also figured in Bialik's poetry – the Hebrew poet rejected the attack on Jewish culture: "Rather than be a *kfir* (lion) among lions, I will die with the sheep/ I was not endowed with teeth and nails/ All my strength is given to God, and God is life!"[25] In a famous verse in "The Dead in the Desert," Bialik cried, "We are the last generation of slavery and the first of redemption!"[26] Bialik saw himself as a definite opponent of Nietzschean influence, but Bialik, like Brinker himself later on, proposed aiding the renewal of Hebrew culture through an assemblage of the best works by Jewish authors in all generations. He pointed out the dialectical significance of this action: the bringing together of the past would facilitate the production of Jewish works by young people.

One could say that Brinker's collaboration in the editing and writing of *New Jewish Time: Jewish Culture in the Secular Age – An Encyclopedic View*, was an attempt at updating, following the example already provided by the literature of the Hebrew revival. In both attempts at a dialectical assemblage, there was the same logic: one must preserve the texts of value and remove the ones without value from archives, libraries and one's memory. This is how Bialik described this contribution to a transvaluation of values: "One must destroy a synagogue in order to build a synagogue in its place [...]. This is the foundation and the root: the need to grow through a new assemblage."[27] Brinker pointed out the interesting fact that Nietzsche's two adversaries in the new Hebrew culture, Ahad Ha-Am and Bialik, exhibited Nietzschean inspiration. Their opposition to his teachings did not prevent them from coining slogans about a transvaluation of values. Nietzsche's criticism, said Brinker, like other radical criticisms, was a radical rejection of tradition and a call for an updating of values in modern times. In a similar way, the literature of the Hebrew revival rejected what it called "ghetto culture," a culture that repressed the instincts, the aesthetic sense and intellectual curiosity of Jewish youth.

Brinker, who did not see these discussions as historical hair-splitting or pedantry, noted that although the remote past was the subject of Berdichevsky's historical studies, in his publicistic writings he was ceaselessly preoccupied by the immediate future. While Berdichevsky the scholar and historiographer edited a genealogy and in so doing interpreted the past, Berdichevsky the intellectual expressed his opinion in the public sphere in order to influence and bring about a change in the collective consciousness. Brinker also traced the affinities between the three aspects of time in Ahad Ha-Am, especially in his controversy with Berdichevsky. Berdichevsky criticized Ahad Ha-Am's view of Jewish culture, a view which in his opinion imposed his personal preference for ethics over aesthetics on the cultural history of the Jewish people in the past and present. The main problem to be dealt with, in Ahad Ha-Am's opinion, was the disintegration of the Jewish nation in modern times. To the geographical and linguistic dispersion of the past were added the differences in way of life and the fragmentation in beliefs and ideas. Brinker regarded Ahad Ha-Am as first and foremost a sociological thinker who called for the creation of a new common denominator like the "spiritual center" or the "national morality" which would bridge the differences in the Jewish people.

Brinker's ideas concerning the controversy between Ahad Ha-Am and Berdichevsky also have a relevance for our own time with regard to the situation in the State of Israel. The "rent in the heart" that existed then still applies to the relationship between the Jewish legacy and the state. Here, Brinker the intellectual fell back on Brinker the literary and historical commentator who scrutinized Ahad Ha-Am's vision for the Jewish communities: the vision of a "spiritual center," as in "from Zion shall go forth the Law," the search for a new unity, a new focus for the national spirit, different from a knowledge of history or the study of Hebrew. Unlike in Dubnow, for instance, or in Graetz, the knowledge of the past in Ahad Ha-Am was something beyond the preservation of the national heritage. Ahad Ha-Am's spiritual Zionism sought to provide a comprehensive solution to the crisis of the secular age. Berdichevsky, on the other hand, who was not a political thinker, was in Brinker's opinion an intellectual, an onlooker and critic, not a sympathizer. Berdichevsky thought that because doubt was preferable to certainty, the problem of the Jewish people in modern times was the unity of the national culture and not the multiplicity of ideas it contained. Because the youth were repelled by homogeneity rather than assimilation, without a national and cultural rebirth the Jewish people would cease to exist.

Existentialism: Jews, Judaism and Jewishness

After the Uganda crisis and the crisis in Hebrew literature at the beginning of the twentieth century, Berdichevsky thought that there was no longer any chance of transvaluation of values in Jewish society or any likelihood of becoming a nation. Consequently, he ceased to be an intellectual fighting in the public sphere through publicistic articles and was henceforth a scholar, a collector and an editor of Aggadot. As Brinker expressed it, he began to build a "literary monument" to a culture he had rebelled against in the past, and "from a rebel became a custodian."

In his rebellious national period, he had recognized the connection between Jewish self-consciousness in the present and an understanding of the past, a connection that created a new consciousness that could mold the present and the future. In Nietzschean terms, it was "monumental history," a new subversive history of the Jewish people which could be the means of transvaluation of values. What was required was not just an explanation of the past but an evaluation of it. The ideal one should strive for was that of the Jewish rebels against foreign powers and the spirit of the zealots in the time of the Second Temple and not "Yavne" and intellectualism. Because the tradition of "Gerizim" and Joshua was older than that of "Sinai' and Moses, "the importance of the land in the faith of the ancient Israelites took precedence over the Torah covenant." In Berdichevsky's opinion, those who saw the "Sinai" revelation as the founding event of Judaism falsified the history of the people of Israel, and in this way institutionalized the contemptuous attitude of the Jews to spatial values for generations to come.

Berdichevsky's profound knowledge of oral law and Midrash gave him an advantage in determining the order of preferences. Like Ahad Ha-Am, he preferred "historical truth" to "archaeological truth." If the tradition of "Gerizim" preceded that of "Sinai," then the "land of Israel" preceded the giving of the Torah. One cannot ignore the analogy drawn by Brinker (who was a left-wing Zionist intellectual) when he noticed the affinity between Berdichevsky's historical studies and his ideological outlook. Brinker reached this conclusion from reflecting on Berdichevsky's ideas as expressed in the assertion in his essay "Sinai and Gerizim" that "Israel takes precedence over the Law." The subversive meaning of this was that the Israelite nation is the continuous factor in Jewish history: "Only the historical bedrock – the people of Israel – is permanent, and it supports [...] the changes in the various Judaisms."[28] This was a supreme challenge to the tradition whose outstanding representative was Saudia Gaon, who said that "our people is only a people by virtue of its Torah." Berdichevsky is revealed once again as a tireless subverter of that tradition.

But the human content in his stories appears to contradict his theoretical position. His call for the individual to liberate himself from the dominance of the collective ("the tyranny of the majority") also entailed the liberation of the present from the past. These two liberations condition one another: the liberated individual looks towards the future. The transvaluation of values and forgetfulness of the past were both necessary for the liberation. Brinker solved the apparent contradiction between a radical individualism and the communal spirit by saying that the liberty of the individual was seen by Berdichevsky not only as an objective, but also as an opportunity for the collective to renew itself. Brinker discerned this point of view in the way that Berdichevsky stressed the liberation of the individual as an aim in itself in the hope that the affinity between the liberated individuals would eventually make possible the founding of a nation.[29] But Brinker also proposed a deep consideration of the fictional characters in Berdichevsky's stories, characters that are surprising with regard to his theoretical demands. They are sometimes like robots unable to break with their past.

The contradiction between the rational demand for liberation and this spiritual inability to be liberated was the final nail in the coffin of belief in a national rebirth on the basis of a transvaluation of values.

The idea that there is a contradiction between "Jews" and "Judaism" became a whole philosophy of history in Berdichevsky's national thinking. The revolt against the rule of *halacha* made him distinguish between the needs of the present and the individual and the spirit of the past and the collective, "the priority of the living man over the legacy of his ancestors." The individual Jews of the present bore the burden of the past which weighed upon them, and he came to the conclusion that the fixed element in Jewish history was the nation, and all the teachings, the ideologies, the theologies and the beliefs – the "Judaisms" – were changing elements in the history of the Jews. Berdichevsky discovered that belief in the religious-cultural continuity of the people of Israel was an ideology that did not correspond to the real history. The belief in continuity, which Brinker also thought was a false idea, had preserved the nation, but the collective of the people of Israel which produced a variety of teachings and beliefs was the only continuous factor. The formula, "Israel preceded the Torah" has a double meaning: precedence in time and precedence as a value. The people is more important than its Torah, and consequently there is no problem with a selective reading of the early Torah. This acknowledgment by Berdichevsky of the role played by suppressions and contradictions in the history of Jewish culture was a pioneering position that preceded that analyses of many later thinkers and historians.

In 1905, seven years after the publication of "Age and Youth," Berdichevsky declared that he had returned to the faith of his youth: "The Torah precedes Israel."[30] He returned to it from the position that the body of the nation, the people of Israel, was more important and worthy of literary celebration than historical Judaism. The new formula, the contrary of the previous one, expressed his despair of Zionism and of the continued existence of the modern Jew. The controversies following the Uganda crisis, the lack of Zionist achievement and the shrinkage of the Hebrew-reading community which caused the closure of all the Hebrew journals except for Brenner's *Ha-Me'orer* in the first decade of the twentieth century, were seen by him as proof of the failure of the attempt to change the values of the nation, a change he had hoped for and believed in. His next question was hypothetical: what would remain of Jewish culture when the Jewish people had left the stage of history? Perhaps Judaism would remain as a "spiritual force" when there were no more Jews. He even wrote in his diary that in the absence of the Jewish people, some other people might adopt Judaism. Berdichevsky held the position that the Jewish culture he had rebelled against – the halachic-rabbinic culture – had a universal significance and was worth perpetuating.

Brinker believed that Berdichevsky's preoccupation with historical research and Bible criticism was not the cause of the lack of interest he showed in the problems of the Jewish people in the years of the First World War, but its result. Berdichevsky neglected, according to Brinker, the publicistic writing which was his main activity in the first decade of the twentieth century; he lost the passion of the period of the "transvaluation of values" and the hope of a renaissance of Jewish culture.[31] Unlike Brenner, who accused Berdichevsky of dramatizing the rents in his heart and exaggerating them unnecessarily, Brinker said that the rents endured by Berdichevsky were real and could not be ignored, but only accepted. They were not stylistic features but authentic expressions of reality. These rents – between the desire for renewal and the appeal of tradition, between the subjective necessity of rebellion and the objective perception of the continuity of the past, between Zionist-political freedom and the yearning for spiritual salvation, between contentment with what exists and the wish for total redemption, between the writer and thinker and the struggles in the public sphere – were at the heart of the experience of this intellectual fighter for values. In this, in Brinker's opinion, Berdichevsky displayed "a voluntarist, anti-deterministic outlook of which there is no other example among the historians and thinkers of the Jewish people." Brinker also pointed to the fact that most of the prose-writers in Hebrew and Yiddish, with the exception of Berdichevsky and Brenner, were skeptical about the future of Zionism, but all the Hebrew poets supported the Zionist movement. The reason, in his opinion, was that the poets believed in ideals and the writers of prose gave an impartial description of the real complex situation. They were skeptical about anything to do with changes of values or spiritual revolutions. While the poets enthused about their dreams of improving the world, the prose-writers were realists and more like collectors than pioneers.

A spiritual school or extended family?

Brinker saw Berdichevsky and Brenner as two critical readers of Ahad Ha-Am. A text in *Slavery In Freedom* served them as an inspiration: "I can take a sentence I like on the beliefs and ideas that my forefathers have bequeathed to me without feeling that this will break the connection between me and my people."[32] Ahad Ha-Am claimed that the modern Jew is entitled, like the enlightened European, to a freedom of choice which is a capacity to choose certain elements of a tradition, a choice that represents his freedom and his Promethean self-creation. The process of secularization was seen by him as a development in modern times which could not be reversed, and at the same time as a process in which there were dangers. As a follower of the European Enlightenment, Ahad Ha-Am wished to find the qualities of freedom, secularism and enlightenment in his own people, and he finally found them in the Jewish national movement. This was a radical idea, because as an admirer of the European Enlightenment which was the inspiration for the Haskalah, he required all traditions to be subject to testing and criticism.

In the opinion of Ahad Ha-Am, the things the people have in common do not make them a spiritual school, the common denominator of which would be a certain ideology, theology or philosophy, but they can make them into an extended family in which, together with continuity and closeness, there is continual change.

Ahad Ha-Am sought a paradigm, a conceptual system in which geographically dispersed and culturally diverse secular and religious Jews would come together in a modern Jewish nation. The content of this paradigm – a "national culture," a "national morality" or "spiritual Zionism" – would represent a national model in which there was a particular Jewish stratum above a universal European stratum. One had, for example, to find a place for the universal ideas of Nietzsche, ideas based on the achievements of individuals and not on the progress of the average man. The "spirit of the nation" was a concept which involved a process of selection made in accordance with universal criteria.

In discussing the genealogy of the Jewish identity, Brinker said that in modern times, with the foundation of nation-states, Jews were faced with the temptation of joining the new national entities at the price of erasing the foundations of the traditional national consciousness. Unlike in the pre-modern period when there was a symbiosis between religion and nationality, there was an attempt to separate their religion from their nationality, The reactions of Jewish thinkers were varied. The Reform and the new Orthodox, for example, responded to the challenge by recreating their Judaism as a religious community participating in the life of the nation. Secular schools of thought found their Judaism in a cultural community or some supra-national movement. In these modern tendencies, the "universal" moral values of the Jewish religion were stressed and the national or racial elements were disregarded. The most audacious challenge, in Brinker's opinion, came from authors, poets and intellectuals writing in Hebrew in Russia and Eastern Europe, who saw Judaism not as a religious sect but as the culture of a people, the culture of a historical group with a continuous memory, that lived with the sense of belonging to a large family. The fact that this family lived in exile and lacked several elements of "normal" nationhood did not negate its national existence. They regarded the religion as only one of the components of the national culture, seeing that nationhood is a continuous consciousness that would exist even if the religion disappeared. According to this view, all those who feel themselves to be Jews belong to the Jewish people.

This idea, which is accepted in Israel today, was regarded at the time as something new. Human beings are not static entities whose identity is determined in advance. The idea that a man is self-sufficient and not part of a heritage is in Brinker's opinion a Promethean concept among mankind. Judaism would have become a religion without a nation if the Jews had accepted the approach of the Berlin Haskalah and later the Reform, an approach whose meaning was that Judaism was a religion that could exist within the framework of any territorial nationalism whatsoever. The Jews of Eastern Europe rejected this interpretation of their nationhood and withstood the temptation to disavow the national elements in Judaism and reduce it to a religious community. The Jewish writers and thinkers in Russia and Eastern Europe at the turn of the century saw the Jewish people as one that could exist in the future by depending on their feelings, their memories and their historical consciousness.

The undermining of the authority of tradition, which was a prominent feature of the European Enlightenment, also had its repercussions in Jewish intellectual history. The major Jewish thinkers in the national period saw the Jewish collective as a historical family and not as a school of thought or a religious community. A national outlook was seen as the only replacement for tradition, a replacement which assured the unity and continuity of the Jewish people in the past and would do so in the future. Lilienblum defended his denial of the "Torah from heaven," and Ahad Ha-Am said, "We have no fear that the thread that connects us to our fathers and our fathers' fathers will be broken," even if "one's heresy bears the name of Darwin." Brinker said that it is interesting to note that these two moderate thinkers pleaded the cause of radical European Enlightenment principles in the heart of the Jewish community.

The danger that many Jewish thinkers feared was the fossilization of the Jew through a strict observance of the old values, and their hope lay in breaking the stranglehold of conservatism, a "transvaluation of values," radical innovation and a renovation of the basic models of Jewish culture.

Brinker diverged from the usual ideas of scholars who stressed the opposition to the unification of Jewish history and culture proposed by Ahad Ha-Am. The scholars emphasized the affirmation of pluralism in Berdichevsky's teachings and the stress on dualities, both diachronic ("Yavne" after "Sinai") and synchronic (rationalists versus kabbalists). Brinker claimed that in addition to the formulas of opposition, "religion versus life" or "the book versus life," Berdichevsky also saw an opposition between "history" and "nature." The God of nature, of the hills and valleys, was already exchanged at "Sinai" for the God of history. But the revolution in the time of Berdichevsky was the most radical of all. Until then, it had never been a question of leaving the national culture for the surrounding culture. The hope of Berdichevsky and Brenner was that those who abandoned abstract Judaism would nevertheless remain within the Jewish fold, or in the sociological terms used by Brenner, that the heretical would not become assimilated.

The "new Hebrew" who had abandoned historical Judaism discovered that the Jewish past continued to live in him. Not only was the present part of his personality, but past eras also continued to reverberate within him. His personality did not achieve harmony and the break with tradition created a rent in his heart.[33] This was not only a Jewish phenomenon, said Brinker, explaining Berdichevsky's intentions, but it was characteristic of the whole of modern humanity. Berdichevsky did not believe that the Jews would achieve harmony if the sociopolitical problem was solved. The idea that the assimilated would choose to remain Jews if a place was found in Jewish culture was in Brinker's opinion a historical and anachronistic. This idea relegates Berdichevsky's views on modernity, views that were only possible in the national period, to ancient history.

Brenner – "heretical believer" or "tragic realist"?

The Brenner-Nietzsche *amor fati* (love of fate) cannot obscure or hide Joseph Haim Brenner's existentialist distress. And what was the nature of that distress? Aaron Appelfeld gave a good description of the Archimedean point in Brenner's stories and personality: "His weaknesses come together with tremendous force, lifting him onto another sphere which I call the sphere of religious distress."[34] This "religious distress," which involves Nietzschean "damnable questions," confronted Brenner with the paradox of heresy and faith – "heretical religiosity."[35]

In Brinker's opinion, Brenner and Berdichevsky shared the conviction that the Jewish people had a culture that was not built layer upon layer, but was a synthesis of individual contributions in the course of history, a national culture made up of foundation-stones that have stood the test of time. This synthesis was not based on commentary and disputation which bridged the generations but was marked by radical mutations, new perspectives and refreshing examples. Ahad Ha-Am, on the other hand, accepted change, but only as a continuation of the past, an interpretation that did not deviate from the norm. What Berdichevsky, *Brenner and Ahad Ha-Am had in common was a desire to Europeanize Jewish* culture, but Ahad Ha-Am was an evolutionist while Berdichevsky and Brenner were revolutionaries.

Berdichevsky and Brenner did not advocate gradual changes and did not rely on the continuity of the Jewish people, and in some cases they were even capable of overturning things completely. In their opinion, continuity not only existed in harmony and agreement but also in denial and contradiction. Berdichevsky held the opposite view from Ahad Ha-Am, who identified the "Jewish distress" with the fragmentation of Jewish culture and thought that the problem could be fixed by unity and conformity. Berdichevsky saw the "distress of the Jews" and the distress of Jewish culture as two sides of the same coin, and Brenner (who agreed on this point with Ahad Ha-Am) saw them as two different things. Unlike Berdichevsky, who regarded culture as all-important, Brenner supported the movement for settlement in Palestine which was infiltrating Jewish life. As Brinker put it, Brenner revealed the blindness of Berdichevsky, an intellectual aristocrat who refused to consider the motivations of ordinary people and ignored the masses.

Brenner's war on historical Judaism, considered more moderate than Berdichevsky's in the late 1890s, had two aspects: the struggle of an enlightened European for freedom in matters of faith, and an attempt to alter the fate of the Jewish people under the inspiration of the new nationalism. For this purpose, he created a new type of nationalism which could be called "existential" nationalism, dealing with Jewish life, and which was different from "essential" nationalism dealing with ideas, beliefs and values. Unlike Berdichevsky's struggle against historical Judaism, a struggle to uproot Jewish norms in order to create new values, Brenner's struggle had a critical character, and its aim, according to Brinker, was to bring a "genealogical suspicion" (in the Nietzschean sense) to bear on existing values. Brenner did not cast doubt on the validity of Jewish cultural ideals but on the validity of ideological prototypes such as "the Jewish spirit," "the mission of Israel among the nations" and "Jewish morality." He had the impression that this Jewish idealization was intended to provide a protection or cover for life in difficult conditions. These ideal claims for Jewish culture could have been self-deception. The people, which was in no position to be bad, treated its impotence as a positive value, its imposed situation as a free choice.

Brinker saw Baruch Kurzweil's comments on those that rejected historical Judaism – Berdichevsky, Brenner, Tchernikovsky, Jacob Cohen and the Canaanites – as a one-dimensional general criticism which ignored the special character of the individual writers of the Hebrew revival.[36] In refutation of Kurzweil's criticism, he gave one example: Brenner, who in 1920 supported the creation of a "small" Hebrew army in Palestine, mocked the "progressive" argument of pure souls who advocated a life without an army, "a sheepish ideal in which one offers oneself up as a prey out of an excess of benevolence." Brenner's surprisingly hawkish reaction might have been expected from writers like Berdichevsky and Tchernikovsky.[37] Brenner's nationalist side was also revealed in his dispute with Ahad Ha-Am in which he criticized the lack of national spirit in the Jewish people, a lack which he thought distorted the image of the individual Jew: "A people which does not have the capacity for political, military and economic life – a working life – has no right to criticize the behavior of other peoples for the injustice of their lives."[38]

Such statements by Brenner gained him the reputation of being a self-hating individual. Brinker ridiculed this accusation and said that Brenner's cry was directed at all Jews – Orthodox, nationalist, liberal, revolutionary – asking them to be more modest because their collective self-image of being more moral than the gentiles had never been tested. Pre-national Jews did not yet have to deal with political conditions, conditions in which they could demonstrate a national morality. One may assume that Brinker, an outstanding intellectual of the Zionist left in the State of Israel, agreed with these statements by Brenner, but this time retroactively, after the Jews had been dealing with national morality for seven decades of independence.

Brenner, a disciple of the Haskalah, thought that the Jewish people had to act according to universal values, but the very fact of the physical existence of the Jew was a universal value in itself. Brinker identified with this position taken up by Brenner, a Hebrew writer who lived in the midst of his people with its many actual problems and did not adopt Berdichevsky's position of viewing spiritual developments *sub specie aeternitatis* – "under the aspect of eternity." Brenner made it clear that as a committed intellectual he preferred Brenner's attitude to Berdichevsky's.[39] Because the Jewish intellectual lives in the midst of the storm and operates within the turmoil of Jewish life, Brenner claimed that the question of the future of the Jewish people was not one that could be answered. He therefore could not have an a-priori outlook like the new secular *halacha* proposed by Bialik in *Halacha and Aggada*. Brenner knew what was not needed, but he did not know what *was* needed, and he was therefore not ready to provide a fully formed system, a totality of solutions. Brinker, who tried to answer the question of why Brenner was regarded by his readers as more than an "ordinary" writer, answered that Brenner came to Palestine before any other writer of the generation of the national rebirth. In Palestine, he lived as a pioneer in difficult conditions, helped his friends with editing and publication and became an authoritative moral figure for a generation that sought a modern equivalent of a prophet. He regarded his pioneering-literary activities – the editing of *Ha-Me'orer*, *Revivim* and *Ha-Adama* and his social involvement – as an extension of his role as an author. "The special personality," wrote Brinker, "seen by those outside literature was simply an emanation of his literary personality."[40]

Brenner's writings, which Brinker called "a rhetoric of honesty," were described by Dov Sadan as a struggle between art and faithfulness.[41] Faithfulness is said to take no account of art, and art is always detrimental to faithfulness. This real or imagined struggle also characterized Brenner's contempt for literary rules, for artistic disciplines and for the drawing of boundaries between literature and life, fiction and reality. By "the discourse of a rhetorician," Brinker meant, for example, Brenner's speech as the first congress of the Histadrut (the Federation of Labor), in which he asked for "the right to shout."[42] It was not as a silent author but as a shouting and denouncing actor that Brenner held forth on the Hebrew language, Jewish morality, theater and the "Bund," hassidism and Haskalah, assimilation and Jewish studies.

The "rhetoric of honesty" characterizes both the form and content of his books and stories – *In Winter*, *Around the Point*, *Out of the Depths*, *From Here and There*, *Breakdown and Bereavement* – in which one may see certain characteristics of the phenomenon: autobiographical hints, pragmatism, a literary text represented not as literature but in the form of a diary, notes, or a monologue, creating a deliberate distance from classical works. These things represent a confrontation between "literature" and "life" in literature, exemplified, for example, in Brenner's statement to Uri Nissan Gnessin that one should "avoid mysticism and the imaginary" and cultivate "realism and sanctity." Brenner in his youth thought that as a writer he had to concentrate on his own experiences, for he had to link his faith to the social and spiritual struggles of his time. What Vissarion Belinsky, following Hegel, called "sanctification," in Brenner became "honesty," honesty that is not self-explanatory and not well formulated, but is rough, warm and direct. This direct personal perspective examined in a critical filter all the dominant ideologies and orthodoxies. Brenner's rhetoric of honesty made a critical examination of Zionism, territorialism, autonomy, socialism, Tolstoyism, Marxism, Nietzscheanism, social revolutionaries, seekers of God, skeptics and penitents.

Brinker, who wrote ironically about the "death of the author" as described by the school of Barthes and Foucault, gave the case of Brenner, a writer who broke conventions, as negative proof. Although a writer is usually a representative of the intellectual climate of his time, influenced by the artistic and intellectual tendencies of his time, by his readers and by the books of his contemporaries, inwardly he overcomes the generalities, the structures, the reductions and the other requirements. Brinker emphasized Brenner's special character as a writer who was a committed intellectual, and he believed that "his literary works and articles were the most important part of Brenner's life, and his life outside literature was a continuation of his life as an author and critic."[43]

After they met in 1908, Berdichevsky wrote about Brenner in his diary: "This man is no longer a Jew in his soul, for he curses Judaism. He sees the destruction and perhaps wants it."[44] Brinker was surprised that Berdichevsky, who distinguished between "Judaism in the abstract" and "actual Jews" and separated the question of a man's Jewishness from the question of his attitude to Judaism, could be so dismissive. Brenner himself saw Berdichevsky's distinction as a major contribution to a modern understanding of the Jews, especially the youth. But Brenner added fuel to the flame and continued his depreciating remarks, speaking respectfully of Jews who honored the Christian faith in the Son of God, calling it "religiously uplifting." At the same time, Brinker approved of the common idea that there was a similarity between Brenner's thought and Berdichevsky's, and suggested that perhaps Brenner was not a religious heretic but what Amos Oz called a "tragic rationalist":

> I think that as a tragic rationalist speaks about a tragic rationalist, so Brinker spoke about Brenner and Berdichevsky. And that is how Brinker spoke about the complex and painful romance between Hebrew literature and European literature. And then there was the complex and terrible romance between our parents and grandparents who loved Europe so much, and Europe, which at best despised them and in a worse case, murdered them. Yes, this was a tragic dialog. This dialog must be conducted from a position of tragic rationalism, and Menahem Brinker's book *Hebrew Literature as European Literature* is the wonderful novel concerning this dialog.[45]

Sartre and Brinker – the existentialist from there and the one from here

The self-hatred Brenner is accused of has a long history. The term originated with the German-Jewish philosopher Theodor Lessing, who used it to condemn assimilated Jews' denial of their religion and culture. Jean-Paul Sartre gave the term "self-hatred" an important place in his book *Reflections on the Jewish Question* (1946).[46] He distinguished between "Jewish authenticity" and a lack of authenticity. Authenticity was the adoption of the identity imposed on a person even if he is not responsible for it, and which he accepts voluntarily. For instance, the fight against antisemitism or an adoption of Zionism were in Sartre's opinion authentic reactions to the "Jewish condition." The lack of authenticity led to a denial of anything that had a Jewish association, a distancing from a Jewish environment and the sanctioning of antisemitic prejudices. Sartre called this "Jewish masochism." A lack of authenticity led certain Jews to repress certain elements in their personal identity, to abandon cultural traditions and to deny the collective Jewish identity.

The intellectual closeness of Brinker to Sartre can be understood if one realizes that an involvement with existential questions out of a deep commitment to life does not depend on any metaphysical truth or philosophical idea. One confronts reality without hope but also without despair. One acts out of the total responsibility one has for one's world and for the world of others. Brinker dealt extensively with Sartre's thought. He translated and edited two volumes of his

Selected Works (1972), and wrote *Forms of Creation – On the Writings, Philosophy and Politics of Sartre* (1992), and a number of articles on his thought.

The essay *Reflections on the Jewish Question* was written in October 1944, a short time before the liberation of Paris. Brinker, who translated it into Hebrew, regarded it as a "model essay" because of its excellent style, the dramatic way of writing and the goodwill it shows towards the Jews. He wrote:

> How many essays of the friends of the Jews are ready to dare to criticize the behavior of the assimilated Jew, to reveal the impasse of all partial, personal or social solutions of the Jewish question, to define the hatred of Jews in terms of the situation of the antisemite and not in terms of the situation of the Jew?[47]

He discerned in the essay deep analysis, an ability for reflection, and a capacity for generalization, emotional expression and engagement in intellectual controversy. All these things justify the special status of the essay and give it its power and vitality.

The essay was not a psychological or a socio-academic study. Brinker thought that the matters it dealt with were known to Sartre personally. His close-up experience and knowledge added to his knowledge of the literary sources in France like the writings of Maurice Barrès, Charles Maurras and the antisemitic journals and newspapers. This was the antisemitic social milieu in which Sartre grew up and was educated, like many other members of the middle class. The subject of the essay – the encounter of the antisemite and the Jew – was more or less a photograph of the time and place in which Sartre lived.

Brinker claimed that Sartre was not interested in a rational disputation with an antisemite, an assertion also made by Ahad Ha-Am.[48] Sartre understood the antisemitic position as a reaction to the situation of the antisemite in the world, not as a reaction to the situation of the Jew. The antisemite wished to intensify his hatred and anger, and so he needed the Jew. Through the ostracism of the stranger, the antisemite could preserve his appearance, his place in society, his status and his property, and through these actions against the Jew the antisemite became the master of France. Sartre's thesis was based on the Hegelian dialectic of master and slave. The antisemite, being a master, creates in the slave an autonomous consciousness of being his own master. At the same time, in the case we are dealing with, the master remains the focus of the slave's identity, and that, on his part, does not encourage an independent identity. Another aspect of this dialectic is the positive consequences of negative phenomena: for instance, the founding of the State of Israel as a result of the murderous antisemitism of the twentieth century.

Brinker did not accept Sartre's idea that with the suppression of antisemitism, the Jew would disappear from the world in a utopian future of "a people without frontiers," just as the worker would lose his special status in the classless society. In this respect, the Jew is like the worker in that both of them are products of society and consciousness, and neither resemble woman, who is a natural product and not a social one.

Two years after the publication of the article, Sartre acclaimed the founding of the State of Israel in which, in his opinion, modern Jewish nationalism was revealed as an autonomous Jewish product of a new kind. Brinker criticized Sartre's focus on the Jewish memory of pogroms and persecutions and his failure to consider the collective cultural continuity throughout the generations. Sartre, in his opinion, ignored 2,000 years of Jewish history and the entry of the Jews into the modern world as a new nationalism. The Sartrian dialectic, which was the product of the French philosopher's poor knowledge of Jewish history and culture, was inadequate. This was not the first time, said Brinker, that Sartre's sympathy for oppressed groups was overcast by his philosophical principles.[49]

Sartre's existentialist outlook was reflected in his claim that the modern Jewish individual could "invent" himself by his own efforts, whereas the Jew of the past was the victim of historical circumstances. He saw Jewish history as a sphere of repetition. Jewish history consisted of unchanging phenomena without renewal or enrichment: in other words, it was a history without a history. In a late interview, Sartre showed he had changed his mind and said that if he had to write about the Jewish question again, he would not neglect the historical, social and economic aspects of the Jews.[50] But in any case, he said, he would remain true to the distinction he made between the autonomous Jew and the Jew who was not autonomous. Brinker challenged Sartre, saying that the Jewish identity drew its memories from the remote past, a past in which there was no confrontation between the Jew and the antisemite. The Jewish identity was never anchored solely in the present or could be understood as such. Atheist Jews explained to Sartre that their atheism was directed against Christianity and not against the Talmud. Brinker added that many of the writers of the Haskalah and the literature of the Hebrew revival opposed the Talmud not on theological grounds but on sociological ones. But there were some who took the opposite view, like Brenner, whose condemnation of Jewish society derived from a condemnation of Jewish theology.[51]

The antisemite saw himself as the authentic representative of a historical nation, the "real" France rebelling against "official" France and its laws. The antisemite rebelled against the legal country in the name of the "real" country. He asked for the laws of the state to be suspended, for above them there was something more genuine than the legal establishment. This analysis by the French intellectual caused the Israeli intellectual, Brinker, to draw a parallel with the "official" (civil) Israel and the "real" (Jewish) one.

The antisemite believed in "redemption through sin." He does evil, but with a pure intention, like a messenger who cures one evil with another for the sake of the good. The preservation of the authenticity of French culture sometimes required ostracism, humiliation and killing. Sartre said that these were the things that led to the legitimation of the murder of the Jews. This was the ethical and metaphysical basis of murderous antisemitism in the name of the "real" France and the "real" Germany, a basis different from the religious character of historical antisemitism – the Jewish guilt for the murder of God.[52] Brinker saw

Sartre's denial of the religious element in modern antisemitism as an essential weakness on the part of Sartre. In his opinion, there was a strong tendency in the French philosopher to stress the modern secular antisemitic ideology and to overlook the simple, ignorant antisemites who collaborated with the Nazi murderers. Another weakness that Brinker pointed out was Sartre's focus on French antisemitism only in the two world wars. He also claimed that the opposition between a civil state that gives equal rights to all citizens and the desire to restore a tribal and racial society not only existed in France. In other places, in Eastern Europe, for example, it was impossible to explain antisemitism in the way in which Sartre analyzed antisemitism in France.

Are we still secular?

Brinker did not accept the idea that the problem Zionism was supposed to solve had not yet disappeared. In 1981 he wrote that the Zionist movement had reached its peak long before, and the Israelis may by then have been living in the post-Zionist period.[53] In the near future, he said, there would be no justification for the Zionist movement to exist side-by-side with the State of Israel. Zionism was not "a piece of eternity that fell into time" but a movement that arose in a specific historical context to achieve a particular historical objective. The achievement of that objective removed any justification for its existence, its preservation or its artificial implementation. Many Zionists were content with less than the idea of founding a state, which was considered a maximum aim. In the past, less ambitious aims were proposed such as a spiritual center, a "healthy" Jewish community in Palestine or a territorial entity without independence.

The idea of founding a state of the Jews, which was the aim of Zionism, was accomplished in 1948, and Brinker believed that the more ambitious aim of concentrating the majority of the Jewish people in the State of Israel was also on the way to being achieved. However, he regarded this as Pyrrhic victory. It would have been better, he thought, for Zionism and Israel if the Jewish people in the diaspora had not been weakened.

A literary critic who was hardly mentioned by Brinker was Baruch Kurzweil, who did not believe Jewish existence was possible without religion. Kurzweil sought to reveal the Zionist ideology as a terrritorialization of Judaism and wished to unmask Israeli nationalism with its pretension of being the heir to the Jewish religion. He claimed that the Canaanite movement was the continuation and conclusion of cultural tendencies which began with the Haskalah and the extreme wing of the culture of the Hebrew revival.[54] The "Canaanites" did not represent an original ideology but were an Israeli strain of a Jewish anti-religious phenomenon that existed in the European exile.

Kurzweil was present behind the scenes in Brinker's writings, as was Gershom Scholem, who did not believe Jewish existence was possible if completely divorced from religiosity and messianic expectation. Already in his earliest works he claimed that the connection between nationalism and mysticism was not merely arbitrary, technical and historical but possessed a profound existential affinity. Only a people that had experienced the suffering and shock of the Spanish exile could believe that God had given a promise of total release from captivity as a special message to the Jewish people. This meant that the meaning of the Kabbalah was particular, a meaning that related to the Jewish people alone and that others could not understand. To such a degree was it impossible to cut the Gordian knot between the national and the mystical.

Unlike Kurzweil and Scholem, Brinker had an immanent secular point of view.[55] In *Hebrew Literature as European Literature* he described this Jewish immanent school of thought as having something profound to say about Hebrew literature, or at any rate the literature of the Hebrew revival. If Kurzweil saw in the secularism of Brenner and Berdichevsky a danger of degenerating into Canaanism, Brinker and writers like A.B. Yehoshua and Amos Oz saw secular Israeli sovereignty as an opportunity for a total realization of the Jewish identity. Kurzweil passed judgment on Hebrew literature and said that its achievements were poor in comparison with European literature. He did not see its productions as remarkable with the exception of the works of Agnon, and he ascribed it to a neglect of the classical Jewish legacy, but he failed to understand that it was precisely this distance between European literature and its Hebrew counterpart that reflected the special inner quality of Hebrew literature. Gershom Scholem also criticized the new Hebrew literature because he did not find in it a messianic religiosity which is sometimes anarchistic, and it did not succeed in solving the riddle of secular Jewish existence. That is why Kurzweil and Scholem seized upon Agnon: Kurzweil because he felt that Agnon described the life of religious Jews and showed the impossibility of a non-halachic Jewish existence, and Scholem because he regarded him as expressing the living Jewish myth.

Brinker also engaged in a debate about religion and secularism with Yeshiyahu Leibowitz. Leibowitz was considered by Brinker "one of the most important representatives of Jewish thought in recent generations," who offered "a meaningful and comprehensive challenge to the secular."[56] In Brinker's opinion, Leibowitz spoke with four voices: that of a religious Jew, that of a scientist and strict rationalist, that of a Jew with a national and Zionist consciousness, and that of a modern humanist and an enlightened person. At the same time, Brinker criticized Leibowitz because in the analysis he made there was nothing that could justify seeing the people of "Gush Emunim" (the "Bloc of the Faithful" who were settlers in the territories) as abandoning the yoke of Torah and the commandments. And while Leibowitz sought to demonstrate that Judaism and nationalism were mutually exclusive, thousands of religious Jews succeeded in showing that acceptance of the yoke of Torah and commandments and the national culture were by no means contradictory. Brinker objected to Leibowitz's way of amassing negative historical facts, which he did brilliantly, in order to show that the State of Israel could only be seen in two ways: as a continuation of historical Judaism, or as a mechanism for creating an artificial nation characterized by nationalism and a cult of statehood. Brinker of course saw many other possibilities for the State of Israel, such as that of a secular Jewish life in which there is a continuous Jewish dialogue on the one hand and in which universal humanist values are cultivated on the other.

Brinker thought that both the view that the Jewish collective was a religious community, membership of which corresponded to membership of national bodies, as claimed by most thinkers of the Haskalah in Germany and the west, and the national view that religion was only one of the characteristics of a culture, as was claimed by most of the thinkers of Russian Judaism including the representatives of the Haskalah, were modern "inventions" that reinterpreted Jewish history. Only when there was a new theoretical basis for a partnership of all the Jews, only after the status of religion had declined, was a strong, open expression of secularism possible. The particular conditions necessary for the development of Jewish secularism only came into existence when the belligerent representatives of the Haskalah, including those who rejected *halacha*, repudiated their commitment to ancient traditions. "Declarative" Jewish secularism arose in Europe as a social phenomenon, not as a phenomenon of individuals (like that of Spinoza, for example) with the emergence of national romanticism, while the national movements of other peoples were bound up with a return to religion. Brinker claimed that Zionism was largely the product of a secular mentality which had already taken root among people. Unlike Berdichevsky, who adopted a radical secular position at the first Zionist congress (in his "transvaluation of values" phase), Herzl wanted a coalition of a majority of the Jews and therefore invited to the congress a group of "Mizrahi" rabbis. The founder of political Zionism refused to make the movement a matter for cultural war in the Jewish street.

The idea of a contract gave the European peoples the possibility of creating a territorial citizenship without ethnic or religious criteria, but when this rationalist-secularist idea reached the Jews, the Jewish social contract obliged the secular Jews to compromise with the religious.[57] According to Brinker, the idea of a social contract of the Jews as a divided people prevented the State of Israel from creating a civil solidarity among all the inhabitants of the state. The stress on Jewish continuity rather than on Zionist-secular renewal revealed Jewish secular culture to be a thin crust without historical depth. In many cases, the modern Jew is unable to express his loyalty to his nation or his humanistic outlook without using symbols with a religious connotation. Brinker therefore called on the modern Jews to create a new language which would be used from that time onward and not to renounce their special modern character in favor of an ancient identity. In his view, this represents the struggle of the individual identity of the modern Jew against the automatic identity bestowed on him by Jewish history and the language of religious symbols. Only an independent tradition of Jewish secularism can release the secular Jew from his personal conflict with Jewish history. The secular man lives more from his thinking than from his sense of belonging, and he accepts the modern imposition of a lack of a single way of life for all.

With his philosophical-existentialist outlook and his liberal approach to literature, Brinker tried to formulate an educational program. In his article, "Jewish

Studies in Israel in a Liberal-secularist Perspective," he showed how a person should be educated according to his principles:

> He can, if he wishes, make the fact of his birth into a Jewish family into a matter of continual choice. The fact of his Jewishness is always something that he can overcome, and only if frequently renewed by an act of will does it cease to be a fact and become a value.[58]

Brinker drew attention to the paradox that "background" is a factor seen as side-by-side with formal education or even in opposition to it, but it also directs and channels it, for in a democracy education requires the agreement of the parents to the instruction it provides. Paradoxically, the background makes the education an ideal image of itself. Parents always expect the pupil to find the golden mean between the "ideal" education and his path in life. An example of this is the difference between Jewish education in non-Orthodox educational institutions outside Israel and education in the State of Israel. The task that parents and educators give to Jewish education in the diaspora is to preserve the pupil's Jewishness in an alien environment. Many Jews are losing their Jewish identity because liberal Western society provides free access to all areas of knowledge, culture, trade and politics. It is hard to see what Judaism has to offer its assimilated sons. But Jewish education in Israel is free from the conflict experienced by the Jews of the diaspora. It therefore has a natural starting point "in its aim of helping, in the most existential possible way, any youth to understand his world: the world around him and the world within."

Because Brinker had a liberal starting point and had the paradoxical aim of educating people towards liberty, education could not in his opinion be based on any predetermined model. "The Jewish past is a basis for future possibilities, models of self-creation and possible examples." The Jewish past is not a store of obligations. It contains no preferred models or proscribed models. One must be acquainted with the sage Hillel and Bar-Kochba just as one must be acquainted with Ahad Ha-Am and Berdichevsky. Pluralism is the litmus-test of liberal education: one must teach the whole spectrum of the history of the Jewish people: from the Bible, the Mishna and Midrash to the liturgical poetry and philosophy of the Middle Ages and a selection of secular Jewish literature. One must start with Ecclesiastes and the Song of Songs, proceed to profane medieval poetry and embrace modern Jewish thought and the new Hebrew literature. All these materials must be brought to the attention of the educator.[59]

Brinker thought that one must create an understanding of the varied aspects of Jewish life, not only out of respect for the student but also from a social point of view. Here one sees Brinker the intellectual at the height of his powers, urging a fight against religious extremism and national radicalism, which in his opinion had nothing to do with personal religious or Zionist convictions.

In Brinker's view, "secular" was not the opposite of "religious." The term required educators to have a liberal openness and not adopt a militant secular attitude. There is no such thing as a secular rabbi and there are no secular articles of faith. One should encourage a free approach to texts and avoid secular holy epistles: "Everything is open, both in interpretation and judgement." The main thing is that the student should learn to distinguish what is obsolete in rabbinic and secular teachings, and what is still relevant. The major texts must give the student the feeling that he is his own rabbi. The task of a school is to awaken a sense of devotion in the student which reflects the choice of a free man, "even a devotion to goodness, truth or beauty, or a devotion to God as the supreme symbol of all these." One must recognize the many aspects of the Jewish people, with the multiplicity of movements it embraced: the Haskalah, hassidism, Orthodoxy, the Reform, autonomism, Zionism, territorialism, the Bund, emancipation, assimilation, and even antisemitism, liberalism, socialism and communism.

These criteria also apply to serious literature. The study of poetry, literature and literary criticism must begin with what is being published now, which can then lead, after the student's love of literature has been aroused, to the study of the poetry and literature of earlier periods. Brinker preferred to begin by teaching works whose subjects were close to the student's world before teaching them about worlds distant in time and place. The Hebrew language is of course a minimal common denominator of the Israelis' Jewish identity. One must therefore ensure a high linguistic level in speech and writing. One must avoid a provincial identification of Israeliness with Jewishness, and one must therefore teach writers such as Franz Kafka, Bernard Malamud and Philip Roth and poets such as Paul Celan and Edmond Jabès.

The method of instruction is no less important than the things studied. For example, teaching though analogies between phenomena in the Jewish world and phenomena outside it is a recommended way of teaching. Maimonides should be taught not only as a teacher of Judaism but as one of the major philosophers of his time influenced by Islamic philosophy. The same applies to Ibn Gabirol's affinity to neo-Platonism, to the Russian-European background to Bialik's poetry, to the liberal and Russian socialist inspiration of Ahad Ha-Am and A.D. Gordon, and to the influence of European philosophy on Rabbi Kook.

Brinker thought that superficiality, vulgarity and materialism were incurable, but so were introversion, lack of independent thought, fanaticism, chauvinism and racism. He said that the task of Jewish studies, like the task of study of the humanities in general, is to place at the students' disposal a wide variety of inspirations in order to enable them to make their lives, their behavior toward others and their decisions as citizens subject to a higher authority.[60]

The landscape of their neighborhood

Brinker, Chaim Beer, A.B. Yehoshua and Amos Oz were to a large extent the heirs of Brenner and Berdichevsky, but they also belonged to a neighborhood (Beer was born in the Keren Abraham neighborhood in Jerusalem). As A.B. Yehoshua wrote:

It seems to me that the ease with which we made contact with one another was partly due to our previous acquaintance, when Mrs. Brinker and Mrs. Yehoshua strolled in the Mekor Baruch neighborhood in Jerusalem with two prams; and therefore the heading of the following will be "Two Prams", in accordance with the famous simile of "Hazon Ish" of Bnei Brak in his celebrated conversation with David Ben-Gurion, of two wagons, religious and secular, that encountered one another on a narrow path. The two prams in the Mekor Baruch neighborhood were both secular, not because of the mothers who pushed them but because of the two children that lay in them, although both were the grandchildren of rabbis. Mehahem was the grand-child of the Ashkenazi rabbi Auerbach, called the "rabbi of the pioneers" because he married couples in the kibbutz even when the woman was in an advanced stage of pregnancy, and I was the grandchild of the Sephardi rabbi Hananiah Gabriel Yehoshua, President of the Beit Din (Law Court) of the Sephardi community in Jerusalem. The two rabbis, who lived at a distance of a hundred meters from each other but hardly knew one another, did not succeed in handing on religion to their grandchildren, who both became the-ological atheists.[61]

Perhaps Yehoshua was hinting at something I have spoken about elsewhere: the dialectical phenomenon I have called "heretical religiosity."

Underlying the call for a transvaluation of values was the longing for a new kind of Jewish religiosity which was not the experience of a fixed order of beliefs and ideas, a religion learned by rote, but a sort of existentialist "other side" of faith in which there was a place for "heretics," from Elisha Ben Abuya and Spinoza to Menahem Brinker. These never asked us to choose between two conflicting approaches to religion, or, alternatively, between religiosity and secularism.

The usual sort of secularism, to which I do not claim that Brinker belonged, is indifferent to the significance of the presence or absence of God. The attitude of the atheist or secular man to the religious phenomenon is one of indifference. The nonexistence of God does not raise a cry or cause pain or longing. The existence of God is a matter of unconcern; his existence or nonexistence does not interest modern man. The normal secularist does not argue with the religious world, unlike the religious heretic, who never ceases to quarrel with the beliefs he was brought up on, with the texts he read in his youth, with the opponents with whom he once shared a *cheder* (religious elementary school) or a house of learning.

Two Jerusalemites of the period of the British Mandate who experienced a different Israelism, an Israelism that is textual and has the quality of a dream, with a close affinity to generations of dreamers, are A.B. Yehoshua in *Molcho* and *Journey to the End of the Millennium* and Amos Oz in *My Michael* and *A Tale of Love and Darkness*. These are encounters which try to make the genera-tions speak. Moreover, one finds in these books the atmosphere of a struggle for an independent national existence. The writers knew the generation of the struggle.

Yehoshua and Oz also have in common a connection with European literature, a connection which Brinker discussed in relation to Frishman, Brenner,
Ahad Ha-Am, Berdichevsky and others. Today, it is a connection that
European literature acknowledges. The works of both these authors are canonical in Europe, and a large number of readers in Europe are aware of them.
Through them, the experiences peculiar to Jewish-Israeli life have become universal. As writers, they are focused on the moment of creation and not on
reflections on their productions. This gap is filled by Brinker's *Hebrew Literature as European Literature*. Brinker does not touch the works of his friends
in the book, but he provides a fascinating theoretical basis for a reconsideration
of their works. Amos Oz wrote about this and described the special status of
intellectual figures:

> Brenner and Berdichevsky made quite a few mistakes in their under-
> standing of the Jewish situation and in the visions they tried to delineate,
> and also, of course, in their pessimistic and optimistic prognostications.
> Brenner was assassinated at the age of forty and Berdichevsky died in
> Germany at the age of fifty-six. Both of them were very significant for the
> Zionist settlement in Palestine at the beginning of the twentieth century.
> What is surprising is that although Brenner was isolated and very extreme
> in his character and in his path in life, and Berdichevsky did not visit
> Palestine even once, the pioneers and the people of the labor movement
> read their works and considered them thinkers of importance for them. And
> not only they did, but also the many members of the generations that came
> after them. [...] Despite the hundred years that have elapsed since the death
> of these two writers and the tragic and non-tragic vicissitudes in the history
> of the Jewish people and the whole world since that time [...], men of spirit
> have a special significance not only in the past but in the present, and not
> only as writers of prose and poetry but as people who say something mean-
> ingful about our lives beyond what one hears from political experts and
> military people.[62]

Brinker quoted the analyses and conclusions of Dan Miron in his article,
"From Pioneers and Builders to Homeless People," concerning the decline in
the status of Hebrew writers from Bialik, Ahad Ha-Am and Brenner to contemporary writers and poets like Alterman. The writers and poets of the
Hebrew revival were in his opinion – to use Ahad Ha-Am's famous term –
"prophets," spiritual guides to the Zionist political leaders, while Alterman,
who was considered an attendant on Ben-Gurion, was a "priest." Brinker,
who acknowledged the decline in the status of the intellectual in the public
sphere, did not think that the phenomenon was necessarily negative: "The
whole business of 'prophet and priest', like 'spirit, vision and action', was
only one of the myths that the seemingly rational thinker Ahad Ha-Am provided his readers."[63] Perhaps the cunning of history was brought to bear on
Brinker himself: this philosopher and literary critic, who devoted much of his

life to studying the works and importance of intellectuals like Berdichevsky, Brenner and Sartre, ended by belittling the capacity of intellectuals to influence life.

The Canaanite intellectuals, for instance, were known to have a marginal status, and their radical leader even prided himself on his marginality. But their sociological marginality was out of all proportion to their influence on the literary and intellectual elite or on the discourse they gave rise to on the option of a Hebrew homeland. The tree that grew in the land of Canaan had many ideological and interpretive branches. In the discourse on the Israeli identity there were many Canaanite possibilities: nativistic and metaphorical Canaanism, Zionist and post-Zionist Canaanism, left-wing and right-wing Canaanism, utopian and biblical Canaanism, ideological and aesthetic Canaanism, and many others.[64] In the following chapter, we will examine the political and social thinking of Boaz Evron, who called for a "civil Canaanism." This was not a mythological and archaic Canaanism like that of Yonatan Ratosh, but a national territorial Canaanism in which belonging and citizenship of the Moledet was not determined by one's historical allegiance, religious faith or ethnic origin, but solely by locality and language.

Notes

1 Haim Be'er, "The Father's Branch," *Literature and Life: Poetics and Ideology in the New Hebrew Literature – To Menachem Brinker in his 70's*, eds., Iris Parush, Hamutal Zamir and Hannah Suker-Schweger, Jerusalem 2011, 15 (in Hebrew).
2 Ibid., 18.
3 Menachem Brinker, *The Hebrew Literature as a European Literature*, Jerusalem 2016, 23 (in Hebrew).
4 David Ohana, "The Secular Perspective of Menachem Brinker," *Haaretz – Culture and Literature*, 4/3/2016 (in Hebrew).
5 Menachem Brinker, "The Hebrew Literature is grounded within European Literature," *Haaretz – Culture and Literature*, 4/3/2016 (in Hebrew).
6 Menachem Brinker, "Brenner's Judaism," *Congress of the Israeli National Academy*, 8 (1985): 211–228; ibid., "'Mahanaim' On the Split Unity of Berdichevsky's Enterprise," *The Hebrew Literature as a European Literature*, 20–98 (in Hebrew).
7 Brinker, "The Uniqueness of the Secular Jew," *Israeli Thoughts*, Jerusalem 2007, 47 (in Hebrew).
8 Yosef Haim Brenner, "To the Approvers and the Readers," *HaMeorer* [London] (November 1906). See: Brenner, *Collected Essays*, Tel Aviv 1985, Vol. III, 144–145 (in Hebrew).
9 George Lindbeck, *The Nature of Doctorine*, John Knox Press, Philadelphia 2009.
10 David Neumark, "Die Judische Moderne," *Allgemeine Zeitung des Judentums*, Bd. 64:45 (Berlin 1900): 536–538.
11 On Berdichevsky's conception of history, see: Ohana, "Zarathustra in Jerusalem: Nietzsche and the 'New Hebrews'," *The Shaping of Israeli Identity*, eds., Robert Wistrich and David Ohana, Frank Cass, London 1995, 38–61.
12 David Ohana, "It Would be a Good Thing if the God of Zarathustra were the God of Israel," *Nietzsche and Jewish Political Thought*, Routledge, London 2018, 31–41; ibid., "Trailing Nietzsche: Gershom Scholem and the Sabbatean Dialectics," *Nietzsche*-Studien (2016): 224–246.

13 Menachem Brinker, "Micha Yosef Berdichevsky (Bin-Gorion)," *New Jewish Time Jewish Culture in a Secular Age: An Encyclopedic View*, Vol. I, Jerusalem 2007, 64 (in Hebrew).
14 Ibid., "'Mahanaim' On the Split Unity of Berdichevsky's Enterprise," 26 (in Hebrew).
15 Micha Yosef Bin-Gorin (Berdichevsky), "Thoughts/Age and Youth," *The Collected Works of Micha Yosef Bin-Gorin*, Tel Aviv 1951, 33 (in Hebrew).
16 Ibid., "'Mahanaim' On the Split Unity of Berdichevsky's Enterprise," 30.
17 Amos Oz, "The Past Belongs to Us. We Don't Belong to It," *Haaretz – Culture and Literature*, 4/3/2016 (in Hebrew).
18 Avner Holzman, "On the Way to the Transvaluation of Values: On the Place of Nietzsche's Influence in Berdichevsky's Work," ed., Jacob Golomb, *Nietzsche in the Hebrew Culture*, Jerusalem 2002, 161–179 (in Hebrew).
19 Oz, "The Past Belongs to Us. We Don't Belong to It."
20 Menachem Brinker, "Hebrew Literature and Zionist Historiography," *Zmanim: Quarterly of History*, Vol. 105 (Winter 2009): 16–23 (in Hebrew).
21 Menachem Brinker, "Nietzsche in the Hebrew Literature of 'the Revival Generation': 1899–1922," *The Hebrew Literature as a European Literature*, Jerusalem 2016 (in Hebrew).
22 Brinker, "The Influence of Nietzsche on the Hebrew Writers of the Russian Empire," in: Bernice Glatzer-Rosenthal (ed.), *Nietzsche and the Soviet Culture*, Cambridge University Press, Cambridge 1994, 393–413.
23 Friedrich Nietzsche, *Geneology of Morals*, trans. Ian Johnston, Arlington 2009.
24 Brinker, "Nietzsche in the Hebrew Literature of 'the Revival Generation': 1899–1922," 140.
25 Haim Nahman Bialik, "On the Verge of the Beth Midrash," 1893, https://benyehuda. org/bialik/bia012.html, taken in 08/03/2019 (in Hebrew).
26 Bialik, "Metei Midbar" (The Desert Dead), *The Writings of H. N. Bialik*, Tel Aviv 1993, 44–46 (in Hebrew).
27 Bialik, "On the Gathering of Spirit," A lecture in the 'Am Ivrit' congress, London 1925, in Brinker, *The Hebrew Literature as a European Literature*, 142 (in Hebrew).
28 Brinker, "'Mahanaim' On the Split Unity of Berdichevsky's Enterprise," 38.
29 Yosef Haim Brenner, *Writings*, Vol. III, Tel Aviv 1977–1984, 743 (in Hebrew).
30 Brinker, "'Mahanaim' On the Split Unity of Berdichevsky's Enterprise," 47.
31 Ibid., 74.
32 Menachem Brinker, "The Jewishness of Brenner," *Narrative Art and Social Thought in Y. H. Brenner's Work*, Tel Aviv 1990, 160 (in Hebrew).
33 Micha Yosef Berdichevsky, "Towards the Question of the Past," *The Writings of Bin-Gorin*, cited in: Brinker, *Narrative Art and Social Thought in Y. H. Brenner's Work*, 167 (in Hebrew).
34 Aharon Appelfeld, *First Person Essays*, Jerusalem 1979, 69–70 (in Hebrew).
35 David Ohana, *Nietzsche and Jewish Political Theology*, Routledge 2018, 41–45.
36 Ibid., 228–246.
37 Ohana, *The Origins of Israeli Mythology: Neither Canaanites nor Crusaders*, Cambridge University Press, Cambridge 2012, 44–45.
38 Brinker, "The Jewishness of Brenner," 183.
39 Ibid., 184.
40 Menachem Brinker, *Narrative Art and Social Thought in Y. H. Brenner's Work*, Tel Aviv 1990 (in Hebrew), 12.
41 Dov Sadan, *A Man of Many Pains*, *Between Verdict and Judgment*, Tel Aviv 1965 (in Hebrew). Also appears in: Brinker, *Narrative Art and Social Thought in Y. H. Brenner's Work*, 227, footnote 3.
42 For the context of this assertion, see: Sadan, 277, footnote 4.
43 Ibid., 25.
44 Ibid., 157.

45 Oz, "The Past Belongs To Us. We Don't Belong To It."
46 Jean-Paul Sartre, *Anti-Semite and Jew*, trans. George J. Becker, Preface by Michael Walzer, New York 1995.
47 Menachem Brinker, "After Thirty Years: Sartre and the Jewish Question," *Israeli Thoughts*, 130.
48 Ibid., 115.
49 David Ohana, "Baader–Meinhoff: A Crusade of Violence," *The Intellectual Origins of Modernity*, Routledge, London 2019, 227–232.
50 Jean-Paul Sartre, *Selected Writings*, ed. Menachem Brinker, Tel Aviv 1972, 190–198 (in Hebrew).
51 Brinker, "After Thirty Years," 129.
52 Ibid., 119.
53 Brinker, "After Zionism," 19–34.
54 Dan Laor, "Kurzweil and the Canaanites: Between Reason and Struggle," *Keshet – Literature, Theory and Criticism Commemoration of Forty Years since the First Publication*, Tel Aviv 1998, 32–45 (in Hebrew).
55 Henry Pachter, "Masters of Cultural History, Gershom Scholem – The Myth of the Mythmaker," *Salmagundi* 40 (Winter 1978): 9–39.
56 Brinker, "The Uniqueness of the Secular Jew," 43.
57 Brinker, "The Analysis and Debate of Yeshayahu Leibowitz," *Israeli Thoughts*, 49.
58 Brinker, "The Jewish Studies in Israel from a 'Secular'-Liberal Perspective," *Talking Vision – An Invitation to Discussion on the Purpose of the Jewish Education*, eds., Shlomo Fuks, Israel Shpeler and Daniel Marom, Jerusalem 2006, 108 (in Hebrew).
59 Ibid., 111.
60 Ibid., 117.
61 A.B. Yehoshua, "Menachem Brinker Proves that there is a Special Meaning to Intellectuals," *Haaretz – Culture and Literature*, 4/3/2016.
62 Oz, "The Past Belongs To Us. We Don't Belong To It."
63 Brinker, "The Hebrew Literature is Grounded within European Literature."
64 Jacob Shavit, *The New Hebrew Nation: A Study in Israeli Heresy and Fantasy*, London 1987; Yehoshua Porat, *The Life Story of Yonatan Ratosh*, Tel Aviv 1989 (in Hebrew); Nurit Gertz, *The Canaanite Group: Literature and Ideology*, Tel Aviv 1987 (in Hebrew); Ohana, *The Origins of Israeli Mythology*.

3   The new Hebrews

The Hebraic or Canaanite idea already formed part of Boaz Evron's intellectual outlook when he joined "Lehi" (Fighters for the Freedom of Israel). Later, for a short time, he was a member of the "Canaan Group"; then, for a longer period, he was a member of "Semitic Action," writing for the theater and publishing books of essays, and he arrived at a political position in favor of a Moledet as a "state of all its citizens," which became a common political idiom he was one of the first to use.[1]

Evron's name came up in David Ben-Gurion's meeting with the intellectuals of the Hebrew University in March 1963. The prime minister complained to them about:

> a youth – a Canaanite, it seems – Boaz Evron, who wrote an article asking why the army assisted the archaeological expedition in the Judean Desert and why Yigal Yadin helped with various arrangements. It would have been better, he said, if the money had been used to provide better food for the reserves.[2]

It was no accident if in his stand-off with the "Canaanite" Boaz Evron, Ben-Gurion confronted him with Yigal Yadin. Yadin and Evron represented two diametrically opposite philosophies of history of Judaism or Hebraism. Yadin represented the Zionist view of archaeology which tried to find an affinity between the biblical past and the new Israel, and the young Evron, who had sat at the feet of Yonatan Ratosh, represented the Canaanite view, which tried to conceive a continuity between the Canaanite past and modern Israel. Biblical archaeology in the country served the Zionist cause which sought a connection between the ancient Land of Israel and the return of the Jews to that land in modern times. Yadin, the second Chief of Staff of the Israel Defense Forces, headed the excavations in the Judean Desert which discovered Shimon Bar-Kochba's letters. Concerning the mythical affinity between him and the messianic Jewish general of the second century BCE, Israel Eldad wrote: "and was it not the finger of God that Bar Kochba's letters reached Yigal Yadin – the letters of one Commander-in-Chief to another?"[3]

In his 1961 article, "Generals and Caves," Evron admitted that he was totally ignorant about archaeology, and described himself as someone who appreciated

Yadin's discovery of the scrolls he found in the Judean Desert.[4] At the same time, if the heads of the army arrived in a helicopter, he wondered whether it was a normal archaeological expedition.

It is not surprising if Evron was annoyed with Yadin. He was disturbed that he, the native-born general, the commander of the Israeli War of Independence, now sought legitimation of his native secular Hebrew identity in an alien, religious and messianic sphere. That it was precisely he, who was naturally rooted in the land and the Hebrew language, that should concern himself with the mythical history of the Jewish religion! In diametrically opposite directions, these two sons of the land, Yadin and Evron, went in search of the imagined starting point of their country.

Evron described how in 1946, when he was nineteen years old, he began to acquire his Hebraic outlook through the "Canaanite" vision of the Ratosh school of thought:[5]

> When I took hold of the book called *Huppah Shehora* (Black Canopy), I found that the obscure words, [...] thoughts and feelings that proliferated in the hearts of many young people at that time found expression. They gave an ideological basis to our feelings about our country, explained the reasons for our boredom with the "Judaism" and "Zionism" they tried to teach us, the feeling that our primary allegiance was to this land and its people [...].[6]

Evron began to hear about Ratosh's views about the new nation arising in the country that did not form part of the Jewish people but was a purely territorial entity, and about the ancient Hebrew culture that was once shared by all the peoples of the area. Ratosh, he learned with fascination, advocated the union of the Fertile Crescent and all its peoples on the basis of the ancient Hebrew culture which they had shared in the distant past and which had been effaced by rabbinic Judaism and Islam. Only the expulsion from the country and the whole of the Middle East of the British imperialists and their European allies – the chief instigators of the dispute between the Jews and the Arabs – would bring peace to the region. These ideas, he later wrote, "were in accordance with the feeling of estrangement which I and most of my friends had towards the Jewish world, the feeling that we, the native-born, were different."

He looked at the part played by "the Canaanite ideology and its metamorphoses" in his life and pointed out several highly significant biographical stations, turning-points which formed his outlook on the world. The first was the blood-feud with the Arabs in 1936, the memory of a nine-year-old child who heard from adults of the murder of a law-court official in Jaffa. He was the first victim of the Arab uprising against Jewish settlement. Evron saw this as the starting point of his Hebrew identity which was molded both by the war against the Arabs and the struggle against the Judaization of the national conflict.

Eight years later, in 1944, Evron joined a Jewish unit of the Mandatory police, for, as he said, "we were all brought up to fight against the Arabs."[7] Cracks began to appear in his nationalist outlook at that time due to the misgivings of a friend.

Were the Arabs really all trouble-makers and murderers? How did they feel when they knew that their country would be a Jewish National Home? Was the motivation of the British in their policy of "divide and rule" among the Jews and Arabs a cold political calculation of imperialist interests? His conclusion, already at that early stage of his life, was that one should unite with the Arabs and expel the British: "We must establish a bi-national state with the Arabs. In that way, we will achieve both peace and the fulfillment of Zionism." And how did the idea of a bi-national state correspond to the fulfillment of Zionism, the aim of which was the establishment of a state for the Jewish people? This inconsistency troubled the young Evron, who was making his first steps towards the crystallization of his national identity.

In addition to the Arab question and the British question, which sowed the seeds of his early Canaanite outlook, there was also the Marxist question. His reading of Marxist literature taught him that his struggle was one of a number of national uprisings against imperialism: "In other words, my nationalism became Marxist." Marxism and the Canaanite outlook fused into a single entity in the crucible of the young Evron.

Between Ratosh and "Ya'ir"

The young Evron hated Jewish history, which was mainly a chronicle of weakness, and he also disliked the Jews' feelings of moral superiority to the gentiles. Such ideas, from which the Hebrew youth concluded that power was the most important thing in life, and certainly in the life of the nation, made the members of the "Haganah" regard themselves as a "protective force" and imbued them with a sense of a homeland and a nativistic romanticism.[8]

Evron said that in the "Haganah," his feeling about the policy the Yishuv had to follow was strengthened, and he gradually understood that only through a struggle against the British could sovereignty be attained. Like many young people of his age, he loathed the moderate circles in the Yishuv and approved of the rebellious activities of the three armedorganizations. Natan Yellin-Mor, one of the three leaders of "Lehi," wrote that Evron "crossed the Rubicon" and came to radical conclusions concerning the Zionist claim that Palestine was given to the Jews by a decision of the nations. He was attracted by the "Lehi" doctrine that the Hebrews were not a people of settlers in the Land of Israel but natives expelling a foreign invader. Even the Balfour Declaration was defective in his eyes because it claimed to give the people of the country the right of ownership of the land, but it was a right that had never been rescinded. The recognition of this fact, wrote Yellin-Mor, was the final nail in the coffin of legal and moral dependence on Britain. Now, it was no longer a matter of attempting to annul the White Paper or of obtaining certificates, but of getting a divorce from the British. The way was open for a war of liberation from them.

In that period, there seemed to be a possibility of a joint Hebrew-Arab struggle which would dissipate once and for all the dark cloud of perpetual war with the Arabs. Principles were enunciated for the first time which would later be developed: neutralization of the Middle East and Jewish-Arab brotherhood. The use of the term "Hebrew" rather than "Jewish" or "Zionist" was a liberation from a heavy historical burden and conveyed the feeling that it was a young country.

The "Lehi" pamphlets he read in his youth, and especially the one titled "We are not Zionists" (a slogan coined by Israel Eldad), which rejected the Balfour Declaration, gave Evron the conviction that the country and its people, both Hebrews and Arabs, had to be liberated from the British occupier.[9] Zionism, he believed, which had gained legitimation from outside, from the League of Nations, had exchanged the aspiration to sovereignty for an attitude of passivity, an atmosphere of intercession and coming to terms with imperialism. In the "Lehi" pamphlets, the Hebrew intellectual atmosphere became a platform for political action: the slogan "We are not Zionists but sons of the land" expressed the self-confidence of the Yishuv. One should remember that the origins of Evron's family in the country (he was born in 1927) went back to the beginning of the nineteenth century. His childhood and youth were the product of the Hebrew educational system in which the term "Hebrew" was sanctified: the police force was the "Police of the Hebrew Settlements" and the Histadrut (Federation of Labor) was the "Federation of Hebrew Workers in the Land of Israel." Industry sprang up in the Yishuv and a self-defense force was created. The members of the Yishuv had the feeling that only by means of the force they possessed could they rise against the British. The Holocaust was far away from them and they had no idea of its horrors. At that time Evron, on his own admission, moved away from Zionism, and over the years he continued to cast stones at it as though he were Ratosh: "The word 'Jew' had a derogatory flavor. It had a flavor of what the Zionists were trying to get away from; it had an exilic odor."[10] The later shift of emphasis from "Hebrew" to "Jewish" took place in his opinion for the ideological purpose of repressing Canaanism.

The pamphlet, "Foundation-stones of a Hebrew Foreign Policy" (1946), declared that the aim was not only to liberate the country but also to expel the British from the Middle East in order to set up a regional federation. Yellin-Mor stated that only the liberation of the entire region from imperialist rule would bring freedom and peace. It was this pamphlet that persuaded Evron to join "Lehi." "Joab," to use his underground title, wished to give equal importance to two factors, the national-Hebrew and the Marxist, in the resolution of the Hebrew-Arab conflict.

Avraham Stern ("Ya'ir") took a bold step when he declared that the Hebrew nation existed because the Land of Israel was its country. By so doing, he "tore to shreds the set of concepts that made us dependent on other nations and set us on our feet as an independent body that could relate in accordance with its interests to any other independent body in the world."[11] At the same period, Evron learned about the "hidden teachings" of "Lehi," Yair's testament, the "Principles of Renewal," which combined messianic vision, the conquest of the "promised land" and the idea of the kingdom of Israel. Evron was surprised at the friendship between Stern – who in "Principles of Renewal" called for an ethnically cleansed Hebrew kingdom in which a Third Temple would be set up, and the subjugation of foreigners – and Ratosh, who rejected Jewish nationalism.

"Principles of Renewal" was kept secret because it was no longer in keeping with the spirit of the movement which had moved leftwards in accordance with an intellectual atmosphere in which movements of national liberation gained inspiration from Marxist ideas. In Evron's opinion there was a certain similarity between Stern's "Principles of Renewal" and Ratosh's outlook, especially in view of their mutual friendship, which explains Ratosh's influence on Stern. There was a parallel between Stern's manifesto and Ratosh's conception: "The promised territory was the same, but instead of a unification of equal parties there was a program of messianic rule." But how did Jabotinsky's vision of a Land of Israel on both banks of the River Jordan, from which "Lehi" was derived, become the "secure borders" of the "Principles of Renewal"? Evron thought that this showed the influence on Stern of Ratosh's "land of Kedem." Although Stern was not religious, he had messianic tendencies due to the influence of Uri Zvi Greenberg, Jacob Cohen and Israel Eldad.

Between Ratosh and Evron

On December 18, 1956 there met in Tel Aviv a group of intellectuals, all of whom expressed opposition to the Sinai campaign, "with its conspiratorial beginning and shameful ending." The founding nucleus of the group, together with other members, wrote a pamphlet of 122 sections called "The Hebrew Manifesto," and set up an organization called "*Ha-Pe'ula Ha-Shemit*" (Semitic Action).[12] The reason for the use of the word "Semitic" was the desire of the founders of the movement, who included Yellin-Mor, Yaakov Yardor, Binyamin Omri, Shlomo Ben-Shlomo and Boaz and Ya'ir Evron, to

> find a cultural basis which can be a focus for a subjective consolidation of the region following a recognition of the objective political and economic necessity for its unification. This is a view deriving from the "Hebrew" conception that the ancient pre-Jewish Hebrew culture should be the myth and cultural cement that binds together the region of the Fertile Crescent.[13]

The members of the group called for the creation of a federation in which, as in all federations, none of its components wields power on its own.

In the years 1960–1967, "Hebrew Action" published a journal, *Etgar*, which came out every two weeks. Five years after the group came into being, its founders held a discussion, and Evron described how it began:

> As soon as I saw the aggression of the three powers [Britain, France and Israel], I knew there would be a national uprising in Egypt. The Egyptians would repel the aggressors, and our partnership in an imperialist conspiracy of that nature was bound to be avenged on us.

This reaction was not unexpected where he was concerned and followed directly from the ideas he held before he was a member of "Lehi," and later of the "Committee for the Consolidation of Hebrew Youth" founded by Ratosh.[14]

In the pages of *Etgar*, there was a bitter, unrelenting struggle between the founder of the Canaanite group, Ratosh, and the rebellious Evron, who had broken his umbilical cord with the Canaanites but still had some hidden inclinations which drew him to the Canaanite idea.[15] Ratosh claimed that while the Canaanites made a distinction between the open, secular Hebrews and the adherents of Judaism, who were a scattered inward-looking community in the country, the members of "Semitic Action" made a tactical use of the term "Hebrew" by which they more or less meant a secular Jewish Israeli. Evron replied that in their manifesto, the members of "Semitic Action" asked for a new Hebrew nation to be created of those born in the Land of Israel, for a separation to be made of religion and state, for the distinguishing trait of the new Hebrew nation to be the Hebrew culture and language and not religion, and for the legal status of the Zionist movement to be annulled. But, in one thing they were different from the Canaanites: in their recognition that the new Hebrew nation had an affinity with the Jews of the diaspora, and it was due to this recognition that Evron left *Alef*, the journal of the Canaanite group.

While Ratosh distinguished between the Hebrew nation and the Jewish people, Evron said that "Semitic Action" desired a confederation or federation of the peoples of the area, with a recognition of the right of each people to have its own culture and nationality. Evron complained that Ratosh did not explain what Hebrew culture was, what the renaissance of Hebrew culture meant, how Hebrew culture would be "purified" from the remnants of Judaism, and how the Hebrew-speaking peoples could accept Hebrew culture without it being imposed on them.

Martin Buber, said Evron, was the first individual in the Zionist movement to take into consideration the fact that Israel is not only the homeland of the Hebrews but also an Arab country, an inseparable part of the Arab-speaking world. Because he saw this he was shunned and considered utopian. From the beginning of his Zionist career he tried to find a formula that would make possible the existence of two peoples in one land, for he realized that there could not be a stable Hebrew entity in the country without brotherly relations with the Arab people.[16] However, Buber, who the members of "Semitic Action" proposed as a candidate for president of the country, was regarded by Ratosh as a professor who had an international reputation specifically in Jewish studies, a Jewish philosopher, a Jew by religion and a Jewish personality, and not simply a distinguished figure of Jewish origin like Einstein or Bergson,[17] and therefore, from the point of view of the proposed political movement, he did not fit the definition of a "Hebrew," as "Semitic Action" claimed.

In other things he wrote, three years before the Six-Day War – things that deepened the split between the right-wing nationalist Ratosh and Evron, the man of the radical left – Ratosh did not distinguish between different parts of the Land of Israel, between that whose borders were established in 1948 and that whose temporary borders were fixed in 1967: "What is the difference," he asked, "between Ein Karem, Jaffa, the mixed city of Haifa, Jerusalem outside the walls or the city of sands built to the north of Haifa, and the Old City of Jerusalem, Hebron, Shechem, Kfar Sumil, etcetera [...]?"[18]

Canaanism, Judaism, Zionism

In Evron's opinion, the task of the intellectual was to decide on social objectives and create a system of values by which they could be carried out. He could do this because an intellectual is not only an enlightened person but someone with a conscience who is willing to follow his moral convictions in confronting society. "Intellectual" and "outsider" are synonymous terms. Evron believed that in Israel men of letters were less respected than men of action because of the reaction against Jewish tradition which emphasized the spirit. As evidence of this, he said that in the time when Ben-Gurion was in power, the intellectuals "stood at attention like soldiers before the politicians."[19]

Evron disapproved of the "artificial" approach of intellectuals, writers and scientists who claimed to see everything in terms of Jewish history, as in the idea, for instance, that "Canaanism is a new Sabbetaiism." Here he was referring to Orthodox intellectuals like Akiva Ernst Simon, Baruch Kurzweil, Yishiyahu Leibowitz, and even Gershom Scholem, who denounced Canaanism, calling it "territorial messianism."[20] Evron thought that cultures should not be viewed in isolation. The works of Bialik and Tchernikovsky should be seen in relation to European romantic poetry and not only to the Jewish poetic tradition. The flowering of Jewish culture took place in periods of openness: the Second Temple period, Spain, the age of humanism, emancipation. In these conditions, something small and restricted can become something large and variegated, and in most cases the final result is different from the origin. For instance, the modern English people are composed of Gauls, Britons, Saxons, Vikings, Normans and French. Similarly, the Jews who came to Palestine founded a new society there and changed their situation. Throughout the world, the Jews are a minority in relation to the dominant religion, but as soon as they lost their minority status, their situation changed, and this was a real transformation. Zionism described this well when it said that it aimed at transforming a potential people into an actual people. It is not surprising, said Evron, that there was an estrangement between those who immigrated to the country and those who remained outside, for that was the aim of Zionism: to leave behind the Jewish diaspora and create a new national entity. Why is a new Jewish ingathering needed if not to create something new?

To Zionism's claim that it constitutes the guarantee of the Jewish people's survival, Evron replied that political existence is no guarantee against destruction: a territorial concentration of Jews could disappear with the changes wrought by history. In fact, the "Jewish nation" is a vague concept. The Jews do not have any of the characteristics of a nation: they do not have a common territory, a common language, secular institutions or a single culture. The Jews only represent a religious tradition. The Jewish settlement in Palestine was not only motivated by Zionist considerations but was part of the mass-emigration of the Jews of Eastern and Central Europe prompted by harsh decrees and anti-semitic disturbances. If a developed and highly populated Arab society had existed in the country, it would not have been able to absorb a large Jewish population, and the congruence of the land of immigration and the Holy Land of religious tradition would have disappeared.

While the Jews are not a nation but a religious community, the Hebrew citizens of the country, who *do* have the characteristics of a nation (language, territory, culture and institutions), have left the theological and ethnic frame-work. In most spheres of life, the citizen does not act as a Jew but as an Israeli, and Israel has a concrete existence and interests which have no connection with Judaism. Where his function and his experience of life are concerned, the Israeli has ceased to be a Jew. There can be a Jewish Israeli just as there can be a Christian Israeli, but an imposition of Jewish religious norms on the state must be opposed. The religious principle and the political principle are essentially irreconcilable because the Jewish religion is in its very nature anti-political. Zionism justifies seeing the Jews of the diaspora as its instruments, mere "raw material" with no life of its own.[21]

Thus, the break between Zionism and the Israeli affinity with the land is highly significant. The Hebrew identity could only combine with Judaism if Judaism pro-vided materials for an authentic Jewish nationhood. Because two national entities could not exist together, many Israelis felt an estrangement and hostility towards the Jewish tradition. But, in fact, their connection with the Jewish people was neither increased nor diminished because they drew their inspiration from Western culture and not from Jewish tradition. Similarly, Arab nationalism had to be opposed because it was not an exclusively Arab region. The only possibility for obtaining a broad framework was to renounce Israeli or Arab authority and create a federated body in a multinational territory made up of a mosaic of peoples.

A year before the Six-Day War, Evron warned against a conquest of the territ-ories, irredentist dreams and the problems with which they would be accompanied:

> A conquest of this kind would be a return on a small scale to the old type of imperialism which would be bound to fail because the acquisition of a ter-ritory with an oppressed and hostile population could only be an addition of weakness.[22]

Evron called for a rejection of the religious common denominator and a rejection of the Jewish basis, two objectives that would achieve a dual goal: a common linguistic and territorial culture and a national territory as the founda-tion for the creation of a people (as against the Zionist idea of a people searching for a territory). A federal structure not on a religious, national or linguistic basis with a recognition of the different character of all the various components would provide a hope for a common organizational principle.

Zionism, according to Evron, sought to create a new Jew resembling a "simple, healthy gentile." The ideal envisaged by people like Israel Eldad and Uri Zvi Greenberg was the Polish or Ukrainian hooligan whom they were afraid of as children. That "Jewish *goy*" who settled in the country bore the original sin of expelling the Arab natives, but Evron said that one should not be overwhelmed by that sin. All peoples are born in sin, for every people settles in a country that was populated by the members of another people. "Almost everywhere there was a conquest, followed by assimilation. That is how it was with the Americans, the Spanish, the French and the English. We too are part of that process." We should not demean ourselves because of the original sin but accept it and try to correct it as far as possible. The condition for a solution is to acknowledge the sin. Evron did not think that the adoption of his point of view would result in "a masochistic self-identification with the fate of the crusaders in Palestine." The main thing, in his opinion, was the absolute security of the nation in its country and a national existence based on territory. The right to live in the country could not be based on historical documents or religious belief, and had to acknowledge the right of the Palestinians as well.

The results of the Six-Day War caused Evron to re-examine the relationship of Israel to Judaism. His previous opinions, he said, were formed on the basis of "certain assumptions," one of which was that the problem of Jewish existence in the diaspora would be solved because the antisemitic potential had been exhausted, but the resurgence of antisemitism in Europe could not be ignored. Most surprising of all was the phenomenon of antisemitism without Jews, as a result of which he now agreed with the idea of the founders of Zionism that the "Jewish problem" was not a socioeconomic matter whose solution would change the situation. The explanation, he believed, lay in the relationship between the creation of the new Hebrew people in its country and the antisemitic reaction to it. If there is indeed a condition of permanent "Jewish distress" as Herzl claimed, it means that the Zionist analysis has proved itself, and the conclusion to be drawn is that Israel is responsible for the fate of the Jews: "I fear that within me there is a refusal to break with my past, which to a large extent formed me. It would be an act of self-rejection."[23]

There is no point, said Evron, in denying the fact of the existence of the Jewish people. The problem was created when that people founded a state, and then the principle of political, territorial and linguistic organization became operative. Just as religion demands an equality before God, so a state demands complete equality of its citizens in a legal territorial framework. A combination of the religious or ethnic principle, which is a voluntary basis, with the political principle, which is an obligatory territorial basis, necessarily creates awkward contradictions, especially in states where there are different religious and ethnic groups. Evron believed that in Israel the political principle would prevail over the ethnic-religious principle. Where he was concerned, his opinions had not changed completely, but he now understood that they were only partial as they related to a situation that was dynamic and changeable: "The Jewish people exists, and there was a need for Zionism and for the creation of a state for the

Jewish people." The Jewish people created its state which must be open to every Jew who wishes to immigrate. It is clear, then, that he now accepted the Law of Return in a comprehensive way and not in a selective way as he did previously. But as soon as the state came into being, it was subject to a logic different from the one which led to its formation. Evron thought it similar to the dynamic of American history which began with the founding fathers who wished to create a theocratic republic and ended with a separation of religion and state.

Evron continued his examination of Zionism, and said that all the distortions were created when the Zionist concept of settlement which claimed that the immigrants to Palestine were people of superior culture who had to supplant the "natives" began to be applied. As soon as the interests of the Jewish community became opposed to those of the original inhabitants of the country, there was a need for Zionist forces to defend the Jews from the local people. This explains the necessity for patrons who would take the Yishuv, the state-in-the-making and the sovereign state which arose, under their protection. The idea that the Jews were a group with a higher culture than their neighbors gave them a sense of power. Zionist dependence on others, like Jewish dependence in history, corresponded to a self-image of victimization, alienation and serving as a scapegoat of antisemitism, and gave rise to the mythical concept of a single Jewish fate. The cure for all this, said Evron, was the healthy national consciousness free from complexes which usually exists in stable, self-assured peoples with an open and positive relation to the world.

The Canaanite idea or Hebrew identity?

In 1984, Evron wrote a review of Jacob Shavit's book, *Meivri to Canaanite* (From a Hebrew to a Canaanite), in which he asked what connection there was between "the direct experience of an intellectual and emotional fever" which the Canaanite group knew in the time of its development and its later treatment as a systematic history. Do the matters described and the scholarly analyses in the history convey "the fever that raged in the Hebrew youth of the nineteen-forties, that revolutionary generation that was burned and consumed in the flames of the war of 1948," and which left behind "despair and ashes" and made possible the victory of conservatism? In the final analysis, the inverted commas around the word "Zionism" referred to the fighters of the Palmach and not to the "Canaanites" who joined their ranks.[24]

Evron claimed that the leaders of the Zionist educational system in the early 1950s were afraid of "Canaanite ideas" because they were aware of the extraordinarily revolutionary character of the Canaanite outlook (and not specifically of the "Canaanite group"), and the continued attachment of the general public, and especially the youth, to these ideas. In the post-war atmosphere there was still a strong rebellious revolutionary potential which found literary expression in S. Yizhar's book, *Yemei Ziklag* (Days of Ziklag), for example, or Moshe Shamir's book, *Pirkei Alik* (Alik's Story). The general intellectual atmosphere, from Yizhar to Moshe Dayan, was imbued with a Canaanite nativistic sentiment that was not esoteric in the early days of the state. Moreover, in the time of the Yishuv before the declaration of independence, there was no real distinction between "Hebraism" and "Canaanism," both of which related to "a great outpouring of feeling for the Hebrew homeland," a feeling that prevailed in all ideological camps. Without an awareness of this and its force one cannot describe or understand the struggle of the Yishuv and the War of Independence. But, in the course of the war, its "spinal cord" was broken and it was absorbed into *mamlachtiyut* (statism). Evron claimed that without the Palmach, the Irgun Zvai Leumi, Lehi, the kibbutz movement and the Haganah, "there would have been no society, there would have been no struggle, and the state would not have been founded." He drew a historical parallel with guiding elites like the Jacobins and the Bolsheviks, without whom historical revolutions would not have occurred.

He went beyond the historical context to a sociological and mythological explanation. Following Claude Lévi-Strauss, he also sought to understand the structural significance of the creation of these myths in the transition from the fall of the Sabbetaian communities and the decline of the ancient religions based on blood and ritual to modern institutions and the nation-state based on territory and civil law. At the same time, he said, the new national movements sought their historical origins in a kind of "restoration of ancient potential and an enshrining of a people and state which had existed in some mythical golden age," although historians had disproved most of the myths. Even Zionism glorified the kingdoms of Judah and Israel and politicized religious concepts such as the Third Temple.

Evron saw "Canaanism" as the product of influences and not as the generational expression of a social-national consciousness with deep historical roots. The idea of a Hebrew homeland required a suitable ideology: Zionism as the ideology of an ethnic group without a territory that sought an area in which to solve the Jewish problem. As soon as an area was found on which to build a society, the inhabitants required a territorial ideology accompanied by a suitable myth. That was why many young people, including Evron, were drawn as if by magic to the Canaanite outlook rather than to the previous "Hebraism."

He spoke of a natural Canaanism, of a state of mind the members of the Yishuv already had before the War of Independence, a feeling that found concrete expression in the Palmach and also in the Israel Defense Forces. These were not intellectual youths motivated by the principles of the Hebrew revolution but fighters for whom it was only natural to strive for sovereignty in practice.[25] The shock of the young people after the war brought some of the members of the underground who were conscious of their nativism to the "Canaanite group." Evron claimed that it would therefore not be true to say that Canaanism was a reaction to the waves of Jewish immigration to the country.

In the chapter, "Canaanism, Its Solutions and Problems," in his book *Ha-heshbon Ha-leumi* (A National Reckoning) (1988) – a book which in a systematic and orderly fashion presented his views about the crystallization of Hebrew nationalism in modern times – he described the "Canaanite doctrine" as "the most audacious and systematic attempt until now to escape from the tangle of contradictions [in Zionism]."[26] Evron identified four main aspects in Canaanism: ideological completion of and opposition to Zionist thought; a generational expression of the people of the land and a direct, unmediated feeling for the homeland as opposed to the acquired sense of the homeland of people like A.D. Gordon and Ben-Gurion; an expression and continuation of the biblical revolution, a return to a direct interpretation of the Bible; and a means of destroying the institution built upon these Scriptures. A preoccupation with the physical and with military activities was not of primary importance in the exile, and the cultural heroes there were the hassid, the scholar, the kabbalist and the man of means. The assimilated Jews were not interested in these heroes and preferred to blend into the gentile environment and adopt European values. The Vilna Gaon and Maimonides were not a source of inspiration for Heine and Herzl, who preferred Goethe and the Nibelunglied, which were translated into Hebrew. The failure of assimilation did not bring about a return to Maimonides but caused Tchernikovsky to translate Greek, Norse and Russian epics and adapt them to the reviving Hebrew culture. Likewise, Bialik intended the redemption of his people in the legend "King David in the Cave" in which the pouring of water on the hands of King David and his men awakens them from a sleep of thousands of years, a mythical story in which there is an echo of a German folk-legend about old Frederick Barbarossa and his knights in the mountains of Bavaria who are asleep until he awakes and redeems his people (and there is also a British version about King Arthur).

In this way, the Jews integrated into the national romanticism of the peoples of the countries in which they lived, but they were alien both to the heroic traditions of the peoples in those countries and to the talmudic tradition which covered the biblical heroes in dust. These heroes experienced a mythical and pagan resurrection: Judah Maccabee, John of Gischala, and the *sicarii* (dagger-men) of Second Temple times were compared to Leonidas, King Arthur and Siegfried. The Zionists and the assimilated abandoned historical Judaism, but in the process Zionism lost its equilibrium. The conclusion to be drawn from the development of Zionism had in Evron's opinion to be a break with Jewish ethnicity and a sole connection with the land and the people that lives there. But Zionism could not break the umbilical cord with the Jewish diaspora which gave birth to it. The Jew who settled in the Land of Israel made contact with those like him before he arrived in the country. He saw the country as a communal-ethnic center, not as a territorial basis for a nation. In other words, Zionism failed to take the necessary next step – a complete break with the ethnic connection. In that sense, and only in that sense, Canaanism was the missing step in Zionism: it went forward from the point where Zionism left off.

Evron said that "a rebel grows up in the conceptual framework he rebels against," adding that the most striking form of rebellion is the one against basic patterns of thought.[27] Canaanism, which called for a complete break with Judaism, decided on its path at the height of the assault on the Jewish people in the Second World War and the extermination of the Jews (Evron on principle refrained from using the term "holocaust"). The Canaanite "declaration of independence" was a provocative call for the Hebrew people to set itself up in the country as a new nation and so to totally disconnect itself from the Jewish diaspora and the "Jewish destiny." Was Evron here echoing Ratosh's call in his "Address to Hebrew Youth" at the height of the campaign of extermination? It was surely no accident that the conscious break with the fate of the Jews took place at that fateful hour of the Jewish destiny, when the carnage was revealed to the world. Evron defended the Yishuv's disengagement which he did not think was exclusive to the Canaanites. The fate of the Jews in Europe was not the priority of the Zionist leadership which was primarily concerned with strengthening the Yishuv. The representatives of "Lehi" even tried to get in touch with representatives of Nazi Germany. The Zionist leadership, and Ya'ir Stern as well, attached the utmost importance to Palestine as the center of national activity.

One should remember that the Canaanite movement, which made its first appearance in 1943, was the most systematic expression of the nativistic frame of mind. A year later, the principles of the movement were formulated in an "Opening Address" which declared that "a Hebrew cannot be a Jew and a Jew cannot be a Hebrew."[28] In Evron's opinion, the meaning of the statement was to draw a clear demarcation line between the experience of the territorial nation and the Jewish experience, "the life of the religious community." And what exactly was the territorial nation? The Canaanite movement held the view that the members of that nation were Hebrew-speaking inhabitants of the "land of Kedem," a land in which Hebrew-speaking peoples existed in the past, comprising Lebanon, Jordan and the present Land of Israel. In this area, there came into being in ancient times a Hebrew nation, a pagan nation which produced a Hebrew civilization and which was destroyed by foreign invasions. Historical evidence of its greatness is provided by the literary legacy of the Bible, the original version of which was distorted and emasculated by later Jewish editing. The new nucleus of this people was the Hebrew Yishuv in Palestine which in the Canaanite vision would later spread throughout the "land of Kedem" and restore the pristine splendor. The Muslim population in the region, on whom Arab invaders imposed an alien religion and language, would in the future return to the original Hebrew culture. This large Hebrew state would grant full civil equality to all its inhabitants and would impose on them the Hebrew culture and language. This old-new nation would have no connection with the Jews of the diaspora.

It therefore follows that, from the Canaanite point of view, the desire of Tchernikovsky or Ben-Gurion to turn the "Jew" into a "Hebrew" was self-contradictory, because underlying it was the assumption that the Jew was a potential Hebrew. In the Canaanite territorialism, said Evron, there could be no common destiny for the Jew and Hebrew. They represented two contrary forms of existence which could not live side-by-side. They were not teleological entities whose objective lay beyond themselves. Zionism saw the "Jew" as the instrument of the "Hebrew." However, Evron pointed out that even if one accepts the Canaanite claim that there was once a Hebrew culture in the whole of the "land of Kedem," that culture came there through Judaism. His conclusion was that even if in the future there will be an Israelite-Hebrew nation separate from Judaism, it will necessarily have a deep connection with Jewish manifestations. Just as one cannot have Arab nationalism without the world of Islamic thought, just as one cannot separate the secular European consciousness from Christian manifestations, one cannot create "a Hebrew nation in the land of the Hebrews" based exclusively on the ancient Hebrew territory. The suppression of the Jewish legacy would distort the spiritual character of the Hebrew culture and give rise to a strong reaction from the suppressed elements.

Similarly, one cannot divorce the Arab peoples from their Islamic legacy and impose Hebrew culture on them. The Canaanite assertion that, because these peoples' original language was Hebrew, they must be liberated from the imposition of Arabic and brought back to their authentic language, was in Evron's opinion imperialistic.

Evron said that there were four political assumptions underlying Canaanism:[29] (1) The state is the political expression of the nation. In this respect, Canaanism does not differ from the Zionist view that Israel is the political expression of the Jewish people. (2) The state must be large and powerful in order to act independently in the political sphere. The success of the nation and its transformation into an independent, sovereign or even international entity depend on the creation of a common political framework. (3) Potential regional independence will only become actual when the political process will take place in the entire area. The needs of the Jewish people outside the country and the needs of the Arab nation outside the Middle East are irrelevant. The abandonment of these external factors will encourage an independent policy in the region. (4) A federal solution for the region cannot be based on the Jewish or Arab people because of their limitations. Canaanism saw them as self-absorbed religious communities, and any attempt by either of them to dominate the region would therefore be repression and coercion. A new structure was needed, not based on the old affinities, one that would be a common basis for all the inhabitants of the region.

Evron saw the "Canaanite idea" as the deliberate creation of a spatial myth to counteract external influences and form a new national entity of equal citizens from different communities, like the national myths that flourished when national movements were arising in Europe. It was perhaps the need for an integrative myth of this kind that gave Zionism and the Arab national movements their autonomous character. The need to create a regional nation helped to form a separate regional consciousness. The Canaanites believed that the Yishuv as a progressive factor in the area would cause a regional Hebraic revolution. This revolution would come about through an alliance with the non-Arab peoples in the area threatened by the Sunni Muslim majority. The Canaanites saw it as a barbaric element, preferring a regional "alliance of peoples." Hence the Canaanite criticism of the Israeli government in the 1948 war for preventing the conquest of areas densely populated by Arabs. The founders of Canaanism repeatedly said that the birth of the Hebrew nation that would impose its culture on the peoples of the area would be through an act of war and not through cultural propaganda.

The "state of all its citizens"

In a 1983 interview entitled "I feel a foreigner in my own land," Evron said that "the State of Israel has not yet been founded." He called "for the creation here of a new national society in which non-Jews will also be accepted" and opposed the concept of Israeli citizenship to that of Jewish unity.[30] With regard to the observation of Hanan Porat, one of the leaders of "Gush Emunim," that "secular settlement has finished its task," Evron replied:

> There's an element of truth in that. The world of Zionist values is exhausted. What Hanan Porat is proposing is a return to pre-Zionism: a closed-up Jewish community with weapons, an armed ghetto. He suggests that the entire Jewish people should come together in the country and fight against the whole world, but that would lead to a disaster. It's an insane approach, a suicidal approach.
>
> When the state was founded, it was possible to move in various directions. After the 1967 war we also had two possibilities – to renounce the territories for the sake of peace or to annex them and call all their inhabitants Israeli citizens. We did not do one or the other. It could have been a revolution.[31]

He was the first to point out the contradictions in the dialectical assertion that the "Gush Emunim" settlements would hasten the creation of the "land of Kedem" in which a Hebrew nation would be formed combining different religious and ethnic groups and communities. These Canaanite ideas based on a Hegelian "cunning of reason" were similar, he claimed, to the pretentious logic of "Gush Emunim" in interpreting the secrets of God's messianic plans. This pretentiousness reveals a lack of understanding of political and sociological processes. Together with examples of a mixing of populations, there are examples in history of failures to create a homogeneous population which only led to wars, the destruction of native populations and the expulsion of settlers. The examples are familiar: the French colonists in Algeria, the British Protestants in Ireland, the Dutch in South Africa, the British settlers in Rhodesia and Kenya. While the negative examples are modern, the precedents for a mixing of populations are ancient: the Vikings in England and France, the Mongols in China and the Franks in Gaul.[32]

Evron equated the colonialist enterprises which failed with the colonialism of the settlers. First of all, the culture of the settlers is radically different from the native culture of the occupied. The Israeli and Palestinian populations have opposing, self-sufficient ideologies, and the friction between them is not conducive to mixing but to hatred. Second, the enmity-producing friction is particularly pronounced in this case because one side has imposed itself on the other. In this relationship of master and slave, said Evron, contrary to the dialectical thesis of the Canaanites, the settlement project arouses the national consciousness of the oppressed. In many cases, such a consciousness is created where it did not exist previously and it was only caused by foreign occupation. And here Evron was mistaken in his forecast (one should remember that it was made in the 1980s): he said that unlike the Canaanites, the settlers had apparently no intention to seek the formal annexation of the West Bank to Israel because then it would be difficult to avoid granting citizenship to its Arab inhabitants. The real aim of the settlers is not the Hebraization of the Arabs as the Canaanites desired, but their expulsion. The American support for retention of the settlements, influenced by the Jews of the United States, reveals the cunning of history in the fact that that in the final analysis the Canaanite program needed the support of elements outside the region.

Hanan Porat and "Gush Emunim" could be described as religious right-wing neo-Canaanites. The political theology of "Gush Emunim" supports a Jewish-ethnic nationhood within the borders of the Greater Land of Israel. On the many occasions when the laws of the Torah have clashed with political requirements, leading activists and rabbis in Judea and Samaria have preferred the physical place (the Land of Israel) to the metaphysical Place (God). They changed the order of preferences of religious Zionism from "the Torah plus the Land" to "the Land plus Torah."

Evron gave an explanation for the support of the Canaanites Yonatan Ratosh and Aharon Amir for "Gush Emunim" and the settlement enterprise.[33] It was a dialectical explanation: the settlers are religious extremists who have designs against the Palestinians, but it is a transient phenomenon which will hasten the establishment of the "land of the Hebrews." Evron specifically drew attention to the relationship of these Canaanites to "Gush Emunim":

> The grotesque dialectical result of this approach was the consistent support of Ratosh and the orthodox Canaanites for "Gush Emunim", despite the fact that they were the contrary of "Canaanism". The Canaanite idea in this matter was as follows: the conquest of the areas of the "land of Kedem" and settlement there would lead to a mixing of populations. Although the settlers are inward-looking religious Jews, they unconsciously carry the Hebrew culture, even if in a distorted religious form. The superiority of that culture will gradually lead to its infiltration to the non-Jewish population and its "Hebraization", as has already happened to a certain extent in the areas of the "old" Israel. The fact that they live side-by-side will lead in the course of time to an increasing closeness between them, even if in the early stages there is a relationship of hostility and conflict, the product of acts of dispossession and repression, but this is a known phenomenon which has long been seen in the settlement of invading peoples […].
>
> The settlements of "Gush Emunim" are a dialectical step towards the creation of the Hebrew "land of Kedem" which is above all ethnic, religious

and community divisions and combines the whole population in the framework of a single nation – the Hebrew nation.[34]

Parallel with the religious right-wing neo-Canaanism of "Gush Emunim," one of whose sources of inspiration was the "Canaanite idea," post-Zionism can be seen as a secular left-wing neo-Canaanism based on a shift from history to geography: a nativistic outlook favoring a civil definition, a territorial nationhood, a separation of religion and state, and the idea that the state belongs solely to its citizens, not to history and not to Judaism.

This civil Canaanism was the outlook of Evron, who wrote in 2002: "The only lasting solution can be the thing which everyone fears, both on the left and right: a state that is democratic and open to all its citizens, sufficiently strong to embrace Christians and Muslims, Semites and Slavs."[35] The ideological basis on which Israel was founded must be rejected. It must be de-Zionized, and from that time onward it must be seen as a state of all its citizens. The Zionist revolution, which translated the Germanic myths and adopted the pagan Greek epics, adapting them to ancient Hebrew formulas, was in Evron's opinion a form of collective assimilation. As soon as Zionism recognized this, it lost its self-confidence and "ceased to be a theory of political, national and revolutionary importance."

The "civil Canaanism" is in a certain sense an attempt to continue the path from the point where Zionism left off. The completion of the Zionist revolution requires the severance of the people from its diaspora and for the citizen to be defined solely by the geographical context of his country. The shift from the old community-based ethnic concept to the new national-territorial concept necessitates the cutting of the ethnic umbilical cord. It would seem that the following words give an accurate description of the Hebrew vision of Evron, a man whose roots went back to his early acquaintance with the Canaanite ideas of Yonatan Ratosh:

> I am not frightened of the future of our culture if it opens its doors to all the inhabitants of the country. It is strong and deep-rooted, and can absorb all that come to it, making them into one people transcending religious and ethnic divisions.[36]

Evron's ideas supporting a Moledet as a civil state were in total contradiction to the idea of a Jewish Moledet to which intellectuals like Robert Wistrich subscribed. One should remember, said Wistrich, whom we shall discuss in the following chapter, that the original Zionists – Herzl, Pinsker, Nordau and others – saw antisemitism as the greatest problem of Jewish existence, and the reason for this was the attitude of the nations of the world to the Jews among them.[37] They believed that a Jewish state could create a situation of "normalization" for both the Jews and the world where antisemitism was concerned. But antisemitism proved to be a much greater problem, deeply rooted in the historical consciousness of Western civilization, than could be solved by a national state.

Notes

1 Boaz Evron, "Political Autobiography," *Athens and Oz*, Tel Aviv 2010, 23–40 (in Hebrew); Shlomo Sand, "A National Reckoning," *Theory and Criticism*, special issue: 50 to 48, ed., Adi Ophir, Vol. 12–13 (Winter 1999): 339–348 (in Hebrew).
2 David Ohana, *Messianism and Mamlachtiyut: Ben-Gurion and the Intellectuals – Between Political Vision and Political Theology*, Sde Boker 2003, 158 (in Hebrew).
3 Ohana, *On Land of Stones: 1967 – The Place of the Israeli Place*, Tel Aviv 2017 (in Hebrew).
4 Evron, "Generals and Caves," *Haaretz*, March 26, 1961 (in Hebrew).
5 Evron, "Political Autobiography," 26.
6 Evron, "A Hymn for Jonathan," *Yediot Aharonot*, January 30, 1981 (in Hebrew).
7 Evron, "Political Autobiography," 24.
8 Nathan Yellin-Mor, *Fighters of Israel's Liberty, People, Ideas, Stories*, Tel Aviv 1999, 363–364 (in Hebrew).
9 Joseph Heller, *Lehi, Ideology and Politics, 1940–1949*, Jerusalem 1989 (in Hebrew).
10 Evron, "Political Autobiography," 27.
11 Evron, "Mixing of Powers, On Yair" (no additional information) (in Hebrew).
12 Niza Arel, *Without Fear or Impropriety*, Jerusalem 2006 (in Hebrew).
13 Evron, "Power and its Perlis," *Etgar*, 133, April 14, 1966 (in Hebrew).
14 Evron, "One Revolution in the Land and the Space," *Etgar*, 22, January 12, 1962 (in Hebrew).
15 Jonathan Ratosh, Letter, *Liberty*, September 18, 1964 (in Hebrew).
16 Evron, "The Character of Martin Buber," *Etgar*, 22, January 12, 1964 (in Hebrew).
17 Ratosh, "The Confessions of a Dumber-Than-Average Guy," *Etgar*, 97, November 26, 1964 (in Hebrew).
18 Ibid.
19 Ehud Ben-Ezer, ed., "Boaz Evron," *Unease in Zion*, Forward by Robert Alter, New York 1974.
20 David Ohana, *Political Theologies in the Holy Land*, London 2010, 54–92.
21 Ben-Ezer, op. cit.
22 Ibid., 174.
23 Ibid., 180.
24 Evron, "The Action – And its Academic Reflection," *Yediot Aharonot – Culture, Literature, Art*, March 2, 1984 (in Hebrew).
25 Yaakov Shavit, *The New Hebrew Nation: A Study in Israeli Heresy and Fantasy*, London 1987.
26 Boaz Evron, *A National Reckoning*, Tel Aviv 1988, 332 (in Hebrew). English translation is available: Boaz Evron, *Jewish State or Israeli Nation*, Indianapolis 1995.
27 Ibid., 335.
28 Ibid., 336.
29 Ibid., 339–341.
30 Rubik Rosenthal, "I Feel Estranged in My Own Homeland," *Al-HaMishmar – Hotam*, September 26, 1983 (in Hebrew).
31 Ibid.
32 Evron, *A National Reckoning*, 344.
33 On similar developments among other "Cannnites," see: Avi Shilon, "The Influence of the Six-Day War on the Cannanite Idea in its Varieties," *Iyunim BeTkumat Israel*, 11 (2017): 66–67 (in Hebrew).
34 Evron, "Political Autobiography," 343.
35 Ibid.
36 Evron, "Democratic, Not Jewish [State]," *Haaretz*, September 11, 2002 (in Hebrew).
37 Robert R. Wistrich, "Max Nordau and the Dreyfus Affair," *The Journal of Israeli History*, 16, 1 (1995): 1–19.

4   From antisemitism and anti-Zionism to Moledet

The historian Robert Wistrich related that when he was twelve years' old, he had an illuminating experience. Two representatives of the British Zionist Organization came to his home in Kilburn in north-west London. They wished to put up a plaque at the entrance to the house, which said, "This is where modern Zionism was born." Theodor Herzl had visited the Anglo-Jewish writer Israel Zangwill in that house to seek support for his ideas.[1] Wistrich said:

> It was the first time I had heard of Herzl […] Looking back later on, it was wonderful to know that as a child I had done my homework in the very room in which there had been a historic meeting with Theodor Herzl – a turning-point, a turning-point of historical significance.[2]

Some time later, in the 1960s, the plaque was defaced by anti-Israeli activists. One can say that this anecdote combining Zionist endeavor with anti-Israel protest was symbolic of Wistrich's intellectual life. The prime conclusion Wistrich endeavors to draw from his research is that the only way to eliminate antisemitism is by having a homeland, *Moledet*.

During his intellectual and public life, Robert Wistrich maintained the motto suggested in Albert Einstein's famous speech. On February 6, 1923, Albert Einstein – shortly after receiving the Nobel Prize for Physics and when he was at the peak of his fame – gave the first scientific address ever to be delivered at the Hebrew University in Jerusalem. In an impassioned speech that testified to his Zionist credo, he declared:

> I consider this the greatest day of my life […]. This is a great age, the age of the liberation of the Jewish soul. And it has been accomplished through the Zionist movement, which has remained a spiritual movement, so that no one in the world will be able to destroy it.[3]

This essence of Zionism was central to Wistrich's research, but also to his way of life in his maturity and his ideological outlook. In which way was his personal outlook reflected in his academic work? How did he arrive at his

Zionist outlook and his study of Zionism? Before Wistrich came to Israel, he wrote his doctoral thesis (in English) on the attitude of the political Left to the Jews in the nineteenth century. For his part, he never believed that scholars are without feelings and that a choice a man makes in the academic field is unconnected with his personal life. Wistrich grew up and was educated in England in the 1950s, 1960s, and 1970s, and claimed to have experienced antisemitism, but of a mild kind. He said that he researched

> the various anti-Zionist ideas of the Orthodox, the socialists, the Communists, the Bund. When you read the things they said and wrote before the founding of the State, most of their arguments against setting up a Jewish state were convincing.[4]

Wistrich, at the beginning of his intellectual and academic development, was a kind of cosmopolitan Jew, a radical youth who dealt with the problems of the world rather than the misfortunes of his people. But later he felt a dramatic change in the attitude to anything to do with the Jews, and first and foremost with regard to the State of Israel and Zionism. In 1968, when he returned to Europe from Stanford in California, he heard of the student revolt that had broken out in France, and immediately, with the reflex of a nomadic revolutionary, he went to Paris and sympathetically overviewed the disturbances. In that same year, he went to Dubček's Prague, where they attempted a "socialism with a human face," and then the Russian tanks came in. By the end of 1968 he realized that all the dreams of the student revolt were no more than dreams. He decided to go to Israel because he felt Jewish.

Wistrich was then twenty-three years old and was appointed editor of *New Outlook*, the English language journal of Mapam, the socialist party in Israel. This was his first encounter with Zionist socialism. He studied at the Hebrew University under professors such as Jacob Talmon and Yehoshua Arieli and returned to England for a decade to finish his doctorate. He was away from Israel for ten years but he knew he would return. But it was not because he was a Zionist; it was something emotional. He had a deep inner conviction that the State of Israel was the future of the Jewish people. He didn't want to live in exile: Israel, for him, was a homeland, *Moledet*.

Wistrich mentioned that Alexis de Tocqueville, the great historian, said that the French Revolution had two very distinct phases – the first, which sought the abolition of everything in the past; and the second, which tried to reconnect with that same past from which the French had cut themselves off. In the case of Zionism, its basic tasks and objectives were not simply to destroy a given socio-political structure, or even to achieve national independence after an interval of 2,000 years.[5] The Zionist revolution derived most of its peculiar features from the fact that it was a revolt against historic destiny itself, or as David Ben-Gurion, the founding father of the State of Israel, once put it, "against the unique destiny of a unique people."

The world of yesterday

In the Second World War, Wistrich's parents fled from Poland and he was born in Kazakhstan. In 1948 the family immigrated to England, where he was raised and educated from the 1950s to the 1970s. He examined the different forms of anti-Zionism among the Orthodox, the socialists, the communists and the Bund, and came to the conclusion that most of the things they said and wrote in the pre-state period against founding a state for the Jews were convincing.

In his autobiographical article, "From Cracow to London – A Polish-Jewish Odyssey," Wistrich further related the story of his life in an attempt to place the vicissitudes of his family within the context of modern Jewish history. In a statement in the article, he described the motivation for his academic career: "From an early age, I had experienced a fairly robust English xenophobia at school and on the streets, which sometimes slid into violence."[6] He eventually became one of the leading world experts on antisemitism. In 2002, he was appointed head of the Vidal Sassoon International Center for the Study of Anti-semitism in the Hebrew University, Jerusalem. Under his leadership, this research institution became a spearhead in the war against antisemitism throughout the world. Wistrich, not content with his many studies of antisem-itism, left his ivory tower for the campuses and parliaments of the United States and Europe in order to awaken them from their sleep, as he said, with regard to the hatred of the Jews which was raising its head once more. He also initiated and authored the exhibition, "People, Book, Land. The 3500-year Relationship of the Jewish People with the Holy Land," organized by the Simon Wiesenthal Center and UNESCO.[7]

The year of his birth, 1945, the year in which the Holocaust and the Second World War came to an end, had a special significance for Wistrich, and it was a reference-point in his academic work. In the preface to his comprehensive study, *Who's Who in Nazi Germany*, containing the biographies of 350 important figures in the Third Reich, he wrote, "May this book serve both as a guide and as a warning to those born after 1945, to guard preciously the flame of freedom."[8] The book, first published in 1982 and written in the framework of his function as editor of the journal *Wiener Library for the Study of the Holocaust and Genocide* in London in the years 1974–1980, was one of his numerous studies, many of which are still relevant today. It is remarkable how many of the things he wrote at the beginning of his academic career are still relevant.

Wistrich was as well-known as an expert on Austria as he was as a scholar of antisemitism, and his major achievement in that field was his book, *The Jews of Vienna in the Age of Franz Joseph*.[9] Milan Kundera observed that in the period before Hitler, the Jews were a cosmopolitan "intellectual cement" that gave the empire a spiritual unity. Austro-Hungarian intellectual figures such as Karl Kraus, Otto Weininger, Stefan Zweig, Arthur Schnitzler, Franz Kafka, Franz Werfel, Joseph Roth, Theodor Herzl and Max Nordau were prototypes of "marginal Jews" (*Grenzjuden*) who were far from Jewish tradition but were not fully integrated into Central-European society. They distanced themselves from the Jewish community, but the Austrians did not welcome them either, even though they contributed a great deal to the culture of their homeland. According to Wistrich, they were characterized by a split identity. Stefan Zweig, for example, found consolation in regarding himself as a "good European,"[10] Joseph Roth became an admirer of Hapsburgian supra-nationalism, Karl Kraus represented the ambivalence of the Viennese-Jewish "master-victim."[11] A biting satirist and a master of the German language, which he used skillfully in defense of moral values, he resembled the prophet Isaiah in denouncing the corrupt society in which he lived. He not only renounced Judaism at the age of twenty-four but was also harshly critical of the members of his people, and to his hostility to Judaism he added radical criticism of psychoanalysis, feminism, Zionism, political laws and sexual hypocrisy. He attacked the Jews especially because they seemed to him to dominate the cultural establishment, but he also had no hesitation in accusing Zionists like Herzl of being "antisemitic Jews." Other intellectuals changed their faith or became Zionists, or assimilated or were social-democrats. They lived in an intellectual climate in which the winds blew in various directions – towards art, ethnic confrontation, assimilation, or Zionism.

Max Nordau was another complex figure in the diverse mosaic of the Central-European Jewish pantheon.[12] He was born in Budapest but his culture was entirely German. He thus changed his name from Südfeld to Nordau, which sounded more Aryan, and was a change that bore witness to his wish to assimilate. Despite his adherence to Zionism, which began in 1895, he remained a "Germanized" cosmopolitan liberal intellectual. His scientific, Darwinist and positivist outlook was reflected in his famous book *Entartung* (Degeneration). Wistrich traced the hidden connection between his cultural criticism and his Zionist vision of a "new Jew." From the pathology he detected in a European society sick from modernization, individualism and nihilism, he drew conclusions concerning his own people. The "ghetto Jews" had to be immunized and to recreate themselves in their old-new country. They therefore had to abandon the Yiddish language and Jewish traditionalism and spirituality. In 1903, he called for the creation of a "muscular Judaism," the antithesis of the antisemitic view of the Jews. In his eyes, a Zionism of strength was the cure for the sickness of European antisemitism.

Nathan Birnbaum, who coined the term "Zionism" in 1890, also attracted Wistrich's attention. Birnbaum was born in Vienna into a family with a religious background but, like many of his generation, moved away from his religious roots which went back as far as Rashi. In his youth, he believed that the Austrian Jews were not Germans but belonged to a different people who were destined to move to Palestine. He founded "Kadima," the first Jewish national students' association. In the first Zionist Congress he was elected general secretary of the World Zionist Organization, but left the movement a year later because Herzl opposed his election.[13] Birnbaum passed through many changes, from developing a theory of pan-Judaism, acknowledging the centrality of the Yiddish language and supporting national autonomy to a return to Torah

Judaism and the religious roots of the Jewish people. He supported a variety of ideologies Zionism, socialism, Yiddishism, cultural autonomy – in an attempt to confront the modern Jewish identity. The cultural historian Carl Schorske described thinkers like Birnbaum as a collage of "fragments of modernity, glimpses of futurity and resurrected remnants of a half-forgotten past."[14]

The figures of Herzl, Kraus and Freud were used by Wistrich to illustrate the Viennese complexity, their sense of belonging together with their estrangement, their Jewish prophetic mission. Freud, a product of the turn-of-the-century anti-semitic atmosphere in Europe, like all his generation was drawn to assimilation but to some extent identified with the fate of the Jewish people.[15] Wistrich gave a good description of this emotional ambivalence which may have been the sensitive ground that gave rise to *The Interpretation of Dreams*, the major text of psychoanalysis.[16]

But of all the Central-European Jewish figures torn between the poles of anti-semitism and Zionism, Wistrich was most fascinated by Theodor Herzl. In the many articles and chapters that he wrote about him, he searched for Herzl's magic secret as a political artist, as a statesman who knew how to make a modern use of myths and the aestheticization of politics, as a charismatic figure who understood the importance of international leadership and as a sensitive Jewish public figure who recoiled from messianic visions.[17] It is ironic that Herzl himself became one of the main symbols of the Zionist movement he founded. In his appearance and behavior, he exemplified the strength and physical beauty that Zionism proposed as an alternative to the "degeneracy," ugliness and despair of life in the ghetto. Herzl was wonderfully in keeping with the Zionist image of a new, strong, upright, aristocratic Jewry advocated by one of his associates, Max Nordau. In his image one saw the very heart of the Zionist dream: a manly, handsome figure with a beard recalling the Jewish prophets and penetrating, melancholy eyes. All this exemplified for many Zionism's promise of resurrection. When he mounted the platform to speak at the first Zionist Congress, many saw him as "as a descendant of royalty steeped in legend, fantasy and beauty." It was as though the Messiah himself had appeared after 2,000 years of exile to inaugurate a new era of Jewish history.

Wistrich, who was a historian of Central-European politics and culture in the modern era, gave a good description of the conditions of life of the Jews at that time who desperately needed a founding myth, and who found it in the figure of Herzl. But the tranquil lives of the Central-European Jews were soon to be over-taken by a storm. A war on a scale that had never been previously known was about to transform their lives from start to finish.

A hundred years after the First World War, Wistrich asked to what degree the war had changed the course of history.[18] He answered that before it, Europe had a tendency to liberalism and parliamentarism, but the war shuffled the cards and gave birth to a reality of extreme ideologies which determined the fate of many Jews in the twentieth century.

The First World War destroyed the cosmopolitan ethos and pluralistic culture of the old multinational European empires. In the countries that replaced the empires after 1918 (except for Czechoslovakia), a narrow nationalism became dominant. This boded ill for cultural minorities like the Jews, who had previously been the cultural glue of Central Europe in the Hapsburg era. The new radical nationalism tended towards a deep ethnocentrism following the loss of the vast territories.

A new period now began of unmitigated violence, barbaric atrocities, ethnic hatreds, deadly national struggles and fanatical racism, which drowned in blood the naive patriotism prevalent at the beginning of the war. The "world of yesterday," as the Austrian writer Stefan Zweig wrote nostalgically, had disappeared. Wistrich drew attention to the fact that not even the terrible price paid by the Jewish victims on the battlefield helped the Jews to be accepted in society or lessened the degree of nationalist antisemitism in Central and Eastern Europe. On the contrary, the hatred of the Jews continually increased. However, the results of the war were mixed: the world war, with all that took place at that time, also strengthened the national sentiment of the Jews and led to the Balfour Declaration issued by the British government in November 1917. Nine years before the establishment of the state of Israel, another war broke in Europe, a war that would be remembered notoriously in Jewish history henceforth.

The Jews – the demon of Europe

At what point did "normal" ethnocentricity become hatred of foreigners, racism and antisemitism? When did family or group egoism – i.e. the tendency to exclude the other – become hatred, aggressive hostility, deliberate persecution or even slaughter? When did ethnocentricity become an alienating xenophobic safety-belt around a particular cultural identity, or, worse, a racist paranoia directed at dangers of infection from within or from outside? How do racial fantasies develop a genocidal dynamic as happened with the Nazis, a dynamic that ascribes qualities of wickedness to a mythical enemy to such a point that he has to be wiped off the face of the earth? Wistrich sought to answer these questions through his studies which dealt with the background, circumstances and causes of the extermination of the European Jews in the twentieth century.[19] His conclusion was that the Nazi hatred of the Jewish other in its tremendous force and lethal insanity undoubtedly exceeded "normal" preconceptions, institutionalized racial discrimination, hatred of foreigners, racial segregation, or the pogroms that took place in the course of Jewish history. At the same time, one cannot and should not separate it totally from other forms of racism, and certainly not from the long history of antisemitism that preceded it. In addition to the basic antisemitism of the Nazis, they made a widespread, systematic use of Christian anti-Jewish stereotypes. For example, they were able to rely on a 2,000-year-old tradition whose roots are already found in the Gospels (and especially in the Gospel of John), and on the description of the Jews in those works as murderers of Jesus and allies of the Devil. They could also rely on the teachings of the Church Fathers who consistently regarded the Jews as slanderers, desecrators of the Holy Name, an accursed and abominated people and members of a satanic sect. The Nazis exploited and secularized medieval images of the Jews as devils, sorcerers, desecrators of the host, poisoners of wells, ritual murderers, rapacious moneylenders, unbelievers and tireless subverters intent on destroying Christian society.

The Protestant reformation in Germany and the mythologization of the Jews as the sons of Satan promoted by Martin Luther provided Nazi antisemitism with an additional supply of images. The demonization of the other, said Wistrich, is of course not restricted to the Jews. It appears that finding scapegoats and ascribing evil to people given diabolical characteristics is a universal human problem. The process not only removes feelings of guilt, creates a separation between accepted groups and proscribed ones and contributes to the definition of social, religious and national identities, but it also helps to create a moral order in opposition to the dangerous, divisive and contaminating other. The other, who operates according to a different social and moral code, is held to be responsible for anything abnormal, and, as in the case of the Jews, the other is also a reflection of oneself, a self who is deficient and even wicked, who is completely out of control and unable to restrain his violently sadistic impulses. The demonization of the other as a means of ethnic purification has played an important role in modern national movements, which stress ethnocentric differences in order to strengthen their communities against a common enemy.

The eighteenth-century Enlightenment went in a different direction.[20] It promoted a cosmopolitan outlook, recognition of the supremacy of the individual and tolerance towards other faiths, universal ideals, reliance on reason and a belief in the oneness of human nature. The Enlightenment proposed a rational alternative to fratricidal hatred, a hatred that had torn Europe apart in the religious wars of the seventeenth century. Most important of all, the French Enlightenment paved the way in Europe for the liberation of the Jews and Negroes, despite the prejudices of even the best of the intellectuals, and despite the problematic long-term consequences of the philosophical attack on the Judeo-Christian tradition. At the height of the Dreyfus Affair, there was a fateful struggle to preserve the rationalist legacy of the Enlightenment and the French Revolution. The supporters of that legacy withstood the attack of all the conservative forces in the country: the Church, the army, and a massive group of antisemites and nationalists. At the symbolic center of this confrontation stood Alfred Dreyfus. It was not only the antisemites who condemned Dreyfus but all those who saw the republic as a satanic power that undermined the traditional Christian character of the state. Wistrich concluded from the Affair that even in the most enlightened, cultured and modern European country, antisemitism could suddenly break out in force through a combination of the old Catholic demonization of the Jews and more recent social manifestations. The Catholic right accused the Jews, the Freemasons, the liberals and the socialists of orchestrating a demonic conspiracy against France via Dreyfus and his German masters.

There was a revival of the myth of the "omnipotent Jew," represented by the Rothschilds and international "Jewish" capital.[21] The medieval fantasies of the

Jew as the Antichrist, as the agent of the Devil and as a corrupter of values took a new form in which Dreyfus, the embodiment of Judas Iscariot, became a modern symbol of the accursed people. Although the Affair ended with the victory of Dreyfus and his supporters, the rule of law and the republican creed of human rights, it was nevertheless a basis for the rise of European fascism and the fabrication of forgeries like the "Protocols of the Elders of Zion" and ushered in totalitarian politics and Nazi-style antisemitism, as Hannah Arendt said. The tendency to associate the Jew and Jewry with the great forces of modernity – democracy, liberalism, world socialism, modernism in art, secularism, and so on had already appeared in France at the end of the nineteenth century. This tendency gathered force in the Weimar Republic and in all parts of European society after 1918. These developments were seen by Wistrich as a reaction to the growing and visible influence of Jewish emancipation and assimilation on the general crisis in European society after the First World War, as due to the fear aroused by the Bolshevik revolution and due to the rise of extreme antisemitic movements which promoted conspiracy theories. Some of these antisemitic movements were Christian, and all of them believed in the central role played by the Jews in Western culture.

National Socialism saw human history as a life-and-death struggle between Nordic Aryanism and the Jewish spirit. In the Nazi world-view, the otherness of the Jew was absolute, and – what was worse – an evil influence, for it had penetrated the very heart of German culture. This was an otherness that could not be contained and which appeared to retain an unchanging racial integrity. The Jew, who was seen as the bearer of evil in all its forms, was regarded by the Nazis as the embodiment of the forces of darkness. Regarded as superhuman and subhuman at the same time, the Jews and Judaism were viewed as bringers of death whose liquidation was a precondition for the redemption of mankind. This "redemptive antisemitism," as Saul Friedlander pointed out, was at the very heart of Hitler's program, and without it, the Holocaust could not have taken place.[22] The satanic Jew returned to life in Nazism as an apocalyptic internal threat to the existence of Germany, to the purity of the Aryan race and to dreams of *Lebensraum* (living space) and territorial expansion. His racial otherness was clearly reflected in the Nazi demonology and was exaggerated to such an extent that the Jew was totally excluded from the human race. The language of the Nazis was a pseudo-scientific jargon that used medical terminology from the sphere of hygiene and pest-control. And, indeed, the war against the Jewish devil was determined by the gas Zyklon B.

The imaginary power of the Jews, said Wistrich, continues to preoccupy antisemites throughout the world, whether on the left or right, whether religious fundamentalists or secularists, or whether they are in the West, the East, or the Third World.[23] From Russia and Eastern Europe to the Middle East and North and South America, the idea that the Jews seek to rule the world still has its proponents and believers. The idea that the Zionists and Jews "invented" the Holocaust became an important part of this post-war variation of the conspiracy theory. The State of Israel is given a demonic image as the very embodiment of evil. By means of motifs taken from classical antisemitism, Israel and Zionism are depicted as a kind of superpower devising mischief and using devious means to subjugate the Middle East and the whole world. Wistrich showed how the Jews and Zionists are constantly pinpointed and accused of being imperialists, racists, Nazis, expansionists engaged in endless persecution of the Arabs. They are said to manipulate and distort the Holocaust in order to whitewash their evil doings. In radical and fundamentalist circles in the Arab world and in Iran, Israel is usually seen in a conspiratorial light as a satanic power seeking to harm Islam. Especially among the followers of Islam, Israel and the Jews are regarded as agents of the "great Satan" America.

In this new fundamentalist thrust of Muslim self-assertion against Israel and the "infidel" West in which the Jew has become the demonic "other," Wistrich shows that there has been a paradoxical closing of a circle. Zionism sought to solve the Jewish problem in Europe by bringing the Jews back to their homeland, but in so doing it produced a Muslim strain of the same sickness, imported from Europe. European-style antisemitism was duly Islamized and decked out with tendentious quotations from Islamic sacred literature, but the Muslims also made use of classical Christian demonology with regard to the Jews. Thus, Arab and Muslim antisemitic propaganda makes medieval-type attacks on the Talmud and accusations of ritual murder, and depicts the Jews as pariahs and an accursed people – concepts traditionally alien to Muslim religion and culture. And, as if to make the paradox more pointed, the Muslim and Arab migrants to Europe to a greater or lesser degree are represented in a stereotypical way. They suffer increasing harassment, and their segregated and alien presence gives rise to xenophobic and racist reactions. To a certain extent, they – together with the Roma, foreign workers and colored immigrants – have taken the place of the Jews as the "other" which threatens multicultural Europe, a continent which has not yet rid itself of the genocidal and colonialist heritage of the past.

Antisemitism as a lethal obsession

In his book, *A Lethal Obsession*, Wistrich summed up his many years of studying antisemitism.[24] He placed before the reader the situation with regard to antisemitism in the world of the twenty-first century, beginning with a series of surveys made until the year 2009 which showed that there had been a rise in the level of antisemitism since the start of the millennium. He then presented a number of facts which disprove the idea that the antisemitism was caused by Israeli actions. He demonstrated that Israel had very little influence on how the European antisemites saw the Jews. Europeans view antisemitic events in a context that is anti-Jewish and not necessarily anti-Zionist. This was the starting point of his great project: to explain the historical sources of antisemitism, and at the same time to illustrate its activity in history. According to him, the international community sees Zionism through the eyes of antisemitism and not the opposite.

Wistrich found the historical roots of opposition to Zionism in the antisem-itism of Stalinist Russia, which inherited it from Nazi Germany after the Second World War. In this genealogy, nineteenth-century Europe (Western Europe and Czarist Russia) appears to have made a number of modern synthe-ses of classic Christian antisemitic themes to serve political purposes. Thus, for example, the writers of *The Protocols of the Elders of Zion*, who were czarist secret agents in France, intended it from the start as an apocalyptic anti-Jewish vision.

The turning-point in Russian antisemitism came after the communist revolu-tion. It went underground for a short time but continued to see beneath the surface of the Bolshevik regime. After the 1967 war, communist Russia saw Zionism as an enemy and began to persecute Jews systematically as part of its anti-Zionist foreign policy. The actions of the communist government were characterized by classical antisemitism internally and an alibi for antisemitism externally, the alibi being the State of Israel.

This combination of a sociological analysis of the twenty-first century Europeans and a genealogy of twentieth-century antisemitism helped Wistrich to reveal the antisemitism that still exists throughout Europe and which some-times assumes sophisticated forms in the academic world. Here one finds Stalinist anti-Zionist rhetoric and a more general "classical" antisemitism which had a great revival in Europe at the beginning of the twenty-first century. A Nazi-style antisemitism mobilized the Islamic organizations against "Zionism," and the European left used a rhetoric derived from the Stalinist foreign policy. In this rhetoric, the Israeli regime was said to resemble South African apartheid, the Israelis were accused of neo-colonialism, Israel was seen as an agent of American imperialism, and so on. The tendency to see the Jews as responsible for the situation – almost any situation – took on an old-new form in blaming Israel for all the problems of the Middle East.[25] The neo-Nazi movements in Europe find the Arabs of the Middle East, and especially the Palestinians, to be brethren in hostility to the Jews. Zionism has become the twin of the international Jewish conspiracy, and thus a suitable target for repeated assaults.

Wistrich demonstrated systematically that major Jewish figures in the polit-ical, intellectual and cultural life of Europe, from the Inquisition to the twentieth-century post-Zionist left, had similar characteristics. The Jew, who almost always experienced repression, internalized it. Assimilation did not in most cases efface the Jewish past of the assimilated person in the eyes of European society: as far as it was concerned, the Jew remained a Jew. An interesting example was the Austrian philosopher Otto Weininger, who committed suicide in 1903 when he understood that the Jews "live from the destruction of other peoples." Hitler called him "an honest Jew."

The common factor of the radical socialist tradition, from Marx's change of religion to the New Left of the 1960s, was hatred of Jewish particularism and its political institutionalization in Zionism. Wistrich saw the conscious universalism of these Jews as a massive attempt to rid themselves of their Jewish identity.[26]

There is no parallel to this phenomenon – a persistent disregard of one's origins in favor of universality – among other ethnic groups. The revolutionary Rosa Luxemburg, for example, replied to a letter from a friend in 1917, asking her opinion about the pogroms against the Jews taking place in Russia, as follows:

> Why do you come to me with this special Jewish suffering? I feel just as much concern for the Indian victims in Putumayo [a province in Columbia], the Negroes in Africa […]. I am unable to find a special place in my heart for the ghetto.[27]

Leon Trotsky, Rosa Luxemburg, Karl Radek and others always denied the exist-ence of a "special Jewish suffering." It seems as if the socialist Messiah could not come unless all oppressed groups in the world *except for the Jews* were lib-erated first, as if the communist Jews denied the needs of their people in order to prove their faithfulness to internationalism, as if describing the Zionist move-ment as "petty-bourgeois" would get rid of it. Wistrich saw this tradition as anticipating the post-Zionist outlook.

Wistrich's profound pessimism with regard to antisemitism stemmed from his historical analysis of the phenomenon: he could find no simple ethnological, psychological or sociological explanation for its scale and complexity.[28] The natural human tendency to hate foreigners does not explain the antisemitic hatred and its durability. He called it "the oldest hatred." Other prejudices generally did not stand the test of time: it always seemed that one could "rectify" people's opinions. Thus, for example, a phenomenon like legal slavery disappeared, as did various prejudices in the national, medical and even racial spheres. But only antisemitism continued to assert its presence in the twenty-first century, in the burning of synagogues, vandalism, violence against Jews. Wistrich pointed out that Christianity gave antisemitism a new dimension that did not exist in other hatreds: the mythical-gnostic dimension which permitted antisemites to see the Jew as the representative of evil on earth, with contra-dictory ideas of Jewish wickedness: e.g. the Jew was idle, the Jew was over-industrious, the Jew was rich and parasitic, the Jew was poor and parasitic, the universalist Jew, the Jew who only cares about himself. The gnostic dimension was also responsible for the Nazi concept of a war of the Aryan race against the Jewish race: a concept at the heart of the Nazi doctrine. From Hitler's point of view, the struggle against the Jews was a struggle of all against all, a struggle for survival.

Antisemitism has taken many forms: Hellenistic, Roman, medieval Christian, Spanish, and so on. What is special about antisemitism is not only its durability, although that is exceptional, but the capacity of the basic hatred of Jews to pass through so many metamorphoses without losing its vitality and energy. But, despite the metamorphoses of the antisemitic idea, it is by no means clear if all these manifestations that Wistrich called "antisemitism" can be placed under one heading. It seems that for him, antisemitism as a concept had an independent life, a life in history.

Old homeland, new antisemitism

In the new antisemitism, in Wistrich's opinion, unlike the one before the Holocaust and its counterpart in Eastern Europe which led to a national awakening, there is an attack on Jewish nationhood and on the right of the Jews in Israel to determine their future by themselves as an independent political entity. This right, the main principle of Zionism, is like a red rag to a bull for progressive liberal circles and leftist internationalists. For them, the abhorred State of Israel is the absolute negation of their vision of a general dissolution, of a world without frontiers, nations, religions or ethnic rivalries. In this respect, the new antisemitism is different from the classic antisemitism before the Holocaust which saw Jewry as an existential threat to internal homogeneity, to Christian values and to the "racial purity" of the nation. Mythical claims of this kind are no longer fashionable in the West, but now there are new libelous claims against the Jewish State. Present-day anti-Zionists see the State of Israel as a greater threat to the peace of the world and the world order than Iran or North Korea. In general surveys, Israel has taken first place among the states accused of endangering world peace.[29] Quite often, wrote Wistrich, one finds in the statements of contemporary Europeans unintentional echoes of fascist myths of the 1930s about "the Jews who are instigating war" and of communist slanders of the 1970s about the expansionist nature of Zionism. International sanctions and isolation are therefore regarded as steps that ought to be taken, not against theocratic Iran or the barbaric Syrian regime, but against little Israel, despite its adherence to the values of democracy, the rights of man and the rule of law.

Wistrich said that many liberals in the West refuse to recognize the depth of the penetration of antisemitism into Muslim political culture. Islamic Judeophobia has a long history which already began in the Koran, and which continued in the Hadith (sayings ascribed to Mohammed), in the Sunnah, and in the long tradition of discrimination against and oppression of *dhimmis* (protected Jews and Christians). Riots against the Jews took place in the Muslim world for generations, although they were generally less frequent and violent than those in Christian countries. The status of the Jews in Islam was nearly always a low one, although there were periods when there was a certain amount of tolerance, tranquility and prosperity. These were usually peak periods of culture like the golden age in medieval Spain or the great age of the Ottoman Empire. But, in the time that the State of Israel has existed, said Wistrich, the hatred of Jews has been more virulent and lethal in the Muslim world than anywhere else. Israel has had a special place as the object of hatred of the Muslim "nation" from 1948 onward, in addition to the basic hostility to Western imperialism, secularism and globalization. Islam's war against the Jew is regarded as a "holy war" against the present embodiment of Satan in the form of the Jews of America and Israel.

The Arab-Muslim world's failure to modernize is one of the explanations given by Wistrich for Islam's pathological attitude to Israel. For over 100 years, the Jews have served in Arab propaganda as a major symbol of the hated West, and are depicted as the supreme personification of its greed and exploitation and as its agent. At the same time, the West itself is often regarded as being under Jewish-Zionist control. This distorted stereotype of the "Jewish-Zionist" West, often seen in the form of "crusader America," is based on an earlier antisemitic legacy from the time of the development of the pan-Arab ideology. From the 1930s onward, Hitler was openly admired by the leaders of the pan-Arab national movement in Iraq, Syria and Palestine. They made an alliance with the Nazis, the main ideological common denominator of which was radical antisemitism and anti-British sentiment. The fingerprints of the Nazis can still be seen in the vocabulary of both pan-Arabism and Islamism. Many years after the defeat of Hitler, Israel is constantly described there as a "cancer." The same applies to the murderous rhetoric towards Israel from the 1950s onward of Arab leaders such as Gamal Abdel Nasser, Faisal, King of Saudia and Muammar Gadaffi, and it has continued up to the Hamas Covenant in 1988.[30]

Although Holocaust denial and antisemitic conspiratorial theories originated in the West, the lethal hatred of the Jews in the Arab media and the Arab street developed independently. Other motifs such as the idea of Jewish dominance in the world, are shared by the extreme right and left in the West and extreme Muslims in the Middle East. The confrontation between the Sunnis and Shiites and the Iranian nuclear threat dwarf the Israeli-Palestinian dispute, but it seems that this does not trouble the millions of Muslims who see the "hidden hand" of Israel as being behind the present chaos. From this radical analysis of the Jewish-Arab struggle over the fate of the Holy Land, Wistrich came to the conclusion that the dispute is insoluble.

In recent decades, there has been a coalescence between the "anti-imperialist" Zionophobia (hatred of Zionism) of the left and the pre-fascist Judeophobia (hatred of Jews) of the *jihad* movement. Wistrich said that both movements are outstandingly anti-Western, "anti-imperialist" and anti-Zionist, and openly or covertly antisemitic. Both of them see the State of Israel as a satanic outpost of the "imperialist conspiracy" and as lacking any legitimacy. He thought that it is doubtful if the radical left has ever made a critical examination of the artificial concept of a Palestinian nationality, whereas the 3,000-year-old history of the Jewish people is totally ignored by it.

Moledet – the destination of Zionism

The messianic link to Zion and the emotional fervor which it generated enabled the Jewish national movement to reawaken dormant energies in Jewish life, which it transferred from the religious to the sociopolitical sphere. But this transference necessarily involved a revolt against Jewish tradition if only because it took many of its ideals from liberal and progressive trends in the non-Jewish world. The secular messianism of marginal, assimilated Jewish intellectuals like Moses Hess, Bernard Lazare, and Theodor Herzl reflected their subjective consciousness of a "Jewish problem."

Nachman Syrkin, the first theoretician of labor Zionism, did not overlook the messianic implications of the new ideology for the Jewish people. "The messianic hope, which was always the greatest dream of exiled Jewry" would, he predicted, "be transformed into political action," by fusing socialism with Zionism in a Jewish state.[31] Ber Borochov, the leading theorist of Marxist Zionism, also saw the goal of a Jewish state essentially as a means to an end – in this case, to facilitate the class struggle of the Jewish proletariat.[32] Neither Syrkin nor Borochov, Wistrich pointed out, went to live in Palestine, unlike Aharon David Gordon, the secular mystic and patron saint of the early Palestinian Jewish labor movement. His "religion of labor," with its revolt against the parasitic economy of the ghetto, strongly influenced the settlers of the Second Aliyah. They shared his belief that only manual labor could create a Jewish national revival in Palestine, based on sacrifice, physical effort, and a life close to nature.

The pioneers of the Second Aliyah had carried the social-revolutionary ideas nurtured in their Russian environment into what was then a decaying backwater of the Ottoman Empire, where there was no industrial base, urban working class, or capitalist bourgeoisie. Everything had to be built from the beginning – the land, the people, the new society. Their opposition to the colonial pattern of exploitation exemplified by the philanthropic paternalism of the settlements run by agents of Baron Edmond de Rothschild is eloquent testimony to this social-revolutionary ethos of early Zionism.[33] They understood that the colonialist social norms which were crystallizing in the old yishuw would undermine their national ideal of regeneration.

The ideology of early Zionism never considered a total rejection of the old world.[34] Berl Katznelson, an outstanding trade union organizer and one of the most representative figures of the Palestinian Jewish labor movement, recognized that Zionism was a "revolt against servility within the revolution." The significance of the Zionist revolution, said Wistrich, did not lie so much in the birth of a new nation as a result of the heroic Israeli War of Independence as in its efforts to normalize the condition and status of the Jews as a people. This either-or attitude was also reflected in a different way in the Israel-centered Zionist rejection of the Diaspora. For a time it really seemed as if the gulf between Israeli and Jew would grow wider, that there was no common identity. Had this happened, Zionism would have succeeded in its most revolutionary aim – to become part of the general history of modern man by breaking out of what it regarded in purely negative terms as the powerless situation of the Galut Jew (Jews living in exile). In that case Zionism might well have produced a new nation of Hebrew-speaking Gentiles, a state in which Israelization (understood as a form of collective assimilation) would inevitably undermine the Jewish heritage. I will return later to this risk of Hebraization or Canaanization of the Jewish state, but another danger lay at the door.

The Zionist movement from its inception regarded assimilation as one of its central enemies, as a morally degrading position for any self-respecting Jew to adopt.[35] Like other national movements, it tended to decry assimilation as an expression of weakness of character rather than to perceive it as a historic process with its own logic and momentum. Thus Zionists all too easily over-dramatized the "spiritual slavery" of the assimilationists. They produced a mythical image of Western Jewry in particular that bore little relation to the realities of Jewish existence in the more open, pluralistic societies of the West. "Assimilationists" found themselves branded as self-hating Jews or traitors to their people even when they were no longer religious, had little knowledge or connection with Jewish tradition, and their self-definition as part of the Jewish people made little sense in the general context of liberal, nineteenth-century European society. It was, moreover, frequently forgotten by Zionist critics of assimilation that without emancipation and exposure to the values of European culture the revival of national consciousness among Jews might never have taken place. The classical Zionist analysis also ignored the fact that much of what it called assimilation was in reality acculturation – the adoption of the cultural values of the general society by a minority group.

Writing in 1906, the president of the Jewish Theological Seminary in America and one of the founders of Conservative Judaism, Solomon Schechter, declared, for example, that Zionism in his eyes was the great bulwark against assimilation.[36] Assimilation meant to him, as it did to most Zionists at the turn of the century, a loss of identity, a process of self-dissolution. The struggle against assimilation was undoubtedly a central myth in the emergence of Zionism and has continued to be one of its major preoccupations. Already in *Rome and Jerusalem*, the work of a German Communist who had once shared Marx's views on Jews and Judaism, the pattern is clear. Self-negation is not only morally distasteful, but it will not work. This was, of course, Moses Hess, the first assimilated Jew to turn to Zionism, who wrote, "every Jew is, whether he wishes it or not, bound unbreakably to the entire nation."[37] Peretz Smolenskin, the Russian-Jewish nationalist, writing at the end of the 1870s, also believed in this unbreakable bond and was equally scathing about efforts by the Berlin Haskalah and the German-Jewish Reform to denationalize Jewry.[38] The young Nathan Birnbaum, founder of Zionism in the Austrian Empire, described the "mania of assimilation" as "national suicide."

None of these early Zionist thinkers made, according to Wistrich, a clear-cut distinction between what is generally regarded today as acculturation (i.e. the adoption by Jews of external characteristics of the majority culture such as language, dress, manners, etc.) and assimilation – understood as embracing the national identity of the dominant majority group. They considered assimilation as a vain attempt to bring Jewish history to an end. By desiring the complete abandonment of Jewish identity, the "assimilationists" were betraying the assumed core value of Jewish history – the imperative of group survival. Zionism, as A.D. Gordon declared, was the answer to this assimilation: only in the Israeli homeland, the *Moledet*, planted in the natural soil and drawing on vital sources from the past, could this ethnic self-escape from the constrictions and the sterility of the Galut happen.[39] The vital force of Jewish national creativity would only reassert itself through renewed contact with the land and through physical labor, enabling a regenerated Jewish people to eventually arise.

All the leading Zionist thinkers vigorously opposed assimilation, just as they negated the *Galut* as a source of spiritual, material, and political dependence. Insofar as Zionism defined itself as a Jewish national renaissance, as a movement of auto-emancipation, a revolutionary transformation of the Jewish destiny, and as a return to the *Moledet*, it was virtually obliged to adopt such an uncompromising stance. Zionism was met with hostility not only from the assimilationist movement, the internal threat, but it also faced hostility and hatred from outside. The widespread libel that Zionism is a "racist" ideology sounds, indeed, like a modern version of original sin. It taints those who support a Jewish homeland in Israel with the stigma of "crimes against humanity." In the view of many of those condemning Zionism, colonialist Jews from Europe brutally displaced a native Palestinian population, supposedly basing themselves on a racist outlook imported from the West. The desire of Israel to be a "Jewish" state is seen as essentially racist, because the Jewish people are viewed as a religious group rather than as a nation. In practical terms, the Law of Return is attacked as being particularly "racist," since it grants Jews from the Diaspora the rights of Israeli citizenship denied to exiled Palestinians.

In striking contrast to the prevailing myths, Zionism showed remarkable indifference to race as a factor in shaping the character and ethos of Israeli society. In contrast to white colonizing societies like South Africa, Australia, the United States, or Rhodesia in the past, color was never of importance in Israel as an indicator of social status. Nor was there any need to use "race" as a legitimizing ideology to exploit native Arab labor. As for the future, Wistrich explains, negotiations will determine the political solution, not discrimination or terror. Unlike the South Africans and white Rhodesians under apartheid or the French colons in Algeria, Israelis since 1948 have been a majority, not a minority, in their own state.

Any analysis of Zionist ideology, Wistrich claimed, will quickly reveal that there is no racism in its mainstream. From Herzl to Jabotinsky, from Weizmann to Ben-Gurion and Berl Kaznelson, there is virtually no hint of racial superiority, no desire to dominate or enslave other peoples, no recourse to mythical-biological explanations of history, society, or culture. As one of the last of the national-liberation movements to emerge in late nineteenth-century Europe, mainstream Zionism combined the humanist and universalist patriotism of the French Revolution with the messianic Jewish tradition of a return to Zion. Unlike most national movements, which arose among people already living in their own land, Zionism was in its origins a movement in search of a territory. It had to resolve a unique problem, the homelessness of the Jewish people, an extraterritorial minority which had lost its sovereignty over Palestine nearly 1,900 years earlier and lacked any independent structure of political authority. The disastrous plight of the Jews in Russia and Eastern Europe in the last quarter of the nineteenth century – an almost defenseless population reeling from pogroms and discrimination – created an increasingly acute "Jewish problem," which required a political solution. In absorbing Jews from the Arab world, the Soviet Union, Eastern Europe, and many other countries, Israel was able to fulfill one of the main goals for which it was established. This was made possible, according to Wistrich, by the Law of Return, which has counterparts around the world from Germany to Greece and Armenia. The Israeli Law of Return provided a secure haven for the Jewish victims of Nazi persecution and other forms of oppression.[40] The Jew who returns to Israel and acquires citizenship is exercising a natural human right to choose his or her destiny, without being under compulsion or being condemned, like his forefathers, to wander as a stranger from one exile to another.

The typical *halutzim* were young middle-class Jews who in going to Palestine turned their backs both on the Diaspora and on bourgeois society.[41] They were seeking personal and communal redemption by becoming workers or peasants. This was closer to the ideals espoused by the Russian writer Leo Tolstoy than to the notions of Western colonialists. Of course, not all Zionists shared this utopian socialist vision. Nevertheless, a common denominator of Zionist ideology was the need to create a healthy economic and political structure for the regeneration of the Jewish people in Palestine.

Wistrich, in *Myth and Memory* and *The Shaping of Israeli Identity* discussed the post-Zionist climate, a debate which is no less about history per se.[42] The focus was not, however, on the Jewish-Arab conflict, but was concentrated much more on those internal Jewish factors which have shaped the Israeli collective consciousness and national-cultural identity in the past 100 years, in all their pluralism, ambivalence, and contradictions. Naturally, these myths, memories, and traumas that have shaped the Israeli identity did not develop in a vacuum nor as the pure product of internal developments within twentieth-century Jewish history.

Even without the devastating blow of the Holocaust and the conflict with the Arab-Muslim world that confronted the new Israeli state, the challenge of constructing a viable Israel would have been formidable. To convert an urban-based diasporic people whose cohesion had already been significantly eroded by cultural assimilation into a "normal" nation rooted in its own land and the Hebrew language was a huge task even under the most optimal set of circumstances. The ideological synthesis of socialist Zionism and the driving myths that shaped Israeli society in its early years reflected many of these imperatives, constraints, and challenges. The emphasis on mamlakhtiut (statism), on national security, rootedness, and the pioneering ethos, as well as the priority attached to a "melting pot" ideology, seemed appropriate to the immediate imperatives of survival under adverse conditions. Similarly, the "heroic" Spartan ethos, so decried by current fashion, was in many respects a functional necessity for a country poor in natural resources, surrounded by enemies, and dependent on a high level of motivation, collective willpower, and an implacable determination to reroot itself in the land. The dominant myths underwent a subtle shift after 1967 as territorial expansion and rule over a large Palestinian population created a new set of problems and dilemmas. The future of the occupied territories, questions of borders and ultimate national goals, the globalizing of the Arab-Israeli conflict, and a changed relation with the Diaspora became contentious and central issues in Israeli politics.

Israeli society was becoming increasingly westernized – more materialistic, individualist, and consumer-orientated. In this de-ideologized Zionism, there was far greater scope for a plurality of identities, for recognizing the validity of the private realm and the needs of the individual. A flourishing Hebrew-language culture and literary experimentation encouraged a new freedom in addressing time-honored ideals and deflating established myths. The era of grand ideological syntheses appeared to be over, and increasingly calls for "normalization" could be heard that reflected a palpable war-weariness and a longing for "peace now." The Palestinian question could no longer be swept under the carpet and increasingly impinged on the Israeli collective psyche as a problem that directly affected the identity of the Israeli people and its state.

The image of the Holocaust as the nadir of Jewish powerlessness in *Galut* (exile) and the stigma attached to it gave way to an increasingly strong symbolic identification with this traumatic memory. The traditional Zionist contrast between tough, resourceful Israelis who make their own history and the passive Diaspora Jews who went like "lambs to the slaughter" has been steadily muted. There is much less need today to dramatize the rupture with the diasporic past, to create a countermodel to the exilic Jew. In its place has come a more realistic and humane approach to suffering, less eagerness to embrace death in the heroic mold, and a much greater interest of Israelis in their own personal and collective roots, which lie after all in Diaspora traditions.

The 2,000 years of Jewish exile in the Diaspora are no longer perceived as a potential threat to the viability of Israeli statehood, but as an integral part of Israel's past, to be integrated into its contemporary history. An Israeli identity, divorced from its Jewish sources, therefore seems increasingly unlikely despite the tension that still exists between the Zionist aspiration and the reality of the Diaspora. Such tensions and difficulties are probably inevitable in the building of a sovereign society and in their own way are the imperfect outcome of the very successes of Zionism in accomplishing many of its original aims. On the eve of the Holocaust, the Jews of Palestine represented a mere 3 percent of world Jewry. Currently, the Jews in Israel are over half of world Jewry.

Wistrich mentions in his writings the Canaanite group. The Canaanites were Israelis in the 1950s who called for separation between Israelis and Jews. They wanted a healthy, vigorous, non-religious culture based on "Hebrew" identity and severed from foreign Diaspora roots. They denied any common ground between Israel and the Diaspora Jews. But the Canaanites were not only a tiny group that appeared on the stage of Israeli history but a narrative and ideology that continues to accompany the Israeli identity. The Israelis, according to the Canaanite narrative, are from this place and belong only here; but according to the crusader narrative, the Israelis are from another place and belong there.[43] On the one hand, the mythological construction of Zionism as a modern crusade describes Israel as a Western colonial enterprise planted in the heart of the East and alien to the area, its logic, and its peoples, whose end must be degeneration and defeat. On the other hand, the construction of the State of Israel as neo-Canaanism, which defines the nation in purely geographical terms as an imagined native community, demands breaking away from the chain of historical continuity. Those are the two greatest anxieties that Zionism and Israel has had to encounter and answer forcefully.

The historian as an intellectual

To use Max Weber's expression, Robert Wistrich was an "ideal type" of the historian as intellectual and the intellectual as historian. This symbiosis was prominent in both his academic work and in his public and private life. His eminence as an historian of international renown who researched the Zionist movement from the end of the nineteenth century was due to his passion for defending the Jewish people and the State of Israel, which had always been subject to opposition and hostility. His stature as an intellectual derived from his historical knowledge shown in the more-than thirty books he wrote and edited and the more than 400 articles he published in academic journals, reflecting his mastery of eleven languages.[44]

But an historian-intellectual like Wistrich could not have gained his international reputation, his academic achievements, and the across-the-board recognition of his contribution to scholarship without his particular biography, which in many respects is a case study of the possible horizons of Zionism. Because he was not born in Israel, the existence of the *Moledet* was not self-evident to him, and he therefore made himself the best-known representative in the world of the fight against antisemitism.

Wistrich claimed that since 1975, with the passing of the United Nations resolution condemning Zionism as racism, the hatred of Israel mutated into the chief vector for the "new" antisemitism. By describing the Jewish state as a "racist," "Nazi" and "apartheid" entity based on ethnic cleansing, its enemies made Zionism synonymous with criminality. Thus, any Jew (or non-Jew who supports the illegitimate and immoral "Zionist entity" becomes an accomplice to an evil on a cosmic scale. In Wistrich's opinion, today's antisemitism is the product of a new civil religion which could be termed "Palestinianism." The official Palestinian narrative seeks to replace the Israeli homeland with a *judenrein* Palestine from the Mediterranean Sea to the River Jordan. In the case of "Hamas," this is stated explicitly and clearly, and in the case of "fatah," the intention is masked for technical reasons. Moreover, the millions throughout the world who are activated by the Palestinian ideology or who support it immediately label every act of self-defense by Israel as "genocidal." Self-defense by Israel is demonized and is seen as part of a wicked Jewish imperialist conspiracy. Thus, one is surprised at the number of pro-Palestinian demonstrations, usually accompanied by antisemitic incidents and by cries of "Death to the Jews!" From the beginning of the twenty-first century, said Wistrich, antisemitism has undergone a process of increasing "Islamization" linked to a holy war against Jews and other non-Muslims.[45]

In his last article, Wistrich asked the Jews of Israel and the Diaspora to reassess their Jewish identity, their Jewish values and their connection to the Land of Israel and their historic heritage.[46] In words in the spirit of the Jewish prophets, which inevitably came to be regarded as his last will and testament, he wrote:

> [...] Let us be worthy of the scriptural promise that "the Torah will come forth from Zion and the word of the Lord from Jerusalem." Here, in the beating heart of the Jewish nation, where its body and soul come together in the City of Peace, we must be true to the national and universal vision of our biblical prophets. Antisemitism, the long shadow of which has for so long accompanied our bi-millennial Diasporic tribulations, and nearly seventy years of renewed statehood, is neither "eternal" nor must it prevent Jews from fulfilling their ultimate destiny to one day become a "light unto the nations".

Wistrich ended his life as an envoy defending the Jewish people. He died of a heart-attack in Rome on the eve of a speech he was to give in the Italian senate. In the speech, he intended to warn of the rising antisemitism in Europe. The Israeli historian wanted to use a quotation from Martin Buber "The past of his people is his personal memory" in connection with his personal experience as the son of Polish-Jewish refugees who fled from the Nazi terror and were exiled in Russia. The history of the members of his family after the Holocaust – returning to Poland in 1946 and then moving to France as penniless refugees, and then England, where young Robert grew up and was educated – left its mark on him, and its influence is seen throughout his academic career. He often did this with an over-emphasis and exaggeration which perhaps were due to the comprehensible fears of a Jew who passed his early life outside his own *Moledet*.

The authoress and essayist Jacqueline Kahanoff also thought, like Wistrich, that Zionism had succeeded in its aim of establishing a homeland for the Jews, but she shifted the emphasis from the "negative" definition of it as a refuge from antisemitism to a "positive" Levantine ethos which she reflected in her essays. The Levantine ethos she proposed was a spatial one: its narrow spatial meaning as the eastern Mediterranean, the meeting-place of east and west, was expanded by her into a model of multi-locality. This ethos included people like the Franco-Algerian writers Albert Camus and Albert Memmi, French poets like Edmond Jabès and Charles Péguy, the Anglo-Indian writer V.S. Napaul and African and Japanese writers. Kahanoff thought that making her Moledet beyond her Levantine identity would broaden the provincial national model into a universal model of multi-locality and meeting of cultures.

Notes

1 On the 1st of November 1895, Theodor Herzl wrote in his diary about his visit to the home of Israel Zangwill in London:

[…] He, too, is in favor of our territorial independence. However, his point of view is a racial one – something I cannot accept if I so much as look at him and myself. All I am saying is, we are a historical unit, a nation of anthropological diversity. That is sufficient for a Jewish state. No nation has uniformity of race.

Herzl Theodor, *The Complete Diaries of Theodor Herzl*, vol. 1, ed. Raphael Patai, trans. Harry Zohn, New York 1960, 276–277

2 Robert S. Wistrich, "Antisemitism and the Origins of Zionism," *Between Redemption and Perdition – Modern Antisemitism Jewish Identity*, London 1990.

3 Ronald W. Clark, *Einstein: The Life and Times*, Bloomsbury, New York 1971, 393.

4 Robert S. Wistrich, "From Cracow to London – A Polish-Jewish Odyssey," in: ed., Slawomir Kapralski, *The Jews in Poland*, Vol. 2, *Judaica Foundation Center for Jewish Culture*, Cracow 1999, 57–73.

5 Robert S. Wistrich, "Zionism: Revolt against Historic Destiny," *The Jewish Quarterly*, 25:2 (1977): 6–12.

6 Robert S. Wistrich, *Between Redemption and Perdition – Modern Antisemitism Jewish Identity*.

7 Ibid.

8 Robert S. Wistrich, *Who's Who in Nazi Germany*, Routledge, London 1982.

9 Robert S. Wistrich, *The Jews of Vienna in the Age of Franz Joseph*, Oxford 1989.

10 Robert S. Wistrich, "Bernard Lazare, l'affaire Dreyfus et l'antisemitisme," *Cahiers Bernard Lazare* (July/August 2007): 23–26.

11 Robert S. Wistrich, "Karl Kraus – Jewish Prophet or Renegade?," *European Judaism*, 9:2 (Summer 1975): 32–39.

12 Robert S. Wistrich, "Max Nordau – From Degeneration to 'Muscular Judaism'," *Transversal*, 2 (2004): 3–21.

13 Wistrich, *The Jews of Vienna*, 349–350, 355–359, 464–466.

14 Carl Schorske, *Fin-de-siecle Vienna – Politics and Culture*, Random House, London 1980, 120.

15 Wistrich, *The Jews of Vienna*, 537–582; Robert S. Wistrich, "The Last Testament of Sigmund Freud," *Leo Baeck Yearbook XLIX*, 2004, 3–21.

16 Wistrich, *The Jews of Vienna*, 538.

17 Ibid., 188–189, 305–309, 370–375, 421–460.

18 Wistrich, "The European Demons the First World War Awake from their Slumber," http://mida.org.il/2014/03/06 taken: 2017.

19 Robert S. Wistrich (co-ed. Walter Laqueur and George L. Mosse), *Theories of Fascism*, London 1976, 284; Wistrich, *Who's Who in Nazi Germany*; Robert S. Wistrich, *Hitler's Apocalypse – Jews and the Nazi Legacy*, London 1985, 309; Wistrich, *Weekend in Munich – Art, Propaganda and Terror in the Third Reich*, London 1995, 176.

20 Shulamit Volkov, "Exploring the Other: The Enlightenment's Search for the Boundaries of Humanity," ed. Robert Wistrich, *Demonizing the Other – Antisemitism, Racism and Xenophobia*, Routledge, London and New York 1999, 148–167.

21 Robert S. Wistrich, *A Lethal Obsession – Anti-semitism from Antiquity to the Global Jihad*, Random House, New York 2010, 107–128.

22 Saul Friedlander, *Nazi Germany and the Jews, 1933–1945*, New York 2009; Robert S. Wistrich, *Laboratory for World Destruction – Germans and Jews in Central Europe*, University of Nebraska Press, Nebraska 2007.

23 Robert Wistrich, *Demonizing the Other – Antisemitism, Racism and Xenophobia*, Routledge, London and New York 1999, 148–167.

24 Wistrich, *A Lethal Obsession*.

25 Ibid., 684–928.

26 Wistrich, *Socialism and the Jews – The Dilemmas of Assimilation in Germany and Austria-Hungary*, London 1982, 435.

27 Ibid.

28 Wistrich, *A Lethal Obsession*, 929–938.

29 Ibid., 494–514.

30 Ibid., 780–829.

31 Wistrich, "Zionism: Revolt against Historic Destiny," 6; Marie Syrkin, ed., *Nachman Syrkin: Socialist Zionist*, Herzl Press, New York 1961.

32 Wistrich, ibid., 8; Ber Borochov, *Selected Works of Ber Borochov*, CreateSpace 2011.

33 Wistrich, *A Lethal Obsession*, 110–112.

34 Dimitry Shumsky, *Beyond the Nation-State*, Yale University Press, New Haven 2018.

35 Ran Aharonsohn, *Rothschild and Early Jewish Colonization in Palestine*, Rowman & Littlefield, Lanham 2000.

36 Cyrus Adler, *Solomon Schechter: A Biographical Sketch*, Andesite Press, London 2017.

37 Shlomo Avineri, *Moses Hess: Prophet of Communism and Zionism*, New York University Press, New York 1987.

38 Charles H. Freundlich, *Peretz Smolenskin: His Life and Thought*, Bloch Publishing, New York 1965.

39 Frances Burnce, ed. and trans., *A. D. Gordon Selected Essays*, Tel Aviv 1938.

40 Wistrich, *A Lethal Obsession*, 522–540; Na'ama Carmi, "The Nationality and Entry into Israel Case before the Supreme Court of Israel," *Israel Studies Forum*, 22:1 (Summer 2007): 26–53.

41 Boaz Neumann, *Land and Desire in Early Zionism*, trans. Haim Watzman, University Press, Waltham, MA 2011.

42 Robert S. Wistrich and David Ohana, eds., *The Shaping of Israeli Identity*, Frank Cass, London 1995; David Ohana and Wistrich, eds., *Myth and Memory*, Tel Aviv 2005 (in Hebrew).

43 David Ohana, *The Origins of Israeli Mythology: Neither Canaanites nor Crusaders*, Cambridge University Press, Cambridge MA 2012.

44 Michael Berkowitz, "Robert S. Wistrich and European Jewish History: Straddling the Public and Scholarly Spheres," *The Journal of Modern History*, Vol. 70 (March 1998): 119–136.

45 Wistrich, *A Lethal Obsession*, 731–789.

46 Wistrich, "Antisemitism and Jewish Destiny," *The Jerusalem Post*, May 20, 2015.

5   A Levantine Moledet

Marcel Proust's book *À la recherche du temps perdu* was of course the inspiration for the title of this chapter, but whereas the French writer investigated the mirages of time, the Egyptian-born Israeli writer and essayist Jacqueline (Shochet) Kahanoff (1917–1979) went off in search of the realms of place. The place in question was the Levant, which in her life and works was the object of nostalgia, a utopian land of heart's desire, the object of social criticism and a metaphor for the home where, after her physical and spiritual exile, she would finally find peace. In the Levant she hoped to close the imaginary circle which began in Cairo and ended in Tel Aviv on the shores of the Mediterranean. The Levant, under Kahanoff's unique outlook, encompasses a rich civilization, human interactions and diverse geo-cultural locations, a dialogue between the East and the West – far surpasses the narrow confines of the familiar geographical Levant.

A hundred years after the birth of Kahanoff has finally gained the recognition she deserves as an intellectual figure of the first rank in Israel and even overseas. Three collections of her essays are now available: *From East the Sun* (1978),[1] her classic work which appeared a year before her death through the good offices of Aharon Amir, the editor and friend who gathered together her essays published in *Keshet; Between Two Worlds* (2005), which revealed her to a younger generation of readers;[2] and *Mongrels and Morals* (2011), a selection of her essays written in English, published by Stanford University.[3] *Jacob's Ladder*, the only novel she wrote, has appeared in Hebrew sixty-four years after it was first published in English.[4] There are university courses on Kahanoff's works, her articles are included in the curricula of schools, in Israel there is a school and a street named after her, radio programmers about Kahanoff's life and work became frequent, a film as part of the documentary series, "The Hebrews,"[5] and an exhibition dedicated to her in the Eretz Israel Museum in Tel Aviv.[6] All these give her place as a writer and essayist who was before her time, the princess of the Levant and the herald of the Mediterranean culture in Israel.[7] A photomontage of Y.H. Brenner, a pioneer of the modern Hebrew literature, and Kahanoff adorning the covers of a series of books about the secularization of the Jewish culture published by the Open University adds an interesting secular interpretation to the embrace of the "Canaanites," the Orientals, the feminists, and the Mediterraneanists: ideologies and movements that clasp her warmly – too warmly – to their bosom.[8] Today it seems that Kahanoff is being acknowledged as a unique Jewish writer who gave a good name to Levantine culture and to her kind of literary essay.

The essays, for which she is best known, are a form of in-depth personal theoretical writing based on an original vision, a genre that has played a decisive role in the history of Hebrew literature from Berdichevsky and Ahad Ha-Am to Amos Oz, and that is now dying out with the disappearance of the literary article. From the end of the 1950s to the 1970s, Kahanoff stood out with a series of essays which revealed the Levantine world to the Israeli-natives, who were unfamiliar with Cairo, Alexandria, Beirut or Istanbul. The subjects of her essays were infinitely varied: Levantism as a concept and as a cultural theory, the status of women, the geographical periphery of the land of Israel, the dialogue between Paris and Tel Aviv, the thought of writers and cultural critics such as Emmanuel Levinas, Claude Vigée, Charles Péguy and Edmond Jabès, to name only a few. She also introduced the readers to aspects of world culture such as the new African literature, poetry from Madagascar, Japanese literature, and so on.

Two sisters from the Levant

In 1963 Kahanoff's name was already known to many people through her writings in Amir's journal *Keshet* and Shlomo Grodzinsky's *Amot*, and the newspapers *Al Ha-Mishmar*, *Davar*, *Maariv*, *Jerusalem Post*, *Yediiot Aharonot*, *Be-Mahanei* and *Haaretz*. Her first essays, written in English, were published in general and Jewish journals in the United States and France. For her livelihood she worked as a freelancer in the *Wizo-Hadassah* journal.[9] It is an interesting fact that already then Kahanoff was an intellectual challenge and source of inspiration for Dahlia Ravikovitch, the Israeli among the women-poets of that time. On May 12 of that year, Ravikovitch wrote a letter to Kahanoff which is published here for the first time:[10]

Rehov Aziel 12,
Ramat Hen,
12.5.63

Dear Mrs. Kahanoff,

Three years ago, when I first read your article, "The Levantine Generation", I intended to write to you, but because I was three years younger than I am now, I was also more shy.

This time – simply – after I read your "French Diary published in *Keshet* 18, I had a clearer idea of what I wanted to write to you.

In all your articles, from "The Levantine Generation" to your latest articles in *Amot* and *Keshet*, there is a basic quality which gives rise to admiration and envy: you are able to write about painful and essential matters without the tempestuousness and bitterness with which people generally write about them. This subdued approach is the correct historical perspective, and because you already have it, you do not know how difficult it is to attain.

Moreover, and perhaps for that very reason, you have a good balance between abstract ideas and concrete details. I have specified the qualities you possess not because you need my appraisal, but because I have a particular interest in them.

You write, among other things, that this country is twenty years behind Europe, and you describe this backwardness not only as a cultural backwardness but a backwardness also connected with the way of life, the outlook and ideas, and tensions in society.

Because I was born in this country and have not been out of it so far, with the exception of one year, this fact has a painful and insulting significance for me. This fact is something irreparable because I have no doubt that the main deficiencies of cultural life in this country also necessarily apply to me. Like all provincials, I too lack a proper sense of proportion in assessing things, and I even find it hard to relate to ills like ethnic or national deprivation as I should. I either exaggerate the evil or I ignore it for a long period.

The matter you described in your last article – the matter of the new way of life in France with a modern but almost anti-revolutionary approach – made a very deep impression on me. I would like to hear more about it, and I would like to hear from you many things about matters with which I am not familiar.

You should realize that every Tuesday I go to Jerusalem to complete my B.A. Owing to the material of my studies and the lively discussions in the classes and the slight excitement of the journey I sometimes refresh my way of thinking, but on the other days of the week I read newspapers and talk about the things that everyone else talks about.

If my Hebrew is too difficult I am ready to translate my letter into English, in which case it will be shorter and there will also be a few mistakes.

I would be grateful if you would answer me in any way whatsoever. My telephone number is 35587 and I live in Ramat Hen, so the geographical distance between us is not great.

Thanking you in anticipation,
Dahlia Ravikovitch

Where did Kahanoff and Ravikovitch stand at the time in which the letter was written? The twenty-seven-year-old Ravikovitch was in a period of intense spiritual awakening. Four years earlier, her first book of poetry, *Ahavat tapuah ha-zahav* (The Love of an Orange) (1959), had been warmly received in the literary world. One critic wrote that the book "We are witnessing a great and a true talent."[11] There were many reasons for her success and they place her at a point of intersection between the generations, a dovetailing of new poetic principles with a certain conservatism and a quasi-biblical language. Ravikovitch humbly acknowledged: "Perhaps the book was sympathetically received because I am less modernistic than other poets and I did not annoy anyone."[12] She received the approval of the doyen of poetesses, Leah Goldberg, and some critics even thought that they not only had a hierarchical relationship, but there was even an affinity between them.[13] As she had not yet obtained her university degree, in 1963 she still traveled to Jerusalem once a week to take part in the courses.

> In the year in which Ravikovitch's letter was written, Kahanoff was already known to the readers of *Keshet*, particularly for the series of articles "The Generation of Levantine" published in the same year as *The Love of an Orange*. In October 1962, Kahanoff was introduced to the readers of *Amot* for the first time through her travel-essay "Wake of the Waves" in which she opened a window on the Mediterranean: This is my first trip abroad after living in Israel for seven years. The Mediterranean Sea, which is much bluer than I remember, whips up foam – a dense white foam that thins out, disperses, and disappears. I have often been on voyages like this, watching the ship's greenish wake as it dissolves, amazed again and again by the way these expeditions of ours leave nothing behind them, even the memory of them erased, unless something happens, a tremor that sends bubbles rising to the surface of our minds. How strange it is that we wander over this cast expanse until one day we reach some shore, some place, which carries back to me, like the spray of sand or water, scenes of our life together, and now we know that everything we have assembled scatter like a wave, and soon our fragments will be cast up at random. I try to find some shape in those scatterings, like the fortune-teller on the beach in Alexandria many years ago, who with her henna-strained hands would toss shells onto the sand to read our future and would say, as we children listened in rapt attention: 'Long journey… sorrow… good luck…love…' And indeed, who among us did not know all of these?[14]

In her Mediterranean article she recalled the year 1937, when she received in Cairo the invitation of the family of her good friend Sylvie to take part in her first visit to Palestine. The train journey took a whole night, and she woke up to the intoxicating scent of orange-blossom: "The people working in the groves waved and called 'shalom', and my heart lifted at the thought that this was the fruit of Jewish labor, and this was the fragrance of Palestine."[15] She forgot the names of the kibbutzim, but she noticed the cleanliness and order of the Jewish villages as compared to the dirt and neglect of the Arab villages. In place of the Arab cactus there was the Jewish eucalyptus, in place of apathy there was energy and initiative. She was sad when she heard people speak of the British colonialist attitude of the native-born, but she nevertheless admired their spirit of socialism and equality. The colonialist reality in Egypt left its mark on her: "They were unable to decide in what category to place the Zionists: whites, native-born, Jews. They were surprised that the Jews in Palestine did not feel any affinity with the Arabs, their brothers of the Semitic race." It was strange, she thought, that the Zionists disregarded their common origin. Jacqueline and Sylvie, pampered children of the Cairo Jewish aristocracy, never ceased to wonder at the pioneering spirit of the Sabras (Israeli-natives), who seemed to them at the same time "reactionary" in their attitude to people.

Post-colonialist ideological thinkers like Edward Said or Homi Babha do not help in understanding the colonialist naivety exhibited by Kahanoff.[16] Inner tensions and contradictions in her developing identity affected her literary image and her life as an adult. Thus, for example, she was surprised at the short skirts of the Arab girls in the West Bank immediately after the Israeli conquest in 1967.[17] Thirty years earlier, she had witnessed the arrogance of the guides who had shown them their kibbutzim. They were unable to let their achievements speak for themselves: their sense of superiority was expressed in the comparisons they made with other peoples. Sylvie said that the Sabras suffered from some kind of distorted vision and short-sightedness, and they lectured all the time about learning the Hebrew language: "They all say exactly the same things. It's so boring!"[18]

Later, Kahanoff said that she did not trouble to explain to Sylvie that there was no reason why people from Eastern Europe needed to know the French language, but it was natural that they would want to revive the Hebrew language. She had a good understanding of the political theology underlying Hebraism: "For them it's like the Gospel, the commandment of spreading the good news. They believe it's forbidden to miss any opportunity."[19] This early sense of perspective which testifies to the clear-sightedness of this twenty-year-old girl from Cairo, in 1941 brought her to San Francisco, Chicago and New York rather than to the kibbutzim of the Hashomer Hatzair (a socialist-Zionist youth movement). The eleven years she spent in the United States gave rise to the literary novel *Jacob's Ladder*.[20] In New York she made friends with French intellectuals such as Raymond Aron and Claude Vigée, and with the anthropologist Claude Lévi-Strauss, with whom she had an affair which influenced her in terms of her intellectual statue until the day she died. After studies at Columbia University in New York and three years in Paris, in 1954 she put her wanderings behind her and made her place of residence in Israel. About a decade later, the paths of the essayist from Cairo and the young Sabra poetess, twenty years younger than herself, crossed: Ravikovitch, in the company of her husband Yitzhak Livni, finally met Kahanoff. We have no details about this meeting, but there is evidence that it took place. Eva Weintraub, a good friend of Kahanoff's, who at that time was working as a librarian in the American Cultural Center in Tel Aviv, remembers it distinctly. One can only regret that no account remains of the meeting of these two key figures of Hebrew culture.

With regard to the fascinating subject of "Ravikovitch and Israelism," the young poetess was exposed to the intense three-cornered relationship between Gershom Scholem, Baruch Kurzweil and Yonatan Ratosh. Each of these spiritual giants proposed his own orientation to Israeli society as it started out. In

Gideon Tikotsky's groundbreaking work *Dahlia Ravikovitch in Life and Literature* (2016) Ravikovitch in the three years she lived in Jerusalem was described as someone drawn to intellectual worlds and influential guides. Before she published her first book, *The Love of an Orange*, in 1959, she had published poems in *Orlogin*, *Achshav* and *Haaretz*. In addition to the poems that had been published until then, she had written about 100 more. The book *Dahlia Ravikovitch: the Poems and Archives*, a collection of rich and mature poems, came out at that period.[21]

An interesting and in our opinion important glimpse of the influence of Scholem's outlook on Ravikovitch – an outlook in which there is an affinity between kabbala and Zionism – is provided by two of Ravikovitch's poems of that period. Her brief marriage to Joseph Bar-Yosef, who taught philosophy and kabbala at the Hebrew University and was the son of the author Yehoshua Bar-Yosef, known for his writings on Safed and the sixteenth-century kabbalists, undoubtedly influenced Ravikovitch's ecstatic and mystical poems as in *The Love of an Orange*. In the poem "Spots of Light," components of dark matter become, through a direct experience, spots of light which moved with a free movement, not chained to reality, and were infused with charm and loveliness, as in the words of another poem, "There did I know a delight beyond all delight."[22] The poem, which begins "And so dark is steeped in sparks of light," says towards the end, "And the light keeps streaming and kissing the dark on the mouth."[23] Within the depths of this dark matter, love is revealed, turning the darkness to gold.

Unlike Tikotsky, who saw the poem "Death In Light," which was not included in *The Love of an Orange*, as the "twin" of "Sparks of Light," I think that "Death in Light" is the reverse mirror-image of "Sparks of Light." Here, the light comes down into the valley: "And lofty visions come down to the valley/ and the body of a dead man climbs up from the valley like a snail." Unlike in the previous poem in which the light climbed up and raised up, here it exemplifies a fall. One must remain facing the light in which there is infinite height but also depths and valleys: "And a man who falls from the height to the valley has a limitless fall." In the words of another poem by Ravikovitch, "If a man falls from a plane in the middle of the night/God alone can raise him."[24] In place of the harmonious world evoked in "Sparks of Light," in "Death in Light" the depths are assimilated, as are the relationships between the upper and lower worlds, which are those between life and death.

It is possible that one can see here the influence of Gershom Scholem, who described the disharmony of the cosmos as follows:

> "Life" here is a free and frequently changing growth which is not bound by any law and is not chained to any authority. That is what "life" is as it bubbles up from the depths within which mysticism is called upon to plunge and within which it is destined to be submerged.[25]

Unlike in Ravikovitch's first poem in which the light is revealed which illuminates the darkness, in the second poem all the dangers of the messianic aspiration are seen. In these poems we see a reflection of Scholem's ambivalent attitude to messianism. This being the case, it is wonderful to see how the young poetess, who was not a philosopher, perceived the duality and complexity of the messianic temptation.

Ravikovitch could be said to be a mediator in the tense relationship between Kurzweil, her esteemed teacher in high school, Scholem, the greatest scholar of Jewish mysticism in her "Jerusalem period," and Ratosh, who attracted her by "his terrible and wonderful vision of the world."[26] Kurzweil, a representative of orthodox Judaism, attacked Scholem's secular Jewish interpretations which in his opinion were the result of the disintegration of Jewish faith due to mysticism, kabbala, messianic movements, Sabbetaianism and Frankism. Kurzweil saw Scholem as the first scholar who picked on nihilistic mysticism in order to attack halachic-rabbinic Judaism. The literary scholar from Bar-Ilan University spoke of Berdichevsky, the "Young Hebrews" and Gershom Scholem in the same breath as profanators of the true interpretation of Judaism, as heralds of the "Canaanism" of Jonathan Ratosh and as people who laid a path to secular Zionism. Finally, he predicted, the political theology of secular Zionism would authorize the "Canaanite messianism" that arose with the conquest of the territories in the 1967[27] war. When the journalist Yaron London asked her what drew her to Kurzweil, to whom she dedicated the poem "Frozen in the North," Ravikovitch replied,

> Perhaps he represents a world of old morality which he already began to see was being undermined. I had a feeling that one had to run towards him to ask for help because [...] he is the last formulator, or one of the last that I recall, of the true world.[28]

Despite Kurzweil's attack on the "Canaanites," Ravikovitch was also attracted to the nonconformist world of Ratosh. Although it was the world of the Bible, it was an archaic Bible, a nativistic world, the product of an imaginary Canaanite modernism, remote in character from orthodox Jewish commentary. One example of a possible influence is the poem "Those who Behave Arbitrarily," whose title echoes Ratosh's "Those Who Go in Darkness." This inflection was intended to confer an archaic charm, and it was related to other poems that evoke a distant poetic cosmos, the world of Canaanite myth. But it must be pointed out that the affinity to Ratoshian poetics was more a matter of style (linguistic archaisms, naivety, literalness) than of anti-Jewish, nationalistic and heroic content. Ravikovitch herself admitted that what attracted her in Ratosh was the wonderful succinctness which portrayed "death without lamentation, rape without a sigh, despair without commentary."[29] With the publication of her second book, *Hard Winter* (1964), she declared that she had abandoned "poets I loved excessively," among whom she named Ratosh.

In view of the thunder and lightning that Ravikovitch had foreseen in the triangular Scholem-Kurzweil-Ratosh relationship, one can understand her remark in her letter to Kahanoff about "an essential quality that arouses admiration and jealousy: you are able to write about painful things of vital importance without the turbulence and bitterness with which they are usually accompanied."[30] Kahanoff's calm way of writing which portrayed the Mediterranean Sea as a bridge between east and west attracted Ravikovitch, especially in view of the crusader discourse taking place at that time among the writers of the "state generation." "Crusaderism" revealed the war of civilizations of that time between Europe and the Levant, Christianity and Islam, east and west. Ravikovitch also imagined the world of the crusaders in her poems.

In the poem "The Horns of Hattin" published a year before the Six-Day War, there is a poetic description of a crusader sea-voyage to the Holy Land before Saladin's victory at the battle of Hattin (1187):[31]

> With morning, strange ships were espied in the seam
> prow and stern of primeval allure.
> In the eleventh century the crusader companies sails forth,
> kings and a mixed throng.
> Arks of gold and booty rolled into the ports,
> ships of gold,
> expanses of gold
> Ignited by the sub with wondrous fires,
> a forest ablaze.
> With the flashing of the sun and the heaving of the waves
> their hearts were drawn to Byzantium.
> How cruel and simple the crusaders were!
> They plundered all…

The voyage of the crusaders is identified with the voyage of Jason and the Argonauts to steal the golden fleece, the image of the kingdom of Jerusalem. The crusader pirates are depicted as bringing with them an Apollonian wisdom, but Christian compassion, which they came to preach, changed into lawlessness, and they were carried away by their madness and simple cruelty. The Christians were soon defeated by the Muslims under the leadership of Saladin, who "passed judgement on them at the battle of Hattin." Finally, justice was done, as is seen in the sound of the poem. In Hebrew, the meaning of Saladin (*Salah Ed-Din*) is "the success of faith" (*din* is religion or faith). Ravikovitch switches roles in this poem. Contrary to Jewish tradition that warns that kindness to the cruel is likely to end in cruelty to the kind, the poetess pitied the crusaders far from their homes, exposed to dangers, disillusioned and deprived of their good name. In the line "the sun ignited by the sub with wondrous fires, a forest ablaze," the poetess hinted at the burning forest in A.B. Yehoshua's story, "In Face of the Forest."[32]

All the major figures in Israeli culture have written works of importance dealing with the Zionist-crusader analogy. In 1963, the year we are concerned with in this article, Yehoshua's story appeared in *Keshet*. In the story, a student, a guardian of the forest working on his doctoral thesis on the crusaders, fails to notice a fire that breaks out in the forest. Did Yehoshua think, in writing about the Arab who passed by like an evil wind and set fire to the remainder of the forest with a torch, of Baruch of Magenza, who in the disturbances of 1091, when the crusaders slaughtered the Jews on their way to liberate the Holy Land from the Muslims, looked half-crazed at a fire consuming a city's gentile inhabitants? A year later, Yizhak Shalev's story, "The Gabriel Tirosh Affair" was published. In that story, a history teacher, who had fought against the British and the Arabs, in order to demonstrate the rightness of his path, brought the precedent of the crusaders to the notice of his pupils as a negative proof that the fate of the Israelis was not the same as that of the Christian invaders.[33]

Three years after the 1967 War, Amos Oz published "Unto Death," perhaps his best story. It was a fictional account of the journey of the crusaders to Palestine.[34] On one level, the Jewish one, the roots of the extermination of the European Jews in the twentieth century are revealed against the background of the persecution of the Jews in the crusades. On another level, the Israeli one, Oz, like Yehoshua before him, wondered whether a transformation had taken place in the Israelis, modern crusaders, after 1967, and they now exemplified cruelty, self-destruction and decadence. In this connection, Ravikovitch's letter to Kahanoff in 1963 provides us with a very significant momentary glimpse of the attitude of the "state generation," secular Sabras like Yehoshua and Oz, to a woman intellectual who had come from far away. Aharon Amir, Yehoshua Kenaz, A.B. Yehoshua, Chaim Beer and Dahlia Ravikovitch all came to Kahanoff to find a bandage for the pains of Israelism. The young Amos Oz, who came from kibutz Hulda with his short stories, met Kahanoff, who was more than twenty years older than him, in the corridors of *Keshet*, and he confesses today that "I didn't have enough sense at that time even to invite her to a café"![35] Yehoshua, whom Kahanoff visited twice at his home in Haifa, described the fascination she exerted on his generation: "She opened a window for us on worlds with which we were not familiar; not oriental folklore but the intellectual Levant. We felt closed in and under siege, and she created openness and exhilaration."[36] Ravikovitch could only be rescued from that closed in Israel through imaginary journeys to the Bible and the world of mysticism, to Canaanism and the crusades, Hannibal and Saladin, but Kahanoff, who came to us from the world-at-large, brought to her new country the scents of the region and the wonders of the West: the streets of Cairo and the pavements of Alexandria, the cafés of Paris, the jazz-clubs of Chicago and the intellectual atmosphere of Columbia University.

In 1954, the year she immigrated to Israel, Kahanoff was free of the spiritual oppression that weighed on Dahlia Ravikovitch and her friends, the writers and poets of the "state generation." She did not feel a "crusader anxiety" about the possible destruction of the state, nor had feelings of "crusader guilt" about appropriating the property of others. She had finally reached her land of heart's desire and the calm assurance of her Jewish identity enabled Kahanoff to publish her essays with a Canaanite editor at *Keshet* without fear of harming her self-image. She rejected Canaanism on the one hand, but also the encomium to exile of her friend from Egypt Edmond Jabès, and she wrote as follows: "In order to be whole we of course need books, but also houses, fields, streets, schools, work, in order not to be simply a race, but a people."[37]

The patriotism shown by Kahanoff in making her home in Israel at the age of twenty-seven was less evident in the writers of the "state generation," who at that time asked critical questions about the authoritarian leadership of the Prime Minister David Ben-Gurion's political messianism, the Israelis' affinity to the "Canaanites" and their crusader-like isolation, their relationship to the Arabs and many matters concerning national identity. They were dissatisfied with their country, but she finally found tranquility in her motherland. They sought ways of escaping from the landscape of their Jewish background and desired a nativistic identity; she was comfortable in her Judaism. They were used to living in a masculine world; she was impregnated with a feminist spirit. The kibbutz and the army were quasi-sacred institutions for many; she scrutinized these foundations of Israeli culture with a critical eye. They closed their eyes to ethnic differences: she made many visits to Beersheva (where she lived in her first two years), Dimona and Kiryat Shmona in the framework of Youth Aliyah and reported on the distress of the new immigrants. She devoted a whole book to documenting Ramat Hadassah, a youth village which absorbed young people from seventy-five countries. They closed themselves up in a Hebrew shtetl and often felt stifled by it; she opened a window on the Mediterranean. The young Levantine woman, who wrote about herself and about many of her generation after their wanderings in the world and in the Mediterranean, "How strange were our wanderings in that vast space!, who went as far as Paris and New York, and who closed the circle and returned to the port of departure, has left us as we go on our way."

Religious existentialism

The few poems of Kahanoff, published here for the first time. She is known first and foremost for her essays, for a novel that was published abroad, for her interviews and for the critical columns she wrote in the Hebrew press. Here, for the first time, she is revealed as a poet as well. What follows is a few of Kahanoff's poems, translated from French:

Life Was
A fabric fabulous
Bolts and bolts
Velvets sumptuous
Cool linens
Warm woollens -
I could choose
I didn't know, I swear.
I'd have nothing to wear
But odds and ends
Hand-stitched end to end

So little to choose!
Take life as it comes?
When it goes?
Nothing is left
But remains
For the graveyard:
There's nothing to choose.

To kiss the light
A child who pranced
And danced
To catch the sun
And bite the light
With such delight!
Remember? The two
of you
The spot of light
That pierced
Through the shuttered room
On that hot afternoon?
You danced and pranced
Twisted in trance
To catch the spot of light
That slipped upon his lips.
You kissed the light
Right on his lips.
He kissed the light
That moved on my lips
Spot of light that slipped
And fell when …
The door opened a crack
creaked
A voice hissed
We no longer kissed
But fled in flight
And dropped the light
I had wanted his son
The son of the sun
I kissed on his lips
Before it slipped
And was gone.

Ciaò
What can one say? What can one say?
It hurts to die

No longer the courage to write
But the wish to feel
Feel life
That, yes! Life
I desire
What can one say? What can one say?
One has to suffer
Before one dies
It's the rule of the game
To die on a low flame
A little every day,
A very little.
What can one say? What can one say?
I love life,
I didn't enjoy it enough
So much the worse! So much the worse!
The world passes and passes me by
Me, it passes by, like
Life itself!
What can one say, what can one say
To the flowers that die?
Flowers that go from red to black
White, blue, pink, then black!
Are the flowers afraid?
Do they know they're dying
A little, day by day?

Nothing to wear
When young, I thought I'd die
Of love.
I tried three times,
But how can one die
Sought out by love?
When life was a sumptuous fabric
Velvet, satin, silk,
Rolled out, unrolled,
Delicate hangings,
Rough wool,
Fresh linen,
Confectionery of all kinds,
Tangible,
Which I loved
To feel
With my hands,
I never imagined

That all that was left
Of all this
Would be odds and ends.
Nothing to wear
But these odds and ends
Sewn and re-sewn!

How
Can one take life aright
When all that remains
Of all these lengths
Are these odds and ends,
A mere nothing
That one has to wear?
I submit myself
To the Lord on high
And in the end
Beyond these scraps
I give back
What remains.

Stitches
They cut me up
They sewed me up
With their little stitches.
Ho! Ho!
I wouldn't give up
They stood me up.
I'm now in stitches!
Ha! Ha!

Ritornello
The surgeons do *petit point*
With their little stitches,
little stitches.
They sew up life with threads
But life slips away, step by step,
with little steps
To the dustbin, my beauty.
Life slips away.

Forbidden Fruit
The good Lord has hung
The pomegranate
With its ruby pips

Crammed with juice
On the tree of life.
Man, you defile
The pomegranate!
You load with lead
The wings of Life
Which explodes
with scarlet drops
Like the rubies
of the pomegranate
On the tree of life.
Ah, if the good Lord knew
That man would load
His pomegranate
With lead,
He would have said, "No, no,
My man. That's not allowed!"
But man would have disobeyed.

The Sound of the Horn
I hear the sound of the horn
The horn in the depths of the woods
the sound
Voice of the body of the body
on wood
Of the billiard …
The sound of the horn of the body
from the depths
Of the hearse.

There is a direct link between these poems and the poems of Haim Gouri pub-lished in *Ha'aretz – Literary Supplement* in February 2017. Kahanoff wrote with a light touch which did not gloss over the difficulties of her life: "What can one say? What can one say? I love life/ I didn't enjoy it enough./So much the worse, So much the worse."[38] Gouri wrote: "You go and fade away in front of my eyes./ From time to time, you are invited to an important consultation between you and yourself."[39]

I met Gouri at Ben-Gurion airport on his way to Paris in 2005, immediately after the publication of Kahanoff's book which I edited, *Between Two Worlds*. I gave him the only copy in my possession. When we met again on the top floor, he told me jokingly that whenever he passed through the electric gate with the book, a whistle was heard. The book was finally confiscated. How ironic, I thought. The ultimate Sabra does not succeed in bringing the Levantine essay-ist through the gate! She remains on the threshold, between two worlds. This state of standing on the threshold between two borders that typified Kahanoff, was also reflected in her deep affinity with cultures outside the hegemonic discourse of Israel in those years. She was particularly attracted to French culture and its poetry. In what follows I will trace her reading of three French poets who had in common what I call a "religious existentialism." Perhaps we can learn a thing or two from her poetic insights which can equip us to read her poems.

The poetry of Charles Péguy (1873–1914) in Kahanoff's opinion was a form of prayer.[40] His poetic cathedral was compared by her to Noah's ark. The ark carried the best of all that the spirit of man had produced and that was worth saving. But his life and poetry, she thought, did not always dwell on the lofty heights of inspiration. His contempt for the modern world, which he felt was lacking in any divine beauty, was in contradiction to his poetry which merged with mysticism. He attempted to rescue the modern world from total degradation, like Joan of Arc, the source of his inspiration.[41]

The two philosophies of Péguy – poet, publisher and editor – were socialism and nationalism. After serving briefly in the French infantry, he was accepted in the 1880s in the École Normale Supériere where he befriended his teachers Henri Bergson and Romain Rolland. He was a socialist, had a bookshop near the Sorbonne that was a meeting-place for intellectuals, and from 1900 until his death, on the day before the beginning of the Battle of the Marne, the battle which saved Paris in 1914, he edited the literary journal *Cahiers du Quinzième* in which he published the works and thoughts of the best writers and poets in France. He engaged wholeheartedly in the campaign for the exoneration of Dreyfus, in the course of which he became a believing Catholic and a fervent patriot.[42] Kahanoff thought that Péguy

> believed in a world in which the elements of emergency and drama of a battlefield were at work, a perpetual campaign of God, whose soldiers were always in a state of preparedness to attack the enemy, to fight a righteous war and a war for the greatness of France.

His patriotism did not contradict a special kind of socialism that in Kahanoff's words was closer to Saint Francis than to Marx. The full greatness of man, he said, would come about when he prepared the soil in his life in this world for the realization of the kingdom of heaven.

Many people laughed at the poet-seer Péguy, but, as Kahanoff rightly observed, few people troubled to read his writings. In his great work *Le Mystère de la Charité de Jeanne d'Arc* (The Mystery of the Charity of Joan of Arc) (1910), he exalted the greatness of France as his admirer, Charles de Gaulle, would do thirty years later. Kahanoff wrote:

> People laughed at Charles Péguy as they were to laugh at another Charles, who not only adopted the cross of Lorraine, symbol of the maid of Lorraine (Joan of Arc) in 1940, but also identified himself with the maiden by declaring that he would fight for France.[43]

The flowery patriotic writings of Péguy and De Gaulle are similar in style. Many lines of Péguy's last poem, "Eve," were echoed in the general's speeches.

The religious poem "Eve,"[44] the climax of his poetry, was according to Kahanoff "a flood of eight thousand lines" written a year before his death, which he foretold in his poem: "Happy are those who fall for cities of flesh and blood/ for they are the body of the city of God." She saw Péguy's religious existentialism as a continuous meditation on the mysticism of God. In his essay *L'Argent* (Money) (1913),[45] he acknowledged his attraction to religion already from an early age: "There is no greater mystery than that of the obscure years of preparation when every man stands on the threshold of his life." Kahanoff claimed that all his life he was on the verge of despair. He felt as a child, as he lay on his back on a hill and gazed up to the heavens, God speaking through France, and he described the scene as follows: "A little man putting his sorrows before God/ with all the seriousness in the world/and consoling himself as though it were the consolation of God." Kahanoff saw his works as an outstanding source of inspiration for the revival of "militant Catholicism in France," and found in them "a spirit both religious and revolutionary."[46]

According to Péguy, militant Catholicism refuses to distinguish between the world of the spirit and the world of matter or to recognize the distinction between body and soul. This in Kahanoff's opinion was the reason for the poet's identification with Joan of Arc, who fought for both: this world, which can degenerate (*politique*) and the next world (*mystique*). Péguy prophesied that in the future the *mystique* of Jesus would become *politique*. He was to be identified with these two concepts he created.

Péguy's biography exemplifies the historical continuity of France. He was not "an anarchist who mixed holy water with petrol"[47] but, as Kahanoff said, a traditionalist who knew that tradition is only effective when it is active. He was born in Orléans, the town from which Joan of Arc is traditionally said to have sallied forth to rescue the French kingdom. The French national mythology went as far as Greek mythology, concluded Kahanoff, and saw Joan of Arc as a kind of Antigone. Péguy himself thought that the tragedies of Oedipus and Antigone had nothing to do with Christianity but represented an existential situation: "The tribulations of Péguy's Joan of Arc, the pariah of pariahs, are expressed in her cry, 'How will the redeemed be saved'?"[48] Kahanoff believed that these thoughts of the poet and his literary encounters enabled him to anticipate modern literary criticism by some fifty years.

In his second year at the École Normale Supérieure, he suddenly left the institution and returned to his mother in Orléans. At the end of the decade, in 1909, after he had returned to the bosom of the Catholic faith, he wrote his mystical work, *Le Mystère de la Charité de Jeanne d'Arc*. His bookshop was frequented by Romain Rolland, Henri Bergson, Georges Sorel, Bernard Lazare and Julien Benda. He was a footsoldier among the supporters of Dreyfus. Many of his friends and people who participated in the journal he edited became famous, but when his store-office was suddenly replaced, they waved farewell to this strange, poor and lonely man, this Catholic with the anarchic soul, as though doing him a great favor.

Kahanoff saw Péguy as an original thinker, an individualist, a wandering pilgrim of France who was before his time. As a prophet, he warned against a disastrous fusion of mysticism and politics, a combination which foreshadowed the phenomenon of political theology in the twentieth century. As a pioneer, he paved the way for a return to simple values, to a mystical approach to life. As a returning Catholic, his intellectual faculties were unharmed and he criticized the politics both of the Church and of the socialist party. Kahanoff astutely described him as "the controversialist who wrestled in the arena of concrete reality while the poet expressed his vision in another world, but the two were always linked."[49] She explained his support of Dreyfus, for example, by the fact that he thought that the latter was excluded from the national society because he was Jewish and by his belief that the honor of France took precedence over the honor of its army.

Kahanoff's view of his relationship to the Jewish people is particularly interesting. In her opinion, he was able to distinguish between "the Jews," who had capitalists among them, and the Jewish people which, like all other peoples, was unable to justify its *mystique* about itself. He wrote: "Israel has given to the world innumerable prophets, saints and warriors, but in normal times the children of Israel do not raise their eyes, are not enthusiastic as in periods of great and wonderful deeds."[50] In periods of Jewish messianism there is a tension between the *mystique* and the *politique*, a tension which characterizes the history of the Jewish people.

He acknowledged in his book *Notre Jeunesse* ("Our Youth," 1910) that, where the Jews are concerned, "to their exile of many years is added the exile of modernity." Kahanoff exonerated Péguy of the charge of racism even when he spoke of the "Jewish race," on the grounds that he also spoke of the "French race" and the "Christian race." Of course, Pétain's disciples gave the concept a Nazi racial interpretation, the opposite of that intended by the poet. But it should be remembered that Péguy rejoiced when the First World War broke out. He viewed it as the end of a "gray" period and the beginning of a heroic period, a period in which France would regain its greatness. He was also pleased when a nationalist murdered Jean Jaurès. These facts did not decrease Kahanoff's sympathy for him, and she failed to ask a critical question: did Péguy's "mystical" outlook contribute to pro-fascist politics in France, like the influence of Georges Sorel, for example?[51] Although Péguy never accepted the view of Charles Maurras, leader of the national-monarchical movement *Action française*, that the Republic had to be completely uprooted, the poet became a source of inspiration for the nationalist and Catholic circles which contributed to the establishment of the Vichy regime. Did Kahanoff, who was able to distinguish between patriotism, which she supported, and nationalism, which she rejected, consider this?

Like Joan of Arc, said Kahanoff, Péguy believed in freedom which came from God, and this faith gave birth to his poetry. She saw it as a prayer of the heart which no one hears except God. In a marvelous passage in his play *Les Saints Innocents* (The Innocent Saints) (1912), he compared prayer to a huge fleet made up of ships and boats sailing towards God, and he "receives the vessels, inclining his ear to the slightest intentions hidden in the recesses of each man's heart."

For Kahanoff, Péguy was "a prophet who remembered the future,"[52] and who, like the "anti-intellectual intellectuals" of his generation, preferred myth to reason. His critique of progress derived from his belief that "the most marvelous inventions and discoveries could be made by man into instruments of destruction and ruin."[53] According to Kahanoff, his mystical poetry was directed against technical progress, party politics, the corrupt bureaucracy, the intellectuals, the "dukes of the Sorbonne," a church only for the rich, and the socialist leaders.[54] All of them in his opinion belonged to the same party, whose members were "on the right side of the table." Kahanoff saw them all as his enemies who stood in the way of the religious existentialism of the believing poet.

If with Péguy Kahanoff revealed a taste for mystical poetics and singular personalities, with her friend Edmond Jabès (1912–1991) she shared a common country and legacy. The national landscape of Kahanoff and Jabès, who were born in Egypt and absorbed the Levantine culture, was identical.[55] Kahanoff discussed the question of why the Jews of Egypt, who lived in the cosmopolitan Egyptian cities, hardly produced any literature. With surprising honesty, she said:

> It seems to me that we looked upon ourselves as too inferior – or as they say in Israel, too 'Levantine' – to express ourselves in writing. Gide and Malraux were our idols, but it never occurred to us that our task was to tell our story in our own words, not to imitate them.[56]

Someone who did tell his story in his own words was Edmond Jabès, whom Kahanoff regarded as the best of the Jewish writers from Egypt. The members of his family were resident in Egypt, traditional Jews with Italian nationality who looked up to French culture and had a cosmopolitan Mediterranean outlook. Jabès worked in the Cairo stock-exchange, was active in the Jewish community and played a prominent part in anti-racist and anti-fascist political activities. He was finally expelled from Egypt after the Suez crisis. Kahanoff remembered Jabès ("Eddie") as

> a handsome young man, a dreamer and charming, whose blue eyes strayed far into the distance. He first wrote a book of poetry called *Je bâtis ma demeure* (I'm Building My Home). At that time he thought it was possible to build a home. All that remained of all this was these broken people in the memory of the writer.[57]

The theme of Jabès's works is religious existentialism, which he expressed as "Judaism after God." In his allegorical and symbolic writings there is a discussion of apocrypha and of the literature of questions and answers. In his book, *Le Livre des Questions* (The Book of Questions), surrealism and kabbalah coexist with dialogues and the sayings of imaginary rabbis concerned with the misfortunes of the Jewish people.[58] Although Kahanoff considered the book "an exceptional achievement," she thought it depicted a barren world, a world of total isolation in which there was no trace of the vitality which had enabled the Jews to survive. Everything led to nothingness, and the human cry of despair, well expressed by Nietzsche's "Where shall I feel at home?," reverberated in emptiness and received no reply.

The need to identify the Jew with the East from where he came, said Kahanoff, is seen in the Mediterranean names of the rabbis in his work. It was no accident if the path of Yankel and Sarah crossed the Mediterranean world in Corfu, Cairo and Marseilles. According to Kahanoff, a reading of Jabès reveals the code connecting the Mediterranean world and the Jewish world:

> I again see with the eyes of my spirit these names, these landscapes, these streets, these buildings, these faces, issuing from *The Book of Questions* and reflected there. I know the place of the tear where the pages of his life were torn out, and I know that there are many wounds that will never be healed.[59]

This tear and this wound caused her to consider the meaning of Jewish existence: "Can we do otherwise than to ask ourselves to explain the insoluble equation of Jewish existence, due to which we are here but also there, everywhere and nowhere?" Kahanoff rejected the "nihilistic conclusions" of the hymn sung by Jabès to exile and hoped that the wandering pilgrim would at last find his dwelling-place: "His very foundation is the fulfillment of the Jewish soul in the harsh and gentle concrete reality of the land of Israel."

In the second half of the twentieth century, Jabès exemplified the image *par excellence* of the alien in French literature. This basis of foreignness, refugee-status or exile, which Nietzsche and Camus called "homelessness," was very characteristic of the culture of the Mediterranean Basin in the period of colonialism.[60] The changes which took place in the Maghreb and Mashrek forced thinkers, writers and political activists to be exiled from their country. The paradox is that many of them felt good in exile and were comfortable in their alienation, perhaps a central principle of the cultural and political history of the Mediterranean Basin. Jabès expressed it well: "My mother tongue was a foreign language. Thanks to that, I have both feet in alienation." This formulation is also valid for the political exiles who had to continue their anti-colonialist activities outside their country.

The work of the French poet Claude Vigée (born in 1921), an Alsatian Jew who went to Brandeis University, settled in Israel, and now, in his ninety-sixth year, lives in France, is also characterized by religious existentialism. Kahanoff wrote essays on his works, befriended him, and interviewed him in 1963, the year when Dahlia Ravikovitch wrote to her. Kahanoff regarded him as "the most outstanding of the Jewish poets in France,"[61] who struck roots in Israel. Through him, she examined the nihilistic and narcissistic roots of the modern sensibility as reflected in the poets, writers and philosophers of her time.

The title of his book *Les Artistes de la faim* (The Artists of Hunger) was inspired by Kafka's story "The Artist of Hunger," in which a character deprives himself of food as a way of refusing the duties of life.[62] Through examining man's experience in modern life and his relationship to the world and to God, Vigée came to the conclusion that Christianity is a life-denying tradition, whereas Jewish tradition honors life and sees it as a blessing. In the Book of Genesis, God blesses his creations, but Christian tradition stresses rejection, the duality between spirit and matter. Augustine's "city of God" is not located in this world, and in his *Confessions* he hopes for salvation in the next world. For modern man, even this hope is not in the realm of possibility.

Kahanoff examined the way in which Vigée exposes the modern heroes or anti-heroes who cling to their arrogant personalities, hating them and worshiping them at the same time.[63] The Don Juans, for example, only feel they exist when they humiliate other people. An ego of this kind can only be victorious through contempt of the "other." Vigée's knowledge of European literature and thought leads Kahanoff to follow him into the depths of the hell of suicidal Werthers, Fausts whose lusts cannot be satisfied, and "accursed" poets (*poètes maudits*), for all of whom the heavens are cold and gray, as if they needed a roof over the dungeon in which they are condemned to live. This is the voice of modern poetry.

Kahanoff looked at Vigée's poetic prism: romantics like Alfred de Vigny who only admired God's eternal silence, Stoics like Baudelaire who described life as "an oasis of horror in a desert of boredom," and who finally locked himself up in a darkened room in order to escape from the hellish fire of the outside world, poets like T.S. Eliot who said that the curse arose when the embryo was created, poets like Mallarmé who claimed that women are no more worthy of respect than the dead, Valéry who declared that his love was narcissistic, the love of a man only curious about himself, and Rimbaud, who ceased to write poetry and became a slave-trader. The conclusion of all this was that the negation of life ends in the degradation of the human personality and of poetry itself.

But, in contrast to this onslaught on the part of Vigée, Kahanoff noticed his hymn to life in his book *Révolte et louanges* (Revolt and Praise), in which he celebrated real people who lived in the real world.[64] The supreme example was the Spanish poet Jorge Guillén whose poetry heralded the morning after the malignant disease that had overtaken Europe. It is as though this poet discovered in his first steps in nature the sunrise, fragrant scents, birdsong and the human voice. This Spanish poet took each of the *poètes maudits* ("accursed poets") and turned them on their head.

Vigée was on the verge of adulthood, like another poet of the same age, René Char, when the Second World War broke out. A new generation of poets looked with horror at the former cultural tradition motivated by an abhorrence of life and hatred of the human race. This, wrote Kahanoff in her reading of Vigée, was an abyss in which some poets were still ensconced. Samuel Beckett's human puppets waited for Godot in vain. He was God, who would never come.

These terrorist poets of emptiness enjoyed degradation and rolling about in the muck, but Vigée is one of those who prefer songs of praise. This vital Jewish ethos does not reject the world or distinguish between the real and the spiritual. Kahanoff understood Vigée's attempt to reconcile man with the world in which he lives. More recent poetry has taken off the roof in its language in order to show that the skies are not only gray, but one can also find an abundance of light. That is the greatness of the Jewish tradition which has never betrayed the world, not even the one known to Job.

In a conversation I had with Vigée in 1997 in view of a conference on Albert Camus, he told me that Camus was the person who persuaded the publisher Gallimard to publish his first book of poetry, *L'Été Indien* (Diaries of an Indian Summer).[65] He befriended the famous author and they sat together in the Brasserie Lipp, amused spectators of the flattery that surrounded the circle of Sartre in the Café de Flore over the road. The lesson he took from Camus's tragic death in a motor accident was not to question fate, to realize the fragility of life, and to conclude that the desire of Doctor Faustus to be master of the world and of Don Juan to prove his superiority to other people finally ended in nihilism.

From the Levant to Africa

The poetic journey that we have undertaken with Kahanoff, which begun with Dahlia Ravikovitch's letter to her, and continued with her few poems influenced by the religious existentialism of French poetry, has now reached its final port of call: her dealings with African poetry and literature.[66] In the works of writers and poets from Africa and other countries, which she analyzed in the 1960s, two contradictory yet complementary principles of the cultural theory Kahanoff was developing were discovered: on the one hand, something she called a "literature of social mutation" and on the other hand, something she called "black literature."[67]

V.S. Naipaul, for example, an Anglo-Indian writer who was born in Trinidad and lived for many years in Jamaica, is not an English writer or an Indian writer, nor is he a Jamaican writer.[68] As a displaced person, he reflects a "mutation," a transitional situation: he has one foot in his community and the other in England. The connection between them is his writing. India has likewise produced a number of writers who do not feel at home in their motherland: the authoress Santha Rama Rau, the writer of *Gifts of Passage*, an Indian emigrant writing in the United States; the writer Dom Moraes, an Indian Christian, and Ved Mehta, brother of the conductor Zubin Mehta – Oxford graduates. The Tunisian-French-Jewish writer Albert Memmi was also given by Kahanoff as an example of what she called the "literature of social mutation."[69]

In 1963, the year in which Ravikovitch wrote to her, the book *Modern African Writing*, edited by Kahanoff, was published in Hebrew. It was an anthology containing stories, poetry and essays, and its aim was to introduce the then-new culture of the peoples of Africa to the Israelis. It did not represent the whole of Africa. For editorial reasons, South Africa, where apartheid prevailed, was not included, nor were the countries of the Maghreb and Mashrek, but it presented the writings of the new African countries south of the Sahara. Examples were also given of the work of Caribbean writers, who, together with those from the former French colonies in Africa, played an important part in the creation of a new literature which is African in inspiration and French in expression. According to Kahanoff, past suffering and hopes for the future are to be found in this literature.

Kahanoff found that the preparation of this anthology was a kind of "voyage of discovery towards what is perhaps one of the most exciting human adventures."[70] In the comprehensive introduction she wrote, she witnessed the birth of "something especially hopeful in an old and weary world." In her words, it revealed the African "essence" which neither slavery nor colonialism could suppress, an essence that was expressed first and foremost in new languages. Historically, there were hundreds of spoken dialects in Africa, but there was no regional written language except for Arabic. In modern times, French, English and Portuguese were the main languages. The colonial cultures had some influence on the literature, but the style and content were typically African, expressed via the European languages. For instance, a syncopated African rhythm runs through the poem "Rama Kam," by the Senegalese poet David Diop: "I love your look, a wild look/ and your mouth which tastes like mango/ Rama Kam/ And your body, black pepper/which makes desire sing out/Rama Kam."[71]

When the writer Camara Laye from Guinea told the story *L'Enfant Noir* (The Dark Child) about a boy's longings for the lost world of his past, Kahanoff felt she was present at an invocation of the mysterious life-forces and magical atmosphere of his adolescence. The evocative phrases, repetitive, chant-like, sounded to Kahanoff like a hymn. The child had gazed spellbound at his father who fashioned gold into a jewel but was unable to do what his father did. He dared not fondle the black serpent, the embodiment of the spirit of the ancestors of the tribe, from which his father gained his strength. The child, who went to a French school, felt he could never be at home in his father's world. The ceremonies for his coming-of-age, which he recalled as a student in France, were associated in the story with his long absence from Africa.

Aimé Césaire (1913–2008), a French poet born in Martinique, studied in the École Normale Supérieure and opposed French colonialism. He was one of the founders of the Francophone "black literature." Kahanoff relates that when he was asked to write a sonnet, he replied, "Believe me, it would be better for us to beat on tom-toms as we have always done."[72] Together with Léopold Senghor from Senegal, he wrote the essay "L'Étudiant noir" (The Black Student), in which he coined the term *négritude*, meaning black identity. As a surrealist poet whom Kahanoff saw as representative of the Africans who emerged from a pre-literary culture, Césaire broke through directly into the modern world. He sought in his poems to speak of the kernel, the root, the beginning, claiming that the Africans were truly the "firstborn of the world" because they had not cut themselves off from their roots: "Possessed, they are inebriated with the essence of all things/ They are truly the firstborn of the world."[73]

Senghor, Césaire's partner in the *négritude* movement, was the first president of Senegal, the first African appointed to the Académie française and a permanent candidate for the Nobel Prize for Literature. Kahanoff was impressed by the comparison he made between the intuitive and sensory ways of Africa and the anti-rationalist tendencies of science and philosophy in our time. Senghor stressed emotion as a way of knowing the world, in which subject and object are not separated but connected. Césaire and Senghor represent what Kahanoff called "integral humanism." The changes that took place in tribal Africa occurred against the background of the trials and tribulations of slavery, colonial exploitation and racial oppression. The phenomenon of the new culture embraced the whole continent, the entire race: "Africa possesses an abundant and joyful self-confidence which is as refreshing as the dew after the excessively pessimistic intellectualism of contemporary European literature."[74] There was new life, she felt, in the African literature, and the Africans confronted their future with an almost mystical sense of awe, as though Africa was able to build itself up as a result of its martyrology.

Césaire from Martinique and Senghor from Senegal represented *négritude*, a new form of universalism and integral humanism, a literature which according to Kahanoff was permeated with ambiguity: on the one hand, elements of the technological, individualistic and rationalistic white civilization, and, on the other, elements of the tribal and poetic black civilization. Yet, nevertheless, there was a synthesis between them. The best example she gave was the journal and publishing house *Présence africaine* in which there were French-speaking writers and poets from Africa, the West Indies and Madagascar. They were jealous of their artist-friends, came together like them in Paris immediately after the Second World War, and then created a journal. Among the contributors were Senghor, Césaire, André Gide, Sartre, Camus, and others. The journal, which fostered nativistic self-awareness (somewhat like Aharon Amir's *Keshet*), provided a platform for many writers who promoted an understanding of the dark continent, its values and problems.

Kahanoff discerned in the journal something of the existentialist idea of *engagement* (commitment) in the African poets writing in French. The attitude of the African poets writing in English was perhaps more healthy and rational, but the "French" in her opinion attained a higher degree of intensity, power and compassion in works like those of Césaire and Senghor. The colonial cultural differences were reflected in the African works of literature. The French wished to pass on their culture to their disciples, and the ideals of the French Revolution played a crucial role in molding the educated African elite, but because this happened in a colonialist regime, it was not fully accepted, and the consequent frustration produced the reaction of *négritude* – black radicalism. The British, who to a certain extent were idealistic, sought to be honest though distant rulers, and thus left their African protégés less divided and hesitant about identity, race and legacy than their French-speaking counterparts.

Jomo Kenyatta (1891–1978), who hid from the yoke of British colonialism and became the first president of Kenya, had a practical approach, unlike the abstract and intellectual approach of Senghor, the disciple of French culture, and most of the French-educated writers were the same. Kahanoff, whose sympathies in the matter are obvious, thought that she detected something false in the facile optimism of English-educated writers such as P. Dai Anang, who wrote, "I will die for the world,/ a wonderful world./ There is no other country/ in the East or West/ that will give me continuation here./ Only Africa can do that."[75] In contrast to him, the black and colored inhabitants of South Africa, where there was an intense racial conflict, produced literature which in her opinion was the most polished in form and the most Western in its ideas and concepts. Top-ranking South African writers such as Peter Abrahams and Can Themba[76] were shown to have a real obsession with the subject of racism. Abrahams wrote about a Zulu child who retained the memory of the glory of the black kings who reigned before the coming of the white man. This child, a proletarian, cut off from his tribal society and dwelling in slums on the outskirts of a city or in mines, refused evacuation to a native reservation. Themba, for his part, gave an excellent description of African aspirations in his introduction to *African Voices*, a literary anthology published by the African journal *Drum*: "Here we are, Africans addressing Africa and the world,/ Dreaming of the great things we will do in the future:/ a new civilization,/ a new African culture."[77]

Kahanoff opened a window on the literature of the dark continent, a world born in a violent, ambivalent dialogue between black and white, between the neolithic and the technological. The continual tension between the two could lead to a symbiosis, to what Kahanoff called a "literature of mutation," or it could lead to the adaptation or isolation of "black identity." Kahanoff saw the various ramifications of multiculturalism very early on, several decades before it was discussed in the postmodernist discourse.

The tales of the African people, which were told from generation to generation, were regarded both as instruction and entertainment. Kahanoff saw them as a special blend of morality, humor and common sense. The Nigerian writer Amos Tutuola (1920–1997) succeeded in rendering this literature in English. In his story *The Palm-wine Drinkard*, a man is observed wrestling with death. It is an example of an African narrative full of imagination, which, like surrealistic poetry, blurs the Western boundary-line between external reality and subjective feelings. In the story by the Ghanian writer Andrew Opoku *Over the Wild River*, the hero of the story, who leaves his village in order to create a cocoa plantation, justifies his action before the members of his tribe with popular sayings.[78] These modern African writers did not break away from their popular roots, but Kahanoff noticed that the traditional foundations of their stories and poems underwent a change in the transposition to European languages.

The African thread was entwined with another, far from Africa, in the Caribbean and on the eastern American seaboard, among the descendants of African slaves.[79] The collective Afro-American memory has been preserved despite the attempt to efface it. The former Africans made an impact on America which is seen in jazz, in negro spirituals, and in the combination of African art and Christianity found in the Haitian cult of Voodoo. After the American Civil War, when a need was felt to rehabilitate the liberated slaves, there was a debate about whether the education of the Negroes should be based on professional instruction or whether it should be given a broader humanistic character. If in the history of the Negroes in the United States after the civil war there was much hope for assimilation, already at the beginning of the twentieth century one could perceive a desire to strengthen the African roots of the Negroes. Kahanoff called this "African Zionism." In his book *The Souls of Black Folk*, W.E.B. Du Bois already in 1903 declared,

> The problem of the twentieth century is the problem of the color-line, the relations of the darker to the lighter races [...] The American Negro [...] would not Africanize America. He would not bleach his Negro soul in a flood of white Americanism [...] He simply wishes to make it possible for a man to be both a Negro and an American.[80]

Kahanoff said that these sentences express a "black humanism," an outlook developed by African and Afro-American writers a generation later.

Writers from the Caribbean islands under French rule – Haiti, Martinique, Guadeloupe – and writers from Guiana, played an important part in the flowering of the new literature, producing an impressive list of authors and poets. In an interesting insight, Kahanoff pointed out that the colonial status and the consciousness of color were often less pronounced in Catholic countries than in Protestant ones. The French, she said, had less racial consciousness than other European peoples. This cultural tolerance permitted young writers to give expression to their *négritude* and their revolt against the artificial order that the white man had imposed in Africa. Many of them played central roles in the continent, both in the colonial administration, in the revolt against colonialism and in the post-colonial society which they created.

In the 1930s, writers from the Caribbean founded a journal in Paris called *Légitime défense* (Legitimate Defense). Kahanoff followed up a few of the many African contributors who participated in the cultural revolution in France, a revolution encouraged by French men of culture, including André Breton, the French "pope of surrealism." Senghor declared that this "would not be just a journal, but a cultural movement." He wrote a poem, "Femme Noire" (Black Woman), about a mother whom he feared was lost. Longings for the good old order of life are aroused by the black mother who also represents the earth, the principle of the renewal of life – Africa itself. The mother, who embodies simple, unsophisticated life, is contrasted with the cold, corrupt world of the west. As a soldier, Senghor had been crushed by columns of tanks in Europe and had rotted in prisons where "the sheets were white and cold." He prayed for recovery and for a consciousness of his value as a human being to be restored to him. In the 1960s, Senghor sought to heal this breach in the article "The African

Path to Socialism," in which, in an almost mystical way, he reconciled traditional African values with the thinking of his time.

The reconciliation reappears in the work of Gabriel Okara (born in 1921), who represents this dual legacy, of which he does not renounce any part. In the poem "Piano and Drums," he listens to the drums of the jungle together with a piano concerto. The African, according to Kahanoff, is not only a man "who has lost everything," but also one who has acquired new tools. His literature touches people's hearts and influences them through its spontaneous joy and poetic enthusiasm. He longs to rediscover a lost magic, seeks pure waters to quench the thirst of modern man who feels alienated from his world because contact with the cosmos has been taken from him. Here, Kahanoff's existentialist discourse reaches a climax, but it is a discourse that says "yes" to life. Like the ancient Hebrews, the African believes that life is good and holy, in the spirit of "God saw all that he had done, and, behold, it was very good." He does not turn his back on the world, does not differentiate between God and the creation and refuses to see man as an irremediable sinner. African man is in Kahanoff's opinion a pilgrim constantly engaged in a tireless search.

But there is another option in Kahanoff-type existentialism. Jean-Joseph Rabearivelo (1901–1937) is considered one of the most important African poets and Madagascar's leading writer. His poems appear in the anthology *La Grande Ile: Poems malgaches* in which the introductions were written by Kahanoff.[81] Rabearivelo published a few poetic anthologies in French and Malagasy, literary criticism, an opera and two novels. As a young man and as a poet under the French colonial regime, he was deeply humiliated when his request to participate as an artist in exhibitions in Paris in the early 1930s was turned down. He was a sensuous poet who was infatuated with symbolist poetry, adored the "accursed poets," especially Rimbaud and Baudelaire, and translated into Malagasy works by Edgar Alan Poe and Paul Valéry. Kahanoff understood his affinity with the post-Christian and nihilistic Western culture of his time in which the isolation and *sacro egoismo* of the genius lead him into nothingness and suicide.

In his works, Rabearivelo interwove Malagasy culture and Western culture. As he was trapped in colonialism – Western culture which gave him cultural benefits without gaining him social acceptance – for lack of choice, he returned to his sources, from which he took his pick. The humiliations endured by the wounded soul of this writer and intellectual were documented in the 1800 pages of his *Calepins Bleus* (Blue Notebooks). In a letter to a friend before committing suicide, he referred to a fable of La Fontaine in which the death of a grasshopper who had sung all night aroused the pity of the ants. Responding to this, Kahanoff saw a link between Baudelaire and modern African poetry: "What poet of that period did not cultivate with groans the flowers of evil of his despair?"[82]

Kahanoff is known as an essayist, a writer and a critic, and she also wrote poems, but it is also worth considering another aspect of her work, her role as a theoretician of culture. The "literature of social mutation," she declared, reflects a cultural process and social change that has not been sufficiently noticed. A search for identity and a refusal to be confined by a narrow definition characterizes the literature of crossbreeds. In their personalities and writings, these writers mix the various elements that molded them without any desire to renounce any of them. We are not only speaking here of Levantinism, but there is no doubt that Kahanoff's Levantine starting point with its mixture of cultures served as an inspiration for her to develop a universal model of culture. In her opinion, a large part of literature was produced by writers who found themselves at an intersection of countries and cultures, and who therefore cannot be described as "national." These writers and poets were the product of a long period of colonialism, and their works reflected a transitional mentality, a mutation from the traditional culture of their predecessors to a new culture.

A theory of spatial identity

The Levant is a geographical region that embraces the eastern shore of the Mediterranean Sea, a state of mind that embodies a dialogue between east and west and a longing that is both nostalgic and utopian.[83] The term "orient" derives from the Latin word *oriens*, meaning sunrise, and the term "levant" derives from the French word *levant*, also meaning sunrise. In Western Europe, the Levant became a synonym for the eastern Mediterranean where the sun rises, an area that includes countries such as Greece, Turkey, Syria, Lebanon, Israel and Egypt, a region that was part of the Ottoman Empire from the sixteenth century to the twentieth. Kahanoff, who in the course of her life and in her works embodied the Levantine region, longing and state of mind, made the entire Levantine journey. She lived in Egypt in the first twenty years of her life, wandered between New York and Paris, and in her two final decades settled in Israel.

Some recent interpreters of Kahanoff, wishing to explain the term "Levant" in her writings, stress the eastern aspect of her thought to the point of making it the sole principle of the Kahanoffian doctrine. In so doing, these scholars ignore the main idea underlying her thinking, which is the importance of a dialogue between the Levant and the West, or the encounter of the Mediterranean with Europe. Unlike the "new school" which interprets Kahanoff as a thinker who proposed an eastern orientation for divided Israeli society, an up-to-date critical reading of her essays published from the end of the 1950s to the end of the 1970s in newspapers and journals in Israel and outside reveals a clear and methodical scheme for a universal culture not necessarily favoring a particular social sector or ethnic group. Kahanoff's cultural identity was anchored first and foremost in the Mediterranean area in which Israel is situated, an area which bridges east and west. In this, she joins other major Israeli intellectuals who formulated theories of cultural identity such as a modern Western identity, the Canaanite option of Hebrew nativism, the option of the "Semitic space" and so on.

Kahanoff's Mediterranean proposition was before its time, and today it appears the most reasonable proposal for a common denominator in face of the ever-increasing social tensions and fragmentation in Israel.[84] In the hegemonic period of *mamlachtiyut* in Israel until the beginning of the 1970s there was a need for social pluralism and cultural openness, but so much friction has taken place since then between the polarities of Ashkenazi and Mizrahi, religious and secular, hawks and doves, that there is hardly any chance of finding a common platform, points of agreement or the possibility of dialogue. In this situation, the Mediterranean proposition still remains an option for a rapprochement between Israel and the Palestinians in which they could cease to confront one another and accept a regional arrangement involving the two Arab neighbors with which peace has been concluded, the southern European countries and the Maghreb.

In Egypt, it was a generation that had absorbed the influences of many waves of immigration from southern Europe – especially Italy and Greece – from the Mashriq and from Iraq, together with British rule and French culture in a Muslim country wavering between tradition and modernity, a dynastic monarchy and a modern centralized administration, nationalism and a tendency to pluralism. Modernity was not identified, as is thought by many scholars, with the European Enlightenment and the French and industrial revolutions, but was an attempt by many societies, in the non-Western sphere as well, to adopt life-styles and forms of adaptation which enabled people to fashion their lives with their own hands, to abandon oppressive traditions and create syntheses of the conservatism of the past and the modernism of the present. The Levant of the two last centuries represents a special form of adoption of modernity.[85] The cultural heterogeneity of the Levant testifies above all to its cosmopolitan character, or, in the words of the poet and translator (and first editor of Kahanoff's writings) Aharon Amir, to "the cosmopolitanism of Mediterranean-mindedness," of a hybrid region comprising Jews, Italians, Greeks and Egyptians. Levantinism as her home-landscape was for Kahanoff a methodical, well-formulated and highly inspirational concept.

She saw the Levant of the classical period as the apex of the orient, and she displayed an impressive awareness of its history, its cultural context and its universal significance. She saw it not only as a region, but as a concept combining the real and the imaginary, attraction and repulsion, birth and decay – a complexity that anticipates the perceptions of Edward Said in his book *Orientalism*.[86]

Kahanoff's conception of the Levant was spatial and historical. The Levant was the cradle of civilization where, from Mesopotamia and Egypt to Persia and Israel, Western culture grew its wings. The modern world would not be anything without the Bible, the events of which took place in the Levant. The great religions and great empires originated or developed in the Levantine region. The Roman, Byzantine and Islamic empires left their mark on the area, but none of them succeeded in effacing its special quality. The State of Israel has continued the tradition of the minorities in the region which struggled through the years to preserve their special identity in the face of the empires which dominated the area. The Jews, in Kahanoff's opinion, are skilled in preserving their identity in the face of foreign cultures while making the adaptations and compromises which allowed them to maintain a separate cultural existence.

Because the Jews as a minority developed widespread cultural connections with the world-at-large, their outlook was comparatively open to changes. The reaction of the Jews of the eastern countries to the European influence was different from that of the majority of the Muslims. Because the Muslims saw the Europeans as conquerors above all, they felt they had to oppose their influence, but the Jews, like other minorities, saw in them an opportunity for freedom under colonial rule and a means of cultural development (as in the founding of the schools of the *Alliance française*, for instance). In this way, the Jews were the standard-bearers of Levantinism.

The minorities in the Muslim world, said Kahanoff, did not systematically adopt European ideals but became completely westernized and thus aroused the suspicions of the local population. She thought that a similar process took place in Europe when the Europeans felt animosity towards the intellectual and communist Jews, preferring fascist elements. The Jewish and Coptic minorities in North Africa and Egypt were annihilated or expelled as happened to minorities in Hungary and Germany. The rise of pan-Arabism and Islamism effaced any remnant of Levantine culture, a cultural synthesis of east and west such as was found among the Jews, the Copts and the Christians. This ended the possibility that these minorities could act as a bridge to the general population and promote a free and open society for the benefit of all the citizens.

The mythical aspect of Levantinism

Kahanoff deliberately created a myth of Levantiniasm so that it could be a source of inspiration for the Mediterranean society of Israel. At the end of her life when her articles were collected for publication in English in the comprehensive critical perspective of the totality of her writings, it could be seen that Kahanoff perceived a mythical dimension in Levantinism in that it was a narrative that provided the story of an identity. She saw the Levant not only as a mythical territorial space but as a "mythical time," or, as she said, a "psycho-historical time." The renewed historical construction of a culture requires a departure from the present consecutive time and place. A cultural myth is anchored in a starting point, a landmark to which one looks today in order to gain a perspective. Mythical time is total and harmonious while present time is partial and defective. This undoubtedly shows the influence of the theory of archetypes and stereotypes of the school of thought of the psychologist Karl Jung and the anthropologist Claude Lévi-Strauss. Modern Levantinism, according to Kahanoff, not only embraces the "mythical spaces" of different cultural narratives, but also the "mythical times" of many cultures and religions. For instance, the different calendars of the religions create and are conditioned by philosophies of history, hierarchies of values and attitudes to the "other," the unbeliever.

The Six-Day War in 1967 changed Kahanoff's perspective on Israel and the Levant. After the generation of the founders who came from Eastern and Central Europe, there was a new generation which was born in its own country. It looked on the Levant in a different way from its parents. The areas conquered in the war at the same time provided opportunities for direct contact between Israelis and Palestinians. Perhaps Kahanoff was suggesting (with naive optimism in that period after 1967) that the task of Israel in the territories it had conquered resembled the role of Britain and France in the Arab countries under colonialist protection. In other words, without colonialism, modern Levantinism could never have come into being.

That was Kahanoff's view when she wrote her articles, essays which in their time gave off an optimistic aroma of conciliation, reflecting a modern perspective on the world. Human beings create history, and so they can create a different history. This was the generation before the intifadas, before the massive colonialist settlement project. In this way, Kahanoff was able to hope that Israel had changed its approach to the Levant and that from now on it would be open to its surroundings and would not focus unduly on the Jewish ethnic aspect as in the past. Perhaps she ought to have known even then that the attitude of the first settlers who gained a foothold in the occupied territories would not produce a modern Levantinism but would turn the dispute into a fundamentalist, nationalist and cultural confrontation which would only get worse. Kahanoff did not delude herself that the pluralistic possibility she offered (i.e. Levantinism) would prevent future wars. At the same time, in the perspective of the *longue durée* (long time-span) of the historian of the Mediterranean Fernand Braudel,[87] she wrote, "In the long run, Israel will succeed in integrating into the Levant."

What Kahanoff envisaged with her modern outlook was the simultaneous adoption of various points of time and place in the Levant, combining different views, relationships and cultural dimensions.[88] Thus, the Levant was seen as a rich mosaic, a mirror reflecting many different cultural perspectives, a fruitful and productive kaleidoscope not confined within a one-dimensional ideology of east and west. Her constant emphasis on the Levant as the eastern part of the Mediterranean was intended to support her view that the region is a cultural area in which a lively and candid dialogue between east and west is possible. But she not only saw the Levantine option as a cultural possibility but as a concrete political proposition.

The Levant excels in intellectual interactions, mutual influences and common affinities – the consequence of conquests, alliances, expulsions, discoveries and wanderings on the eastern shore of the Mediterranean Basin. The culture of ancient Greece, claimed Kahanoff, penetrated Egypt, Asia Minor and Palestine. In the Hellenistic culture of Alexandria, Jews and Greeks encountered one another, and that dialectical encounter created the basis from which Christianity and Western civilization sprang. Greek, the language of civilization, was dominant in the Levant long after Greece became a province of the Roman Empire. The Greek Byzantine Empire became the center of the cultural world after Rome fell to the barbarians from the north. When the Roman emperors adopted Christianity, Greek became the liturgical language of the eastern churches. Thus, Kahanoff continued to trace the Levantine "mythical time" in the Levantine "mythical space," Alexandria for ever and ever.

Levantinism in Israel as an open wound

In her article, "What about Levantinisation?" Kahanoff made a pointed criticism of the cultural hegemony of the "Sabras" ("the Israelis born on this side of the Mediterranean") and their attitude to the immigrants who came from the Maghreb and Mashriq.[89] It often seemed to her that as long as the Jews of European origin failed to respect or understand their Jewish brethren born of the other side of the Mediterranean, they would use the term "Levantines" for them. A Moroccan Jew who claimed an attraction to French culture was called a "Levantine"; an Arabic-speaking man who tried to appear "European" instead of what he really was, was suspected of "Levantinism" – "a mysterious threat to the existence of Israel." Levantinism was a term for a false Europeanism or a pretension to Europeanism. This controversy about Levantinism and Levantinization began in her opinion at the time of the mass-migration of Jews from the Islamic countries to Israel, many of whom came without anything and had no modern skills. Despite this situation at the start, their hopes and ambitions brought them to Israel. To be called "Levantines" when they reached their homeland was a traumatic reception for them. Levantinism was "the hidden thorn in the bouquets of welcome to the country."

On her immigration to Israel in 1954, Kahanoff doubted the possibility of creating a Levantine culture in Israel. Her new acquaintances in the country tried to reassure her that they did not regard her as a real "Levantine." Although she was born into a Levantine society in Egypt, she was told, the derogatory remarks that were made about Levantinism did not apply to her because she had "a real European education." She was more and more surprised. Was "Levantine" a term only used for those who did not have the possibility of obtaining a modern education, those who found it hard to integrate into the new world because they had lived for long periods in isolated and remote communities cut off from the main currents of modern life? Where she was concerned, she had no intention of denying her Levantine origins, just as she did not deny being a Jewess. These two identities were part of her, as they were an essential part of many others. The Levantines had a different past from people from Europe, a past that involved its own benefits and disadvantages, and there was no point in denying or rejecting it.

What hurt her particularly was the thought that this was an Israeli version of European antisemitism. The antisemites in Europe feared that their society would be "Judaized" by the Jews. a foreign element, and one of which they had only a superficial knowledge. Attaching the label of "Levantinism" to immigrants who had only just arrived in the country seemed to Kahanoff a cultural rationalization of prejudice. This could be seen, for instance, in a series of articles by the journalist Aryeh Gelblum in the newspaper *Haaretz* in 1949 concerning the great migration: articles (exceptional, it should be said), which expressed a disdainful attitude to the "Levantines" who were regarded as representing a primitive culture.[90]

This approach seemed to Kahanoff dangerous for a country like Israel whose development depended on the absorption of Jews who had immigrated from different places. Each immigrant brought with him the special characteristics of the region from which he came, the traditions and customs and also the scars of the Jewish past. The attitude of the people of the Yishuv to Levantinism was a historical. The Jews from the eastern countries had their own history in which there were movements which had certain principles that resembled those of the Western Enlightenment. Many people are unaware that a parallel to the Haskalah existed in the urban Jewish communities in the east. Because of Arab nationalism, which became fanatical, and the outbreak of the War of Independence, many members of these communities immigrated to Israel. The Jewish immigrants who had acquired Western culture were regarded as "inauthentic," "Levantine," and a mere imitation of the real thing. The prevailing prejudice prevented the old-timers from having an enlightened view of the Levantines, and this intolerance caused bitterness among those who needed sympathy and understanding on arriving in Israel. If they wished to integrate, into the country, they had to undergo a cultural mutation.

Kahanoff thought that when people speak of Levantinism, they mean a hybrid culture in which there are elements of a more advanced foreign culture. There are some, she believed, who are attracted to a culture that is not their own, although on a superficial level, in order to possess the facilities of that culture, and there are some who are unable to do so and who degenerate together with their culture. The capacity of a culture to renew itself depends to a large extent on the qualities of its members and their ability to adopt elements of another culture, one not in process of degeneration. Primitive peoples have disappeared because they were unable to make the necessary adaptations to the cultures around them.

Kahanoff put forward interesting arguments in favor of what she called the "cultural mutation" of Jews from eastern countries who seemed to have adopted superficial characteristics of the colonialist power which ruled in their area. In her analysis, which anticipated the ideas of Homi Bhabha in cultural studies, she went so far as to develop a theory of the genealogy of culture. According to her, when a culture degenerates – that is to say, when it no longer satisfies the expectations of its members – it is a sign of vitality if its members search out another, more dynamic culture. In the "adoption" of a culture, they are attracted at first by what appears on the surface: styles of dress, food, pop music – things easy to adopt. One cannot gain a deep understanding from the start of something one has not previously known. Only gradually can one expose oneself to an advanced new culture while retaining elements of one's old culture, a combination which creates a new cultural synthesis.

Already in 1959, three years after the Sinai Campaign, Kahanoff wrote that the wars in which Israel was engaged swept social problems under the carpet and appeared to bind the Israelis, Westerners and Orientals, together into a single nation.[91] Israel's success was due among other things to the agreement between the oriental Jews and the Jews of the "old Yishuv" (the term was Kahanoff's) on the need for modernization: technology, education, housing, the war on poverty and so on. These achievements were in her opinion nothing less than a revolution which placed Israel on the threshold of the modern world. The Israeli old-timers were fearful that the Jews from the eastern countries would drag Israel down to the level of the Arab countries so that it would be weakened and unable to defend itself. This fear caused the old-timers to make many mistakes such as the rapid integration of the Jews from the eastern countries in a way that showed no consideration for their beliefs, their feelings or the respect due to them as human beings. Kahanoff's social criticism drove her to put forward a new vision, an up-to-date Levantine ethos.

Kahanoff hoped to see Israel as a vanguard in the dissemination of Levantinism. In that naive period there were thinkers like her who saw Israel as having the potential to defend the rights of the minorities in the Middle East, so that the state would help the Kurds to gain independence from Iraq, protect the Christian minority in Lebanon and serve as a counterbalance to the pan-Arabic and pan-Islamic influences in the region. In Kahanoff's opinion, the answer lay in the mythical context in which the Levant had always been placed and whose source was in the mythical dispute between Isaac and Ishmael. The solution was a compromise in the mythical-symbolic sphere that would lead to a compromise in the actual political sphere. Each side would have to take over a certain inheritance: not everything, which is an idea that reflects hubris, a kind of imperialism. Kahanoff wished to replace Zionism with Levantinism, a multicultural philosophy, a way of life that would facilitate new and original solutions for the area. A modern and critical Levantinism was from her point of view a cultural possibility of that kind, an option for a comprehensive solution for the Mediterranean region above and beyond the interests of the great powers.

Epilogue or prologue?

Kahanoff's writings have followed a long and tortuous path from the time they first appeared in the 1950s in English in the United States and in Hebrew in Israel, to the renaissance they have experienced recently in the academic ivory tower and in the literary world in Israel and overseas. Kahanoff now has a secure place in the literary pantheon as the exponent of Levantine culture, as is shown by the three volumes of her essays (*From East the Sun, Between Two Worlds,* and *Mongrels and Marvels*), the appearance of her novel *Jacob's Ladder* in Hebrew in 2015, academic conferences discussing her ideas, and fruitful studies of her writings representing her as a Levantine mystic, a Mediterranean intellectual and a linchpin of the dialogue between east and west.

In an interview she gave in 1967, Kahanoff declared once again that the term "Levantine" had been distorted in Israel to the point of being unrecognizable. Her aim was to reclaim it from its negative connotation and make it the standard-bearer of a rich civilization which draws on its historical sources. One should remember that the Levantine controversy did not emerge in a vacuum. The Levant, both as a geographical region and as a cultural entity, had been disregarded by the Israeli elites who grew up in the west, in Europe or the United

States. The broadening and deepening of the Levantine narrative has made it into a Mediterranean option for a synthesis between east and west which now, in the era of globalization, is available to young Israelis.

Many people make claims to Kahanoff's legacy. Is any one reading of this original Levantine thinker to be preferred, or can one already speak of "Kahanoffism"? In her analyses, insights and criticisms, Kahanoff anticipated many matters pertaining to the Israeli Moledet: regional identity, cultural roots, varieties of modernity and conservatism, locality and globalization, ethnicity and post-colonialism. One sees the vast scope of the commentaries on her writings and the readings of her cultural universe by cultural scholars, writers and critics. All this reflects the living, relevant and vivid intellectual countenance of one of the most fascinating figures in Israeli culture whose image has been increasingly respected in recent years. To Israel's realms of memory and identity were added the Levantine identity and memory.

Notes

1 Jacqueline Kahanoff, *From East the Sun*, Tel Aviv 1978 (in Hebrew).
2 Jacqueline Kahanoff, *Between Two Worlds*, ed. David Ohana, Jerusalem 2005 (in Hebrew).
3 Jacqueline Kahanoff, *Mongrels or Marvels: The Levantine Writings of Jacqueline Shohet Kahanoff*, eds. Deborah A. Starr and Sasson Somekh, Stanford University Press, Stanford 2011.
4 Jacqueline Kahanoff, *Jacob's ladder*, trans. Ophira Rahat, Jerusalem 2014 (in Hebrew).
5 "Jacqueline Kahanoff – Levantinit," a film by Raphael Balulu, Scientific Consultant: David Ohana.
6 "Jacqueline Kahanoff: The Levant as a Parable," exhibition curator: Sara Turel, Scientific Consultant: David Ohana.
7 David Ohana, 2015, "Jacqueline Kahanoff Between Levantinism and Mediterraneanism," *New Horizons. Mediterranean Research in the 21st Century*, eds. Mihran Dabag, Dieter Haller and Nikolas Jaspert, Schoeningh Ferdinand GmbH, Bochum 361–384.
8 Moshe Shperber, ed., *Secularization Process in the Jewish Culture*, Raanana 2013 (in Hebrew).
9 Jacqueline Kahanoff, *Ramat-Hadassah-Szold: Youth Aliyah Screening and Classification Centre*, Jerusalem 1960.
10 Ravikovitch's letter to Kahanoff, 12.5.63, The Gnazim Institute of the Writers Association in Tel Aviv (in Hebrew).
11 HaNeomi (Zinger) Moshe, "Dalia Ravikobitch Poems Collection," *Ma'ariv*, 11.12.1959 (in Hebrew).
12 See especially: Giddon Ticotsky, *Dahlia Ravikovitch: In Life and Literature*, Haifa 2016, 68–86 (in Hebrew).
13 See especially the critics Ya'ara Shchori and Dana Olmert in Gidon Tikotsky, op. cit., 56–57.
14 Kahanoff, "Wake of the Waves," *Amot*, year A, booklet B, Tel Aviv 1962, 44–53 (translated from Hebrew in *Mongrels or Marvels*, 136).
15 Ibid., 138.
16 Edward Said, *Orientalism*, Penguin Books, New York 1978 and Homi Baba, *The Location of Culture*, Routledge, London 1994.
17 Jacqueline Kahanoff, "With the Return East," *From East the Sun*, 68–77; Dolly Benhabib, "Skirts Are Shorter Now: Comments on Levantine Female Identity in the

Writings of Jacqueline Kahanoff," *Theory and Criticism – An Israeli Forum*, 5 (1994): 159–164 (in Hebrew).

18 Kahanoff, "Wake of the Waves," 140.
19 Ibid.
20 Kahanoff, *Jacob's Ladder*.
21 Daliah Ravikovitch, *Daliah Ravikovitch: Complete Poems*, eds. Gidon Tikotski and Uzi Shavit, Tel Aviv 2010 (in Hebrew).
22 Daliah Ravikovitch, "Delight," *Hovering at a Low Attitude: The Collected Poetry of Daliah Ravikovitch*, trans. Chana Bloch and Chana Kronfeld, W. W. Norton, New York 2009, 69.
23 Ibid., "Sparks of Light," 67.
24 Ibid., "In the Right Wind," 119.
25 Ohana, "J.L. Talmon, Gershom Scholem and the Price of Messianism," *History of European Ideas*, Vol. 34, No. 2 (2008): 169–178.
26 Tikotski, op. cit. 44–48, 47–49, 107–109.
27 David Ohana, "Nationalizing Land: Gershom Scholem's Children and the 'Canaanite Messianism'," *Nationalizing Judaism: Zionism as a Theological Ideology*, Lanham 2017, 95–130.
28 Interview of Daliah Ravicovitch with Yaron London, The Israeli Television, 1.2.1987 (in Hebrew).
29 See especially Daliah Ravikovitch, "Accounting of Cruelty and Compassion," *Yediot Achronot*, 11.1.1963 (in Hebrew).
30 Ravikovitch's letter to Kahanoff, 12.5.63.
31 Daliah Ravikovitch, *All the Poems So Far*, Tel Aviv 1995, 133–134 (in Hebrew).
32 Abraham B. Yehoshua, "Facing the Forest" in *History and Literature: New Readings of Jewish Texts in Honor of Arnold J. Band*, eds. William Cutter and David C. Jacobson, Providence 2002, 409–418.
33 Yizhak Shalev, *The Gabriel Tirosh Affair*, Tel Aviv 1964 (in Hebrew).
34 Amos Oz, *Unto Death*, trans. Nicholas de Lange, Boston 1978.
35 Ohana's interview with Amos Oz, February 2017 (in Hebrew).
36 Nurit Baretzki, "The first lady of the Mediterranean," *Ma'ariv*, 15.3. 1996 (in Hebrew).
37 Kahanoff, "Edmond Jabès, or 'The book of questions'," *Between Two Worlds*, 128–135.
38 Jacqueline Kahanoff, "Ciao," Poems in the Gnazim Institute of the Writers Association in Tel Aviv.
39 Haim Guri, "Burning of Memory," *Ha'aretz – Literary Supplement*, 22.02.2017 (in Hebrew).
40 Jacqueline Kahanoff, "Charles Péguy," *Amot*, booklet 6–7, June–July, I, 1963, 44–58; II, 1963, 50–65; Reprinted in *Between Two Worlds*, 235–288 (the following references would follow the reprinted version).
41 Charles Péguy, *The Mystery of the Charity of Joan of Arc*, trans. Jeffrey Wainwright, Manchester 1986.
42 Charles Péguy, *Notre Jeunesse*, Paris 1957.
43 Kahanoff, "Charles Péguy," 242.
44 Charles Péguy, *Eve*, Paris 1913.
45 Charles Péguy, *L'Argent*, Paris 1913.
46 Kahanoff, "Charles Péguy," 240.
47 Ibid., 246.
48 Ibid., 249.
49 Ibid., 262.
50 Ibid., 266.
51 David Ohana, "Georges Sorel and the Rise of Political Myth," *History of European Ideas*, 13:6 (1991): 733–746.

52 Kahanoff, "Charles Péguy," 275.
53 Ibid., 276.
54 Ibid., 278–281.
55 Shimon Shamir, ed., *The Jews of Egypt: A Mediterranean Society in Modern Times*, Boulder CO, 1977 (in Hebrew).
56 Jacqueline Kahanoff, "Culture In Becoming," *Davar*, 16.4.1973 (in Hebrew).
57 Ibid.
58 Jacqueline Kahanoff, "Edmond Jabès or The Book of Questions," *Davar*, 30.4.1965 (in Hebrew).
59 Ibid.
60 Steven Jaron, "French Modernism and the Emergence of Jewish Conciseness in the Writings of Edmond Jabes," PhD. Dissertation, Columbia University, New York 1997.
61 Jacqueline Kahanoff, "Claude Vigée: A Portrait of a Poet," *Ma'ariv* (in Hebrew).
62 Claude Vigée, *Les Artistes de la faim*, Paris 1960.
63 Claude Vigée, "The Crooked Bridge of Man to the World," *Davar* (in Hebrew).
64 Vigée, *Révolte et louanges*, Paris 1962.
65 Yehuda Koren, "Relevant Even Today – Albert Camus," *Yediot Aharonot* (in Hebrew).
66 Jacqueline Kahanoff, *Modern African Writing*, edition and introducing by Jacqueline Kahanoff, Tel Aviv 1963 (in Hebrew).
67 Ohana, "Otherness, Absence and Canonization in the Discourse of Literary Historiography: The Case of Jacqueline Kahanoff," *Times of Chane: Jewish Literature in the Modern Era, Essays in Honor of Dan Miron*, eds. Michal Arbell and Michael Gluzman, Sede Boker 2008, 235–257 (in Hebrew).
68 Ajay Kumar Chaubey, ed. *V. S. Naipaul: An Anthology of 21st Century Criticism*, New Delhi 2015.
69 Jacqueline Kahanoff, "Albert Memmi, or Wilding Road to Israel," *Ma'ariv*, 18.11.1996 (in Hebrew).
70 Kahanoff, *Modern African Writing*, 7.
71 Ibid., 8.
72 Ibid., 9.
73 Ibid., 10.
74 Ibid.
75 Ibid., 11.
76 Ibid., 16.
77 Ibid., 17.
78 Ibid., 11.
79 Ibid., 12.
80 Ibid., 12.
81 Jacqueline Kahanoff, ed., *La Grande Ile: Poems Malgaches*, Tel Aviv 1964, 2 (in Hebrew).
82 Ibid., 3.
83 Philip Mansel, *Levant: Splendor and Catastrophe on the Mediterranean*, Yale University Press, New Haven 2012.
84 David Ohana, "The Mediterranean Option in Israel: An Introduction to the Thought of Jacqueline Kahanoff," *Mediterranean Historical Review*, 21:2 (2006): 239–263.
85 David Ohana, *The Intellectual Origins of Modernity*, Routledge, London 2019.
86 Said, op. cit.
87 Fernand Braudel, *The Mediterranean and the Mediterranean World in the Age of Philip II*, University of California Press, Berkeley 1972.
88 Jacqueline Kahanoff, "Afterword – From East the Sun," 1968, Kahanoff Archive, Gnazim Institute, Tel Aviv.

89 Jacqueline Kahanoff, "What about Levantinization," 1959, Kahanoff Archive, Gnazim Institute, Tel Aviv.
90 David Ohana, *Israel and Its Mediterranean Identity*, Palgrave Macmillan, London 2011, 92–95.
91 Jacqueline Kahanoff, "Israel's Levantinization," 1959, Kahanoff Archive, Gnazim Institute.

6 Israel's realms of memory

A sociologist and his world

The French historian Pierre Nora, who is known for the concept "realms of memory" which he introduced, recently declared that in the last twenty years there have been significant changes in the relationship between memory and identity.[1] According to him, the new place of memory in our lives is due to two developments. One is the "acceleration of history": there is no longer a slow development of events but quick changes which require an adaptation to an situation of uncertainty. The other is our capacity to recreate our relationship to the past. What is called "memory" today – the reconstruction of past events – was in the past called "history." This change in the nature of memory has a dual significance: first, the use of the past to justify social and political measures has increased dramatically, and, second, there has been a decline in the belief that the historian has a monopoly over the past. In a world in which one speaks of "collective history" and "personal memories," there is a tendency to turn to the judge, the witness, the media, the legislator, and, one may add, the sociologist. A reading of the studies of the sociologist and anthropologist Michael Feige reveals a similar phenomenon in Israel, in which there is a correlation between the memory of the Israeli collective-in-formation and the emerging national identity.

Do the phenomena and test-cases observed by the scholar reflect, each in turn, individual beams of light from his torch, or does the great searchlight of a comprehensive theory color his perceptions and conclusions? Feige was far from being a scholar who allowed a world-embracing theory to color all sociological phenomena, including the contradiction-filled Israeli "project." He saw the world of humanity as quite simply the earth and its fullness which cannot be reduced to dualities like oppressors and oppressed, employers and workers, occupiers and occupied, Ashkenazim and Mizrahim, men and women. His studies give an empathetic view of *la condition humaine*, and at the same time are clear-eyed and critical, sensitive and penetrating, revealing areas hidden from sight: dreams of redemption and the excavation of roots, hopes and fears, the real Israel and the imagined one.

Feige's writings viewed as a whole reveal a broad canvas of the evolving identity of the Israelis: of the changing forms of remembrance – the siren and the monument, the ritual and commemoration, the ceremony and the pilgrimage – by means of which they remember and perpetuate themselves; of the long time-perspectives of Gush Emunim and the short ones of Shalom Achshav; of the great space of the settlers and the confined space of the secular, and of the founding myths of their lives and deaths. Feige sought to reveal the ideal place concealed in the actual Israeli place, and to examine in depth the dialectic of the true Israel and the imagined Israel. He sought to climb above and below the familiar level: to the one above, where great dreams and apocalypses take place, and the one below, where they expose the archaeological roots of the national consensus. These are the hidden sides of our existence: memory and forgetfulness, commemoration and concealment, exposure and repression. These volatile elements, he claimed, are an inseparable part of the true Israel, whereas the more straightforward elements – building and excavation, settlement and uprooting – promote an image of the past and an image of the future and give a mythical picture of the situation. The real conditions the mythical and the mythical initiates the real. The Israeli reality gives birth to and nurtures an ugly and fearful myth, and myth likewise bequeaths to reality its dreams and fears. All this he wished in his academic enterprise to elucidate in small batches, and together they give a great light.

At the time of the withdrawal from Gush Katif, the Israeli sociologists refrained from commenting on these events, and thus shirked their duty as intellectuals – "social critics," as the political thinker Michael Walzer called them.[2] However, Feige not only vehemently analyzed the process of uprooting, but also foretold the results. In contrast to the general belief that the withdrawal would cause a trauma among those evacuated, he claimed that from a sociological standpoint, the 8,000 evacuees would be incorporated in Israeli society without causing more than a "slight tremor." The fact that the transference of thousands to within the green line gained more attention from the media than the immigration of a million Jews and non-Jews from the former Soviet Union, and that their evacuation aroused more interest than the expulsion of poor people from their homes or the demolition of Palestinian houses, did not make the social scientists change their view. Feige's wise prediction was due to his long acquaintance with the settlers.

As a sociologist of Israeli society, Feige dealt with the hermeneutics of the investigation of secular sites like the Dizengoff Center, Mini Israel and the Azrieli Center; with the analysis of sites of disasters and the graves of leaders; with the meaning of the historical "long perspective" and the "short perspective" of the "day of small things"; with the memorializing and commemoration of major figures, pilots and students, a woman settler and a peace-demonstrator; with political groups of shared experience like Gush Emunim and Shalom Achshav; with the privatization process in Israeli society and the globalization here and overseas; and with the traumas and scars starting from the Yom Kippur War, via the evacuation of Yamit, up to the murder of Rabin. He accompanied with his empathetic and critical research many stations on the Via Dolorosa of this country. Feige was a sociologist among historians and a historian among sociologists. If the historian may be compared to the owl of Minerva, goddess of wisdom, which flies with the onset of evening and thus sees historical events in the perspective of a great distance in time, the sociologist sees them in the time when they happen, in "real" time. Feige described the irritability of Israeli society and commemorated those who remembered and the acts of remembrance, the radical political culture expressed in social action, and the elements of the Israeli mythology.

Political "communities of experience"

Feige sought to deeply investigate the nature of the "Israeli place": that is to say, to investigate its dynamic identity, its changing collective image and the self-perception of the increasingly fragmented Israeli society. A place can be described as a fusion of time and space, and these went through his undertaking like a thread. His researches initially focused on two extra-parliamentary movements of the mid-1970s: Gush Emunim and Shalom Achshav.

His acquaintance with the settlement enterprise began with his doctoral thesis in the Hebrew University, which was the basis of his book, *One Space, Two Places: Gush Emunim, Peace Now and the Construction of Israeli Space* (2003).[3] In the book, he made a comparative study of two very important political movements in Israel: Gush Emunim and Shalom Achshav (Peace Now). He began with an analysis of the Zionist movement's domination of the Israeli space through the alienation of exilic Jews and the native Arabs. The presence of the memory of the one coincided with the erasure of the memory of the other, and the creation of the space is the acquisition of the territory or returning it. There is a straight line from "redemption of the land" and the Hebraization of the names of the settlements it contains to the giving of biblical names to the settlements in Judea and Samaria. The forming of the space and the seizure of the moment were interdependent.[4] The conceptualization by the messianic religious right of the territories captured in 1967 took the form of the realization of the covenant with God and the imperative of the promised land, and its success was due to a combination of messianic rhetoric and the national-secular ethos of Zionism. The opposing ideological camp, Shalom Achshav, which wished to avoid ruling over another people, also included its perception of boundaries and space in its conception of Zionism and its place in history.

The land changed its identity. From a promised land ruled by foreigners, it became the motherland. A Zionist, according to Feige, is someone for whom two changes of identity – that of the individual and that of the land – are desirable. A post-Zionist (as distinct from an anti-Zionist) is someone who thinks that these two changes have already taken place. The appearance of Gush Emunim and Shalom Achshav was the result of two essential crises in the Zionist process. The first was the founding and consolidation of the state, following which the question arose: what was the meaning of Zionism when a strong modern Jewish basis had been laid in the country after it had undergone a process of Hebraization? The second crisis was related to the first: if the State of

Israel had already arisen, and in that sense had fulfilled the Zionist idea, what was one to do with the additional areas? Did the Zionist principles apply to them, or was the purpose of Zionism to confine itself to the restricted boundaries of the War of Independence?

Zionism, as a continuous and progressive transformation of people and land, had already run its course before the Six-Day War. But when the new spaces suddenly opened out, there was a discrepancy between the new sphere connected with the mythical past of the nation and the inability to realize the Zionist program there and make it "ours." Between Gush Emunim and Shalom Achshav there was not even a minimal agreement about the perception of time and space. There cannot even be a debate between someone looking for the site of Joseph's tomb in order to sanctify it and someone who says he is not interested in knowing where the tomb is situated.

The same applies to the dimension of time. Gush Emunim relates to a cyclical, mythical time which reverts to ancient days and brings them back to life. The key concepts of their outlook are therefore memory and return. Shalom Achshav and the dovish camp relate to a one-dimensional time that only moves forward. The time of the settlers is the extensive time-frame of Jewish nationhood; it begins with God's promise and ends with the messianic process of redemption. The time of Shalom Achshav and the dovish camp is the restricted time-frame of Zionism. It begins with the Zionist movement and the first waves of immigration and not with the patriarch Abraham. Gush Emunim and Shalom Achshav do not belong to the same time and have no common language with regard to space. Is it surprising that each of them has a different idea of the identity of the same state? When Feige interviewed Benny Katzover at Elon Moreh near Shechem, the latter asked the interviewer where he lived. Feige answered, "Pisgat Zeev" (a Jewish neighborhood in Jerusalem situated beyond the green line). "Fine," said Katzover, "so you too are a settler!" Feige thought at that moment: "they'll evacuate you in order to leave me where I am."[5] In the light of this, one can understand Feige's declaration that the Oslo Accords were an Israeli renunciation of part of the 1967 conquests in return for a Palestinian and international legitimation of the boundaries achieved in 1948.

In the time-dimension, Gush Emunim saw history as a story with a beginning, middle and end, which has chapters delineating events from the mythical starting point (the patriarchs, the exodus from Egypt) to the messianic point of termination: life as it should be lived. Shalom Achshav does not recognize a linear, circular or regressive line in history – that is, a development in which there is a certain logic – but a time that is "empty" or "neutral" in which the life of society or the nation is lived without a framing story or super-narrative. Life just as it is.

The relationship of the two movements to the significance of the space is also different, in a similar way. Gush Emunim relates to the Holy Land with special criteria unique to the people of Israel. The territory is not simply a place but the land of the Patriarchs, a land intended for a messianic purpose, but Shalom Achshav continues to a certain and limited extent the nativistic line which the

"Canaanites" took to an extreme. That is to say, the place is a combination of the space in which the citizens are born live and work, and the language in which they express their culture. It is these things alone that, as in the French model, determine the nationhood of the subjects.

From this are derived two concepts that Feige uses to explain the relationship of Gush Emunim and Shalom Achshav to time and space. Gush Emunim appropriates Judea and Samaria through widespread settlement activity, while Shalom Achshav sees this Jewish appropriation as an estrangement of areas of the land of Israel from the "other" – the foreigner or the native Arab. Gush Emunim creates a Judaization of time and space through the building of settlements, the Hebraization of names and the rejection of the Zionist calendar. Gush Emunim adopted Zionist values with a historical affinity, symbols reflecting the Zionist narrative like "absorption of immigrants" and especially "settlement." But appropriation for the Jew is alienation for the native Arabs: the latter dwell in the space on a temporary basis, guests allowed to stay, while the Jewish settlers in Judea and Samaria are returning home. The relationship of Gush Emunim to space, like its relationship to time, is total because time and space for them are aspects of a theological, meta-historical view of the world. Settlement in the space and a linear or cyclical concept of time are viewed by the settlers within the framework of the story of the *longue durée* (to use the expression of the historian Fernand Braudel) of the Jewish people.[6] On the other hand, the relationship of Shalom Achshav to time and space is "normal," because for them time and territory are concrete, secular, physical, without metaphysical significance. For Gush Emunim, the place receives significance from God, but for Shalom Achshav a place is just a place.

Gush Emunim sanctifies historical time. This relationship makes it a movement of historical memory. The "meaningful" Jewish past in the ancient land of Israel, unlike the "dispensible" historical past of the exile, conditions all its activities in the present and all its plans for the future. The past is the significant point in time from which everything is derived. The Jewish past in the land of Israel is the basis of the restorative utopia (to use Gershom Scholem's expression) of Gush Emunim, as in "restore our days as of old." The members of Gush Emunim described themselves as continuing the modern, secular Zionist enterprise, and, not only that, but as the continuation of their ancestors. Gush Emunim's memory of the past is the reverse mirror-image of the memory of the past of Shalom Achshav. The members of that movement, who preach normality, believe in forgetting as a principle: forgetting retaliation and revenge against the enemy, forgetting the exile, forgetting the mythical past of the land for the sake of a normal, unpretentious life in the present.

Gush Emunim is connected to Gush Etzion. That is where the inaugural gathering was held in 1974, and the leader of the settlers, Hanan Porat, was resident there. For him, the return to the settlement lost in 1948 was a symbol of redemption on its way: 1967 was a correction of 1948. But Feige did not ask the critical political question that now arose: if the people of the four settlements of Gush Etzion returned to their homes by reason of their right of return, what can prevent the inhabitants of the 400 Arab settlements who lost their homes or were expelled, from making the same rightful claim?[7]

The greatest importance was given to the perception of time and space after the Six-Day War. If, for the people of Gush Emunim, the conquest was a return home to the ancient space and the extended time-frame, for the people of Shalom Achshav it constituted a threat of becoming colonialists who ruled lands where others lived. They also saw it as an abandonment of the restricted time-frame, normal time, to which they had become accustomed in the nineteen years between the War of Independence and the Six-Day War. The people of Gush Emunim wanted to continue the Zionist enterprise in the old-new spaces that had opened up to them in 1967, but the people of Shalom Achshav thought that the Zionist enterprise had successfully achieved its objective with the founding of the state. At the present time, the Israelis with their independence should be like the other nations of the world. That is to say, the meaning of post-Zionist time was that the ideology had been realized, and the Israelis were concerned with the day of small things and the construction of civil society.

These opposing outlooks of the two political movements concerning the realization of the ideology and the purpose of the state, and concerning the idea of sovereignty and the importance of history, were matched by different practices. The most important practice of Gush Emunim, that of settlement, was seen as a historical and political copy of the biblical map, a metaphysical return to the land of Canaan and a symbolic duplication of the conquest of the land. As Feige said,

> According to the settlers, they have not come to a land of Arab villages, refugee camps and army camps. They have come to Hebron and Shechem just as the patriarchs did, and to Jericho, Ai and Gibeon just as Joshua did.[8]

The settlers saw the return to the ancient space as a rebirth.

Different places in the Jewish areas in Judea and Samaria represented the different perception of time and space of the people of Gush Emunim. In the self-image of the settlers of Hebron, the town was an outstanding embodiment of the ancient biblical space which had an aura of sanctity because of its proximity to the Mahpelah Cave and because of its association with the relatively recent events of the 1929 riots against the Hebron Jews. The Jewish right of return existed both in the dimension of memory and in the dimension of space. According to Feige, the community of memory in Hebron and Kiryat Arba links "monumental time" to "social time." Hebron, for the settlers, is the vanguard of the Israeli nation and embodies the best Zionist values; simultaneously, it is seen as a peripheral and neglected place by modern, secular Israel. Unlike radical, violent Hebron, Ofra commends itself by its normality. This bourgeois settlement erected by the first members of Gush Emunim is a thriving national-religious community set in a landscape, far from acts of violence – an island of conciliation. For Feige, Hebron and Ofra represent two models, radical and normal. In this way, the people of Gush Emunim gave different expressions to their lives among the Arab population.

In contrast to the political theology of the settlers in Judea and Samaria, the members of Shalom Achshav saw the territories conquered in the Six-Day War as spaces inhabited by a Palestinian population, foreign places outside the time and space to which the "little" Israel was accustomed. This difference led to a call for a separation of the peoples and a separation of the territories, a call expressed politically by large protest demonstrations. The comparative studies made by Feige illustrate the metaphors, symbols and representations of Gush Emunim and Shalom Achshav, examine the different practices of the two movements and describe the political cultures of the opposing ideologies. Shalom Achshav disliked pathos, went in for irony, distanced itself from the memory of the past and represented itself as a liberal, secular and dovish movement. The security-minded former officers among them completely rejected pacifism, however, and the intellectual pluralism and political restraint of the members of Shalom Achshav were in contradiction to the absoluteness of the settlers, who made their homes in distant areas and devoted themselves wholly to the settlement enterprise.

The two political movements also wished to appropriate "Judea and Samaria" or return the "occupied territories" by academic means. The discourse they used could take the form, as described by Ian Lustick in relation to the appropriation of areas, of the use of science for national or political purposes.[9] Lustick, who was inspired by Gramski's idea of a "cultural hegemony" in which the existence of a certain social order was self-evident, thought that if Israeli society saw the "territories" as something foreign, there would be a reasonable possibility of withdrawing from them, and if it saw them as a legitimate part of the State of Israel, there would be a good chance of annexing them in the future.[10] In order to justify their claims, the two movements adopted different practices, different methods of research and a different scientific language. Through an examination of the scientific discourse of these movements, Feige reached the conclusion that the mechanisms of appropriation that had been effective after the founding of the state failed in the period after the Six-Day War. The Palestinians of the territories who embodied the semiotics of the place prevented a similar treatment of the space. The political disagreements about the "occupied" or "liberated" territories did not permit a decision according to a Zionist super-narrative or through an Israeli national consensus. The disappearance of a common national language and the retreat of the humanities and social sciences from a symbiotic relationship to the state precluded the possibility of an official state discourse. The voiding of the center left the field open to Gush Emunim and Shalom Achshav, which promoted their narratives – "territories of the homeland" or "occupied territories" – and mobilized science on behalf of their camps. In this way, official science became political-sectorial science.

The subversive practice of the settlers was to adapt the old to the new through an ideological combination of Land of Israel studies, Bible, history, and geography. The settlers' map was supposed to link up with the biblical map and represented a metaphysical return to the land of Canaan. They therefore struggled over the names of the settlements and their conformity with the biblical texts and their original locations. They took trouble with the renewed codification and imagined geography. They recreated the biblical text in the old-new space and gave the Bible priority over the Mishna and Talmud. Rabbi Jacob Ariel prepared a splendid atlas of the boundaries of the biblical land of Israel; scholars like Yoel Elitzur and Zeev Erlich combined secular sciences with halachic sources; colleges and field schools were set up to study the new settlement; conferences were held and books published on the subject of the land of Israel, and there was also a branch of biblical archaeology. All this was investigated by Feige when critically examining the fusion of science and politics among the settlers.

Feige's book on Gush Emunim, *Settling in the Hearts: Jewish Fundamentalism in the Occupied Territories* (2009),[11] was highly praised for its scope and amplitude, and won the Shapiro Prize from the Association for Israel Studies for the best book in the field. One review declared that Feige excelled in his capacity to make a broad synthesis of historical, political and ethnographical evidence.[12] In another review, it was pointed out that Feige's book filled a gap in the discussion of Jewish fundamentalism, a discussion in which anthropologists had not participated until that time.[13]

Feige regarded Shalom Achshav as a more revolutionary movement than Gush Emunim, inasmuch as it was the first large political movement to place on the national agenda, as an essential matter, the return of territory controlled by the State of Israel. It did this by distinguishing between "us," on one side of the Green Line, and the "other" who lived "there." The movement consequently made a series of reports using social sciences such as demography, economics, statistics and cartography. They examined the government's investments in the territories, the subsidies received by the settlers, and the expansion of settlement. The sociological analysis revealed something paradoxical: this "scientific" examination of the settlement enterprise resulted in a modification in the reactions of the movement and was different from Shalom Achshav's protest activities, which until then had only taken the form of mass-demonstrations. At the same time, the movement published a "true map" revealing facts and figures about the conditions of life of the population in the territories, a map ratified by senior geographers.[14]

There was a division in the use of science by the two movements. Making the area beyond the Green line an object of research was essentially different before and after 1967. The new criticism revealed a close affinity between power and knowledge in modern Israel. The settlers chose the disciplines of history, geography and archaeology, and the people of Shalom Achshav, as we said, chose the social sciences, which were considered more "scientific" than the humanities. The various research practices of the two movements were revealed: the settlers linked the biblical past and the alien space to what was open and known, in this way seeking to prepare Judea and Samaria as a restored national home. The project of nationalizing the territories sought to anchor the Israeli present in the Jewish past, but this time not in "exile" overseas but in the land of Israel, a bowshot from Jerusalem. The research practices of the settlers portrayed the territories as an open and dynamic space, a space undergoing the process of the return of the sons to the womb of the land and of history. The settlers sought to find the magic that lay beneath the surface, while the people of Shalom Achshav tried to do the opposite: to expose all that was negative in the space of the "other," the unknown, and to make it known. They therefore used the positivist sciences and a technical professional discourse of counting, measuring, tables of statistics, graphs of tendencies, and so on. The neutralization of the sanctity and the removal of the magic were accomplished by means of a critical use of science.

Feige's analysis, which was made after the Oslo Accords, ends with the words,

> The success of Shalom Achshav, or, more exactly, the failure of the settlers "to win people over" [...][15] is in agreement with the dialectical process described by Uriel Ram in his review of the book *Two Maps of the West Bank*: Feige puts forward a thesis concerning the irony of history: through its actions, Gush Emunim created the bargaining chip through which the State of Israel could carry out the program of Shalom Achshav – the agreed final fixing of the borders of the State of Israel on the 1967 lines.[16]

Have the theses and analyses of the sociologists Feige and Ram stood the test of time? Time will tell, but a hint of the answer may perhaps be found in Feige's review of Akiva Eldar's and Idit Zartel's book, *Adonei ha-aretz: ha-mitnahalim u-medinat Israel 1967–2004* (Lords of the Land: the Settlers and the State of Israel 1967–2004). From the conceptual point of view, he wrote, the book has already given back the territories. A complete separation has been carried out and the occupation was never an integral part of the Israeli identity. The book tries to reveal an innocent and righteous Israel concealed and camouflaged by the occupation. Did such an Israel ever exist? Does it still exist somewhere? Is there a way or a reason to bring it back?[17]

Living with the trauma

Gush Emunim and Shalom Achshav were born in the shadow of the trauma of the Yom Kippur War. Until 1973, Israel's wars created national solidarity, but the "oversight" represented by this particular war caused protest among the demobilized soldiers. The future activists of Gush Emunim and Shalom Achshav held hands in demonstrations against the Israeli government, but despite their common protest, their ideological difference with regard to the territories led, in a short time, to a political parting of the ways and a separate convergence. Each side took cover in its own outlook. Each side had its own answer to the question: where was Israel going after it captured the territories in the previous war, the war that had united them only seven years before?[18]

The future members of Gush Emunim did not see the war as a special trauma but as a stage in the long history of the people of Israel in its country and as a dialectical step towards redemption. Their self-appointed task of lighting up the way of the weak and despondent derived from their redemptive philosophy of history. Feige claimed tentatively that it was the Yom Kippur War that made possible the rise of Gush Emunim. The young people of the movement said that the political consequences of the war caused a disaster which forced them to act. The wounding of the parachutist Hanan Porat in the war did not diminish his belief in redemption and even strengthened it. The wounding of Yuval Neria, a member of Shalom Achshav, on the other hand, was not accompanied by meta-physical consolations but by an understanding that it was possible and necessary to have prevented the war. Among the people of Shalom Achshav, the "over-sight" created a trauma which was the main impetus for their political activity. The war was seen as an "abnormal" phenomenon: it caused a severe crisis in the political and military establishment, and for those who took part in it, it was of course a deeply traumatic experience. The Yom Kippur War destroyed the sense of self-evident legitimacy with which Israel's wars until 1973 had been received. The fighters among the people of Shalom Achshav concluded from the trauma that they should protest against all future wars. In contrast to the point of view of Gush Emunim, which saw the trauma as part of the historical manifestations of the birth-pangs of redemption, the people of Shalom Achshav adhered to the direct experience, the trauma which they themselves embodied – an experience which in a short time became a critical outcry and a political protest.

The "trauma" of the evacuation of Yamit was an outcome of the trauma of the Yom Kippur War. The results of the war caused the visit of Anwar Sadat to Jerusalem and the signing of the peace treaty between Israel and Egypt. In the treaty it was stated that all Israeli settlement in Sinai had to be removed, includ-ing that of Yamit. Unlike Judea and Samaria, the Sinai region had no sacred significance for the settlers. The Sinai Desert was seen as peripheral, the area of the passage from slavery in Egypt to the promised land. The people of Gush Emunim joined the protesters against the evacuation of Yamit, most of whom were secular, only in the final stage of the struggle. The religious settlers who emerged from the Merkaz Ha-Rav Yeshiva in Jerusalem, the house of study of Rabbi Zvi Yehuda Hacohen Kook, might have been expected to believe in the tortuousness of the process of redemption which they had learned from the writ-ings of Abraham Yitzhak Hacohen Kook. As Feige said, "The teachings of Rabbi Kook recognized the possibility of retreat, delay, birth-pangs of the Messiah, but even if redemption is hidden, it is a temporary stoppage on the way to an assured redemption."[19] It is therefore interesting to ponder the question of why the people of Gush Emunim nevertheless saw the withdrawal from Yamit as a trauma. The answer is that they sought to intensify the trauma in order to prevent the evacuation of Yamit from becoming a precedent for what might happen in the future to the ideological settlements.

Among the people of Gush Emunim, there were two reactions to the trauma of Yamit. One, conciliatory, was represented by Rabbi Yoel Bin Nun, who said that the settlers had not succeeded in winning people over, and they therefore had to devote themselves to work in education and the media. The other, radical reaction to the trauma was that the indifferent Israeli society could not be relied on, and one therefore had to create a radical vanguard in the form of a Jewish underground that would speed up the redemption and be a threat to the Palestinians. The attack on the Palestinian mayors and the actions of the Jewish underground in July 1980, which caused a crisis in Gush Emunim, were a testimony to the dramatic experience of the evacuation of Yamit and also a result of it. The activists of Gush Emunim did not succeed in reconciling the destruction of Yamit with their redemptive outlook. Although, said Feige, "the trauma of the withdrawal [...] was shared by the evacuating soldiers and the evacuated settlers,"[20] the settler camp failed to nationalize the trauma of the evacuation of the region in Sinai and extend it to Israeli society as a whole.

The perpetuation of the memory of the evacuation long after it had taken place, and the experience of the trauma, were expressed in the statement of Sarah Druckman that the sight of the soldiers evacuating herself and her friends made her think of the Holocaust. However, the evacuation of Yamit did not make a great impression on the governments that followed, and they supported further withdrawals, and the proof of it is that the memory of Yamit did not play a special role in the evacuation of Gush Katif in August 2005. The outbreak of the first Lebanon War some two months after the evacuation diminished the attempt to make the experience of the withdrawal from Sinai a collective traumatic memory, and in the 1980s Israel developed a divisive character in which there was hardly any place for national memories.

In the mid-1990s, there was a trauma in Israel comparable in some ways only to that of the Yom Kippur War: the murder of the acting prime minister. Following the murder of Yizthak Rabin, Feige wrote two pieces about it: a study of the commemoration of the man and his work,[21] and a portrait of the murderer Yigael Amir in his social context, with an examination of the relationship between religion and ideology, ethnicity and the center.

Fifteen years after Feige wrote his article on the commemoration of Rabin, he began to investigate the ethnic and radical contexts of the murder. In his article, "The Murder of Rabin and the Ethnic Fringes of Religious Zionism," published some two months before he was killed, Feige asked, "Why Yigael Amir specifically? Why should a man with a certain biography, a defined place in society in Israel, be the one to commit the murder?"[22] Feige explained that Amir was characterized by a stubborn individualism, refused to be defined by the normative ethos of the group he belonged to, and took a radical direction in every framework he entered. He and the other Mizrahim (Jews from Arab countries) appeared to the ideological settlers as the most natural candidates to join them. In Benny Katzover's confession marked by condescension and Orientalism, he said,

> I must say that I feel best when I come into contact with people of the oriental communities. These people have the healthiest attitude to the land of Israel. When you say to these people "such and such", they understand and don't try to philosophize.[23]

The profile drawn by Feige of many of the murderers from the rightist camp showed that all of them were on the fringes of the settler movement: Yona Avrushmi, the murderer of Emil Grunzweig; David Ben-Shimul, who fired a rocket on a bus of Palestinian workers in 1984; Shaul Nir and Uzi Sharbuf, who in 1993 murdered students in the Islamic College in Hebron; Ami Popper, who in 1990 murdered seven Palestinian workers; the brothers Eytan and Yehoyada Kahalani of Kiryat Arba, who in 1994 tried to murder an innocent Arab on his way home; Eden Natan-Zaada who made a shooting attack on a bus in Shefaram; Jacob Teitel, who murdered Palestinians and placed an explosive charge in front of the door of the home of Professor Zeev Sternhell; and the murderers of the youth Muhmad Abu Hadir in 2014. The number of people on the fringes of ethnic groups is out of all proportion among the political murderers in Israel. Next to them, of course, one cannot overlook the members of the Jewish underground, who came from the very heart of the settler establishment.

In the settler camp, as in Israeli society as a whole, not all the individuals fitted in socially or ideologically. Many marginal people remained outside the ideological camp, frustrated by their inability to fit in for ethnic reasons. Religious Zionism did not take responsibility for these ethnic marginals, who according to Émile Durkheim define the boundaries of the collective by their presence. The national-religious public defined its moral norms by thrusting the delinquent elements outside the camp. Thus, the settler camp avoided taking responsibility and placed it on the ethnic marginals who were regarded as "noxious weeds." The failure of that camp to grapple with the problem of social integration also prevented a moral stock-taking with regard to the root of the controversy aroused by the murder of Rabin. The setting of boundaries to the hegemonic identity, the orientalization of the Mizrahim (Jews from Arab countries) and the resulting frustration formed a combination which "contributed to the murder of Rabin and led to other cases of murder," and Feige added, "perhaps it will also lead to another political murder."[24] Feige criticized placing the responsibility for Rabin's murder on Israeli society as a whole. He warned that there is a danger in such claims that they diminish the value of social distinctions and also lessen the severity of the actions of those who were really responsible. One must define the political, religious and socioeconomic background of the murderer and examine the historical context of the act.

Excavating the present

Feige planned to write a book on archaeology in Israel. He conceived a book together with Zvi Shiloni, *A Spade to Dig With: Archaeology and Nationhood in the Land of Israel*,[25] and even wrote a few chapters, but he did not succeed in bringing it to completion. Archaeology reveals the secrets of the past. Feige claimed that the great faiths, religions and nationalisms seek to reveal roots and identity, and archaeology serves them as a metaphor. Archaeology fired the imagination of the adherents of the Zionist movement as it was closely connected with their enterprise. An archaeological excavation is required when historical depth preserves a magnificent past and things are dangerous and hostile on the surface, as was the case with the Jewish community in Palestine in the years before the founding of the state, and is the case with the settlers in Judea and Samaria in our time. The immigrant and the settler make a covenant with their ancestors who lived in the country thousands of years ago, and archaeology is respected as something that rescues them from the past and brings them into the present. Perhaps the true reason for the diminished status of archaeology among the Israelis today is that in the short time that has elapsed since the days of Yigal Yadin and Moshe Dayan the surface has become more comfortable, and the ancestors who once lived in the country have become more strange, distant and alien. Moreover, the findings from the excavations are not in keeping with the myths we have grown up on. Strangely enough, the biblical archaeology that is supposed to strengthen the national narrative reveals the real Israel of the past as against the imagined Israel of the tales of the Bible.

Amos Elon said in his time that Israeli archaeologists not only look for pot-sherds in the depths of the earth, but also seek roots and identity. In his writings, Feige translated this insight into sociological terms. The archaeologist Eliezer Sukenik approached some young people from a kibbutz after the excavations at Beit Alpha and told them that something had been revealed to them that was not only a plot of land, but "history had been revealed to them, and they would see it with their own eyes." The people who in ancient times lived in the place where the excavations were conducted and the young kibbutz members belonged to the same nation! Biblical archaeology was Zionist inasmuch as it sought to delineate and stress the continuity of the Jews in the land of Israel. Jewish history for 2,000 years was seen as a bridge between the loss of national independence in the first century and its renewal in the twentieth. Sukenik saw the history of the Jews in the manner of the philosopher Friedrich Hegel, as a movement towards an end – Zionism as the fulfillment of history. The announcement of the discovery of Bar-Kochba's letters by Yigael Yadin, Sukenik's son, for instance, was deliberately made in the residence of the president, Yitzhak Ben-Zvi. In this way, national archaeology linked the ancient president with the modern president, and "the last commander-in-chief" (Bar-Kochba) as Israel Elded called him, with the first Israeli commander-in-chief, Yigael Yadin.

Zionism represented itself as a movement of return, but its model was not exactly Jewish society at the end of the Second Temple and in the years following its destruction. Plowing the land was more meaningful for the pioneers than excavating it until Skukenik came along and proposed seeing the archaeological remains of the ancient Jewish community as the beginning of the reviving Hebrew community. As in other national movements, the Greek and Italian, for example, in the Jewish national movement archaeology sought to anchor the resurrection of the nation in the modern era in the uncovered past. But what was special about the Zionist movement was the archaeological revelation of the people's affinity to its ancient location despite the fact that for most of the time it had lived outside it. The Bible and archaeology thus had the dual task of integrating the new society in Israel and revealing its roots and identity, and of asserting its initial ownership of the ancestral land in the face of the Arabs. As the journalist Shemuel Schnitzer said: "Zionism has no more effective tool of propaganda than the archaeologist's spade. Wherever he inserts his spade, the historical connection between the people of Israel and its land becomes proven and real."[26]

Feige's researches on archaeology were made at the end of its golden age and at the height of the period when its status was being questioned. The struggle against the *Haredi* (ultra-orthodox) demonstrators contributed to damaging its halo.[27] In addition to all-important questions like whether bones were damaged and whether there was a cemetery in the City of David, there was above all a disagreement over the claim of the archaeologists to own the roots of the nation and their unwillingness to share control of the national past with the ultra-orthodox. Moreover, it was not only the ultra-orthodox who proposed an alternative ideology reflected in their attitude to national archaeology. There were other groups who did not define themselves in accordance with the remote past of the land of Israel, but in accordance with their roots overseas. The many waters that have flowed under the bridges since then – the fragmentation of Israeliness, the criticism of Zionism and the undermining of the national narrative – have revealed an interesting paradox: the findings of national biblical ideology have diminished the greatness of the kingdoms of David and Solomon. Instead of archaeological investigation aggrandizing the heroic past with its discoveries, it has tended to diminish it. Thus, science undermined the past. Which came first: the critical archaeology (and other scientific disciplines) whose subversive findings raised questions about the exodus from Egypt, the conquest of the land and the greatness of the unified kingdom, and which strengthened the Zionism of the new Israelis against the old Zionism, or the post-Zionist way of thinking, the skeptics who in their researches came to conclusions not in keeping with the Zionist ideology? Perhaps a third possibility is the correct one: that there is a mutual affinity between the two.

The annual conferences of the Society for Exploring the Land of Israel and Its Antiquities, from the 1940s to the 1960s, reflected the unquestionable nationalism of the early Israelis. This was expressed in an emotional relationship to the biblical past, in an emphasis on the importance of science, in the absorption of immigrants and in integration into the area. In this yearly encounter, the scholars discussed important matters that lay outside their narrow field of research like the controversy about the conquest and settlement of the country in the biblical period between Yigael Yadin and Yohanan Aharoni. The masses flocking to the conferences, the participation of the country's leaders in them and the holding of the conferences in the periphery testified to the great popularity of archaeology, which reflected in the conferences the core subjects of Israeli nationhood-in-the-making. For the participants, this, according to Feige, "was an unforgettable formative experience, part of a period of personal and collective maturation which they return to and embrace nostalgically."[28] In the 1950 conference, Ben-Gurion said: "In the field of Jewish learning, Jewish archaeology will take its proper place, for all its achievements bring our past into the present and confirm our historical continuity in the country." This key concept of "bringing our past into the present" reflects the harnessing of archaeology to the connection of biblical history with the Zionist claim of returning to the ancestral land. In this way, the ideology used archaeology for its aim of forming a national identity.

With the development of the state, the annual conferences ceased to be forms of identity, a change which reflected a new relationship between Israeli science and the national culture. There was no longer any need for national archaeology and other scientific disciplines or state ceremonies to embellish a meta-narrative of an Israeli society with roots in the distant past. The normalization of the new society was sufficiently strong and sure of its identity to reject the ethos of a magnificent past. The way archaeology was integrated into official frameworks was more important, in Feige's opinion, than any specific archaeological study. With regard to the question of what came first, he thought that "it was not subversive findings that led to the disintegration of national archaeology but a social change that took place in Israel which changed the cultural position of every field of research."

In their first two decades, many of the conferences took place in the development towns, both because of the proximity of Beersheba, Ashkelon, Safed, Beit Shean, Eilat and Acre to the excavation sites, and in order to create a local memory that would connect the inhabitants of these places to the Zionist meta-narrative. These were considerations of fellow-feeling, with the intention of "bestowing memory on the region, and thus to respond to the problem of the symbolic emptiness of the periphery."[29] In their pilgrimage to the periphery, the elites sought to express their symbolic ownership of these distant regions. In this, their attempt resembled the visits, described by Clifford Geertz, of Queen Elizabeth I to her subjects in the periphery to symbolize the limits of her kingdom. The attempt to connect the periphery to the center which was part of the attempt to form a complete Israeli political body, and the attempt to make the inhabitants of the periphery into the nucleus of a pioneering endeavor, prompted Feige to make a critical observation: the elite's pilgrimage to the periphery as a way of symbolically asserting its control never stopped in the "other" periphery of the Arab villages.

The development towns were prototypes for a comparison between the disciplines of archaeology and anthropology. The archaeologists saw going to the periphery as a symbolic act of nationalization, an attempt to create a single national memory through the perception of a special past. The anthropologists, on the other hand, emphasized a variety of spaces, a periphery of memory, and the legitimacy of the "other," with the intention of telling the story of the separate identity of different communities. The metaphor of archaeology was in keeping with a single national memory and the metaphor of anthropology was in keeping with individual community and ethnic memories. The archaeologists were the high priests of civil religion and national identity, and the anthropologists, who believed in the representation of the "other," raised their voice in favor of "the silenced."

Feige wrote about three forms of "otherness": that of the periphery, that of the Haredim (ultra-Orthodox) and that of the settlers. The otherness of the periphery or development towns in the encounter with the archaeologists was seen by the latter as a temporary, illegitimate and denied otherness. The annual congresses of the Society for Exploring the Land of Israel and Its Antiquities boasted of raising the status of the inhabitants of the periphery and giving them a proper local identity as part of a comprehensive hegemonic attempt to annex them to the legitimate national identity. In revealing the remains of a magnificent past lying beneath the surface near their peripheral place of residence there was an intention of showing them that this was their own past and that they constituted an essential link in the chain of national historical continuity. Towards the periphery there was a patronizing attitude of adoption and appropriation on the part of the archaeologists, and towards the Haredim, the second "other," there was an attitude of hostility because they represented a radical ideological otherness which refused to recognize the Zionist narrative. In this case, also, the archaeologists found themselves representing the Zionist hegemony, but this time in face of the ultra-Orthodox, a homogeneous community which rejected the imperative of national transformation and adaptation to modernity. The ultra-orthodox campaign against archaeological excavations and disturbing the bones of the dead reached its climax in the excavations of the City of David in Jerusalem at the beginning of the 1980s. But the dispute between science and faith was thrust aside because of the significance of archaeology for Israeli nationhood, especially in face of the Palestinian otherness.

The conflict was not so much seen in terms of religion versus secularism; it was rather that the ultra-Orthodox were accused of harming the proof of the connection of the Jewish people with its land.

As Israel Eldad wrote:

> The struggle against the excavations in the City of David is not a matter of a dispute between science and faith […] It is one of the links in the chain of struggles over the fate of the city, or, in other words, the fate of the country, or, in other words, our own fate.[30]

Feige viewed this struggle from an interesting paradoxical angle. Between the two narratives concerning the struggle of the ultra-orthodox against archaeological excavations, the national and the Haredi, he thought there was more common ground than division. Secularism, science and nationalism which were open, positive and future-orientated, united in an official framework against a religious belief in the resurrection of the dead, the study of sacred texts, and a religious lifestyle. This being the case, who was more faithful to Jewish continuity: the ultra-orthodox or the archaeologists, faith or science? The outward aspect of Zionism, which demanded of the Jews a transformation to modernity in order to realize its ideology, was different from that of the ultra-Orthodox, who claimed to be the sole authentic representatives of Judaism.

If the otherness of the development towns was a denied one, and that of the ultra-Orthodox was a radical one, the otherness of the settlers was described by Feige as a radical nationalism. Here, in contrast to their attitude to the development towns, the archaeologists seemed to withdraw from their national obligation when the settlers asked them to continue to fulfill their original role as the guardians of the continuity of Jewish nationhood in the land of Israel. The ultra-Orthodox asked the archaeologists to stop their excavations in the name of the Jewish ethos, and the settlers asked them to continue. The settlers, like the earlier Zionists, saw archaeology as a means of contending with the hostile surface of life, but soon discovered that the archaeologists did not respond to their demand. Thus, they criticized the archaeologists who for scientific reasons cast doubt on the reliability of the biblical sources. The settlers claimed that the landscape of Kedumim and the findings from beneath the ground were proof of the Jewish past, while ignoring the Arab inhabitants on the surface.

Just as the settlers condemned the archaeologists for not fulfilling their national role, they criticized the secular Zionists for abandoning the legacy of the biblical past. Some of the scholars among the settlers said that the Zionist settlement which commemorated Zionist leaders in the names of settlements forsook their original names found in the Bible.[31] The settlers created an imaginary map for their own purposes: to legitimize the existing settlements as a continuation of the biblical settlements, to provide evidence of their chronological precedence over the Arab settlements, to give the settlers an identity, to restore the past and renew it, and to symbolically dispossess Palestinian nationalism in Judea and Samaria. The symbolic dispossession was of course intended to counter the semiotic map of the Palestinians, whose presence on the surface ironically recalled the biblical Hebrews.

The settlers said that unlike the Haskalah, whose view of the Bible as a book of history was adopted by the Zionists, they saw it as the sacred record of a past which should be restored. They therefore nurtured what I call a "restorative memory" of the Bible. The settlement movement sought to concretize images of the biblical past of the land of Israel. This concretization embodied various facets of the biblical historical memory. Some stressed the metaphysical principle of the commandment of settling the land, and some were intended to facilitate political compromises with regard to a sacred site or a sacred source. Perhaps Feige's interest in the affinity between archaeology and nationalism not only derived from a wish to examine the separate narratives of the periphery or the ultra-Orthodox or the settlers with regard to archaeology, but principally from a wish to examine the meta-narrative common to all of them, what is hidden from the eye, what is not talked about: the Palestinian otherness and how in a concealed way it formed the Zionist and Israeli identity.

The "old man" and the desert

The archaeologists have denied the biblical account of the children of Israel passing through Nahal Zin on their way to the land of Israel, but archaeological facts are one thing and the creation of a mythical space is another. Ben-Gurion's choice to be buried in the desert on the banks of Nahal Zin, in the place where, according to the faith, Moses and the ancient Hebrews went towards their motherland, has a dual significance. On the one hand, according to the pioneering view, the desert is virginal, a place without history, a place where the future can be written. On the other hand, it is connected with the ancient history of the people at the time of its formation, with the ancient myths that were a central element in the creation of the Israeli ethos. The founding father of the Hebrew rebirth looks out from the cliff at the place where the children of Israel passed on their way to the country. In other words, the reason the place was chosen had nothing to do with family, community or politics: it was the connection with the founding myth of the nation. As he attempted to do in his life, in his death Ben-Gurion defined himself as symbolically part of the monumental history of the Jewish people while avoiding questions connected with the social, political and even physical realities of his time.

I had the honor of being Feige's partner in writing some of the studies of David Ben-Gurion, including the study of the funeral which took place at the Midreshet Ben-Gurion shortly after the Yom Kippur War.[32] The funeral symbolized the maturation of Israeli society in a painful parting from its founder. It can also be seen as a symbolic transition of the State of Israel from an ideological society, mobilized and collectivist, to a fragmented society, polarized and lacking a common vision. It can be said that many of David Ben-Gurion's sanctified principles went down into the grave with him. But this did not stop the Israeli leaders from going southwards every year for the memorial ceremony at the grave of the "old man."

The forgotten funeral was in many ways a key event. Israel lost its founding father, and although he had retired from the leadership of the country years before, his authority overshadowed Israeli politics. Ben-Gurion died a month after the Yom Kippur War, which was a watershed moment in the history of the state. Many saw the symbolism of the moment of his passing at a time when Israel entered a new and uncertain stage. Ben-Gurion's funeral was characterized by a mass of contradictory logic and complex interests which can be grouped under three headings: the personal, the national-governmental and the bureaucratic. The order of the funeral was fixed first of all by the desire of the deceased, as expressed both in his will and his choice in advance of his place of burial. Ben-Gurion is considered a founding leader, but his view of the world was only partly accepted by those who thought themselves as continuing his path, and Israeli society in the 1970s was already a long way from the ideals he represented. The funeral allowed him for a last time to try to represent in a very impressive religious ceremony the values which he felt should guide the nation.

Parallel with Ben-Gurion's desire and in opposition to it, there was the official, national logic of the leaders of the period which placed Ben-Gurion in a context which seemed to them suitable, correct and in keeping with their political interests. Ben-Gurion placed the value of *mamlakhtiut* (statism) at the center of political existence in the early years of the state, but after he left the public arena there were significant changes. The fusion of the founding father with the evolving Israeli ethos was not necessarily in agreement with what he wanted.

Next to the requirements of Ben-Gurion and the state, the bureaucratic logic which ordered the ceremony in accordance with its rules and customs was also very important. The young state did not have much experience of ceremonial occasions of this kind, and the attempts previous to his funeral were seen as failures and not in accordance with the modern image that the young state wished to project. Thus, traditions had to be invented and anchored in hard and fast rules. As a result, the ceremony of Ben-Gurion's funeral and burial had an orderly protocol which imposed a bureaucratic logic both on the will of the deceased and on that of the commemorating state.

The statist principles represented by Ben-Gurion were already anachronistic in his lifetime. He was thrust aside, and in his last years many people saw them as pathetic. The moment of his death was a temporary return of Israel to the leader and his teachings, and Ben-Gurion sought to use that limited opportunity to the best of his ability. He succeeded in giving his death and burial the significance he wanted, but he failed in his death, as he failed in his last years in office, to create a path for the society and state to follow. A connection with the mythical ancient past is not noticeable in the Israel of today; pioneering has died out and arouses reactions of denial and mockery; the Negev and the periphery of the country have not changed much. He, for his part, went to a border area and in his last years remained in the neglected periphery without any real influence, and his grave is a site that many people visit, but few carry out the pioneering ideal it expresses. Once a year, on an official Day of Remembrance, the leaders of Israel come to the grave, and the tiresomely repeated message they pronounce is both negative because they did not carry out his commands and were negative and positive in their commitment to do so in the future. In his decision to be buried far from the Israeli political center, Ben-Gurion positioned himself as a great critical eye looking out at the leaders of Israel and judging their deeds. With a directness this is rare in occasions of this sort but in terms that already sounded anachronistic, prime minister Ehud Barak expressed this in the ceremony for the year 2000:

> Year after year, the "old man" troubles to summon the leadership of the state here, at the site of the grave facing the desert [...] Year after year, the leaders of the state come here to give an accounting. We as leaders must adhere to the path of Ben-Gurion. Say "yes" to the old man.[33]

In practice, however, most of the leaders of the state said "no" to the old man.[34] Together with the physical burial of the leader, his teachings were also buried. The funeral was a flash-in-the-pan, a last attempt to illuminate for a moment the pioneering and statist ideal. Feige who, as the specialist in memorials Vered Vinitzky-Seroussi pointed out, loved to set opposites against each other, revealed the means employed by Begin to make Ben-Gurion bestow legitimacy on his right-wing government. For that purpose, he had to make Ben-Gurion the father of the nation: "Begin changed him in order to change him."[35] Begin used Ben-Gurion in order to impose an agenda on a society that had long ago abandoned his path. Within four years of his funeral, a reversal accomplished by broad sections of Israeli society – the revisionist camp, religious Zionism, the Haredim and the Mizrahim, who felt alienated by the state he set up – was crowned with success. They opposed the universalist pretensions of his statist vision and at the same time wished to stress their particular contribution to the nation. Perhaps this reversal paradoxically was precisely a great victory for the statism envisaged by Ben-Gurion. Broad social groups attached themselves to the evolving Israeli democratic project and joined it, each in its own way. On the fourth anniversary, there stood before his grave the prime minister at that time, Menahem Begin, the declared successor of Zeev Jabotinsky – both of whom had been his bitter opponents – and declared, "In the place where the British flag was lowered, [Ben-Gurion] hoisted the flag of the renewal of Jewish independence."[36] In this way, Begin demonstrated, with characteristic historical cunning, that the change of political parties in Israeli society was also under the protection of the symbolic wings of the founding leader.

The memorial ceremony at the graveside confronts the real Israel with the imagined Israel and Ben-Gurion's vision, and the vicissitudes of the ceremony have reflected both the changing society and its attitude to the figure of the father of the nation.[37] This pilgrimage-like ceremony, in which the ruling elite and political center of Israel disconnect from their base and invade the geographical area of the community living in the Midrasha, puts the founding father in the position of an onlooker and a judge deciding if his successors were true to the high standards he represented and fulfilled the commandment of his legacy. The peripheral site makes Ben-Gurion special and differentiates him from all other prime ministers. But, let us not be deceived! Apart from two hours in one day of the year, Ben-Gurion does not serve as a national compass. The ceremony also frames and domesticates the "old man" and enables the governments of Israel to continue on their way, which can be contrary to his "statist" way, with tendencies to fragmentation, weakening of the welfare state, neglect of the periphery and a political theology aiming to fix the boundaries of the country.

A comparison between Ben-Gurion's and Rabin's memorial days is instructive with regard to both figures. Ben-Gurion is commemorated in an official way due to his status, both official and unofficial, which is uncontested. Compared to other prime ministers, his symbolic status is far above theirs, both because he was the first and because of the general picture of the courage and wisdom of the difficult decisions he made. Yitzak Rabin is not commemorated because he was a chief of staff, minister of defense or prime minster, and others who held these positions are not commemorated in this way or on this scale. Rabin is likewise not commemorated because of his decisions or policies, and the commemorators – the heads of state and the general public – do not have to identify with the Oslo Accords in order to honor his image. Rabin is commemorated because of what was done to him no less than because of what he himself had done.

But the comparison is liable to miss the salient point. The mass-mobilization to commemorate Rabin is due precisely to the weakness of the figure and the ceremony, the continual threat that hangs over them. The success of the commemorative enterprise reflects the failure of the enterprise for which he was murdered: namely, making peace with the Palestinians. It also represents the failure to mobilize the public-at-large in support of the peace process, a failure that found expression in the murder. The supporters of Rabin's path have to fight a ceaseless war for his memory, in which a large part of the public has no interest. The situation with regard to the memory of Ben-Gurion is quite different. Ironically enough, the marginality of Ben-Gurion's day of remembrance shows the success of the historical enterprise connected with his name. In accordance with the opinion of Ernest Renan, who claimed that a nation remembers failures more than its successes,[38] Ben-Gurion's day of remembrance can "permit itself" its marginality as it is an expression of success. Boredom and banality are one of the great achievements of the commemoration of Ben-Gurion. It is a commemoration which does not have many achievements apart from being self-evident. The calm routine of the Ben-Gurion commemorations as against the yearly agitation and misgivings attending the commemoration of Rabin, perhaps shows that unlike Rabin's achievements, which are a matter of controversy, the main achievements of Ben-Gurion are accepted by the majority, including his chief opponents.

The privatization of commemoration

The privatization of the Israeli identity in recent decades has necessarily also led to a privatization of bereavement, commemoration and memory. Each camp has its dead, each group has its commemoration. The change from a social-democratic welfare state to a state with a neo-liberal capitalist economy was accompanied by a cultural logic. The responsibility for setting the agenda, for the national values and the collective ethos passed from the state to the citizen. Bereavement was no exception to the process of privatization, but because it was still seen as a national affair that the state had not relinquished, and the state had not abandoned responsibility for the price in blood which its decisions and actions had incurred, there was a clear discrepancy here. On the one hand, bereavement had undergone a process of privatization, and on the other hand the process was not exhausted as the bereaved parents would not forgo the role of the state and its responsibility, for in this way they neutralized the personal trauma of the fall of their loved ones and divested it of its social significance. Parallel with this, the state also for its own reasons struggled with the privatization of bereavement. Feige, perhaps because of the sensitivity of the subject, did not take his ideas to their logical conclusion and say that the state needs bereavement, and it plays a role of primary importance in social and national integration.

In his study of the privatization of commemoration, memory and bereavement, Feige examined the way in which Gush Emunim and Shalom Achshav commemorated (or did not commemorate) the fallen of their movements;[39] how the bereaved families of the helicopter disaster waged their struggle to commemorate their loved ones;[40] and how the commemoration of the commemoration of Yitzak Rabin eclipsed his personal commemoration. One should remember that Feige's studies of the commemoration of Rabin were made at a time when the representatives of the past in Israel were subjected to a tsunami of negative criticism. A great deal of time passed before the events of the Holocaust and Israel's wars were researched, but the commemoration of Rabin was researched as soon as it took place. Feige wrote: "A case could be made for saying that the study of the commemoration was itself a way of dealing with the mourning and the trauma."[41] "One prophecies and knows not of what." One could put forward the argument that the introduction to this collection of articles by Feige, which was written in the year that he was murdered, was itself a way of dealing with the mourning and the trauma.

The processes of commemoration had gone through many changes from the beginning of Zionism to those days. The mechanism of commemoration acquires principles in keeping with the positions of the ruling group, the hegemonic ideology or the prevailing norm. The retroactive acquisition of selective principles by a leader, an ideology or an established process is the recognized basis of all mythicization. The ethos of settlement and defense in the 1920s interpreted the life and death of Joseph Trumpeldor in a mythological way. The *Gdud Ha-avodah* named after Trumpeldor acquired the socialist-communal principle, while the *Brit Joseph Trumpeldor* (Beitar) acquired the national, activist, anti-socialist principle. An example of the acquisition of a date is the declaration by the National Labor Federation of the second of Tammuz, the anniversary of the death of Herzl, as its festival. And that, of course, was the response to the first of May, the festival of the General Federation of Labor. There is also a selective acquisition of historical figures: Israel Eldad, on the right, saw the Bar-Kochba revolt as a positive myth of a struggle for national liberation; Yehoshafat Harkabi, on the left, saw it as a negative myth of lack of political realism leading to exile and extermination. The biography of Ben-Gurion was retroactively made into a "leader myth." The party-inspired principles of "without Herut or Maki" and the refusal to bring the bones of Jabotinsky to Israel were overlooked on account of the statist principles of "from a class to a people" and the founding of the State of Israel.

The criticism of the heroic cult of state idealism did not, of course, come into being overnight, and its origins are to be found in the perceptions of a critical generation. Little by little, the great edifice of sacrifice began to crumble. In the Yom Kippur War, the last nail was driven in the coffin of the mythological Sabra. That was the great time of significant changes in the Israeli ethos. A fragmentation of the national myths is only possible at such a time, when values change. Israel went from the ethos of a pioneering and heroic society – a compelling value – to the ethos of a consumer and media-centered society, and the myths changed accordingly, from the sacrifice of Isaac to the sanctification of individualism. The Israelis passed from an era of ideology to an era of media, from "what ought to be" to "what is," from Tel Hai to Channel Two, from the hero to the *freier*.

Together with his analysis of the official commemorations of Ben-Gurion and Rabin, Feige also analyzed the changes that have taken place in the forms of private commemoration in the last two decades. The change came from the change in the make-up of those commemorated and in the make-up of the bereaved families when an acceptance of those hit in hostile actions became of great importance in the acts of commemoration in Israeli society. One of the expressions of this – the construction of a monument on Mount Herzl to those killed in acts of terror – was accompanied by an arduous public struggle. Feige wrote:

> The main dispute was about the question: ought one to commemorate a civilian who was killed in civilian circumstances (for example, when he was sitting in a café in the context of his daily life) as if he were a soldier slain in battle?[42]

This controversy about civilians hit in acts of terror, he said, in some ways resembled the debate which took place in the Yishuv about the *Yizkor* book for the year 1911 which commemorated the death of guardsmen and workers.[43] The controversy in the Yishuv concerned the question of whether there was a difference between someone who fell when guarding and someone killed in an accident: for instance, when drowning in Lake Kinneret. The question of the distinction between civilian casualties and casualties in the forces of defense has accompanied Jewish society in the land of Israel from the beginning of Zionist settlement and comes up all the more strongly today.

The commemoration of those killed in hostile actions broadens the concept of commemoration, and brings one to a reconsideration of the question of the inclusion of the Israeli bereaved family. The monuments commemorating those killed in hostile actions were erected among other things because the number of those killed in acts of terror was greater than the number of those who fell on the battlefield. This new form of commemoration, according to Feige, not only represented a change in the landscape of Israeli monuments but also changed the composition of the Israeli bereaved family and included within it groups that until then had been excluded. The monument erected on the shore of Tel Aviv to commemorate those killed in the attack on the Dolphinarium Club in June 2001 who were mainly immigrants from the Commonwealth of Independent States, showed that acts of terror created new communities of bereavement and also new definitions of participation in the Israeli collective. In addition to new immigrants, acts of terror also hit others – Arabs, Haredim or migrant workers – whose sons had not in the past been among those fallen in battle.

The iconoclastic mood of the period deconstructed the figures of the leaders, heroes and fighters of the past. It uprooted the image of the founding fathers and the ethos of a pioneering, heroic, socialistic and secular Israel. In the view of some Israelis, this was a praiseworthy expression of maturation, a healthy and necessary process of adaptation to modernity and acceptance of it, and a liberation of society from the chains of ideology. The demystification of Israeli history was seen as a positive consequence of the peace process, which tended to stress negotiation and compromise rather than heroic values and self-sacrifice. Other Israelis, however, saw this tendency as an undermining of the foundations of the ethos and aims of Zionism, a blow to the collective national effort since the state was founded. The controversy about the founding values was represented as defeatism which could lead to national suicide. The dispute was not about the history as such but about Israeli society and its evolving identity.

At the height of the process of the fragmentation of Israelism, the Israelis suddenly experienced a fateful and fearful moment. In the helicopter disaster of the fourth of February 1997, seventy-three soldiers were killed on their way to Lebanon. Two helicopters collided and fell into a black hole without a witness, without a black box, without an enemy – without even a cosmological cause in the form of the weather – and without the context of a battlefield. The first helicopter came down in the cemetery of Kibbutz Dafna, and the other crashed into a zimmer: on the one hand, the graves of those fallen in 1948, and on the other, the symbol of normal contemporary Israelism. Was the disaster of the seventy-three a turning-point in the self-perception of the Israelis? What memorial would be suitable for this disaster and what would be the proper commemoration of the trauma?

The arbitrariness of the helicopter disaster demanded a narrative around it, a task generally fulfilled by the state. In following up the stages in the commemoration of the fallen, Feige examined the problematic and complex mesh of contradictions between the individual and the state. The state does not easily relinquish the fallen, for the simple reason that they help to unify it even in an age of privatization. In this respect, the interests of the bereaved families and the state coincide: both sides refuse to fragment and to separate. The bereaved parents are not interested in the loss of their loved ones remaining their private possession, and the state, for its part, needs the legitimation of the bereaved families which lends it a halo of sanctity. In his researches into the struggles of the families concerning the character of the monument to those killed in the disaster, Feige perceived the social and cultural changes that had taken place in Israel between the moment of the disaster and the erection of the monument eleven years later.

The privatization of commemoration was not only reflected in the helicopter disaster, but also in the different ways that Gush Emunim and Shalom Achshav dealt with the kind of memorial to be given to their fallen heroes. Rachel Druck, the mother of seven children, was killed in 1991 in an attack on a bus of settlers from Shilo on its way to a demonstration in Tel Aviv. Emil Grunzweig, a student, was killed by a Jewish assailant who threw a grenade on a Shalom Achshav demonstration on February 10, 1983. In the conclusion of his comparative study, Feige wrote that "as understood by the members of their movements, Rachel Druck and Emil Grunzweig had no place in the same pantheon of heroes. Can one speak of such a pantheon at all in our time?"[44]

Some women among the settlers, who included married women and mothers, and who called themselves "women of Rachel," set up a guard around the grave of Rachel Druck in order to build a settlement there. Rachel Druck became a ceremonial object of political memory, involving a mythologization which associated her with the famous Rachels of the biblical and Zionist narratives such as the matriarch Rachel and Rachel the poetess. Although the founding of settlements by women is an appropriation of something generally done by men, this did not exceed the traditional limits of the discourse between men and women. Rachel Druck was not a feminist symbol, and her nationalization and the "women of Rachel" were seen as "a metonymy of the return of the people of Israel to its land."[45] The settlers built up her memorialized image in accordance with the iconic value of her mythological name. In contrast to them, the people of Shalom Achshav were determined not to make an ideological use of the image of Grunzweig and to leave him as "other," individual and unique. He remained an accidental and arbitrary victim of ideological violence, whereas in the mythological treatment of the "settler" and "mother," the arbitrary nature of Rachel Druck's death was denied.

Emil Grunzweig, as a victim of the violence accompanying a demonstration in favor of the resignation of Arik Sharon, Minister of Defense at that time, preceded Yitzhak Rabin, the martyr of the peace camp, by twelve years. The political, secular, practical and "empirical" discourse of Shalom Achshav was in contradiction to the creation of myths by the settler camp. The members of Shalom Achshav saw their task as being to shatter myths rather than to create them. Although they recognized the value of myths in political struggles, they refused to use the death of Grunzweig and make him into a myth. One of their members said, "Shalom Achshav is not a church built on the blood of martyrs."[46] Yaron Ezrahi, who guided Grunzweig in writing his doctorate, said that his death represented a rare case of a political movement rejecting the temptation to turn it into kitsch. But, in contrast with the dominant approach of Shalom Achshav, far from the limelight, there was a political group of social activists which stressed the importance of myth and called itself "the Tenth of February." It combined the vision of peace with a demand for social justice, and coined the slogan, "Money for the neighborhoods and not for settlements!"

Rabin and Grunzweig were both seen as victims belonging to the dovish camp in Israel, but there is no doubt that due to Rabin's status both in his own right and as prime minister, there was a difference between the two. In his researches, Feige focused on the execution of Rabin's commemoration, which was reproduced on a massive scale, and the reproduction of which itself became a subject of research. There was the reproduction of Clinton's saying, *Shalom haver!* (Farewell, friend!); stickers on cars which made them into monuments on wheels; envelopes showing the first day after the murder, in which memorial candles appeared, the words of *Shir La-shalom* (The Song of Peace), and the phrase "Shalom haver"; the site of the murder designed by David Tartakover in which there was a basalt monument and a wall showing the framed graffiti of the first month and a list of the stages of Rabin's life; and the annual ritual of an official day of remembrance on Mount Herzl and a political day of remembrance in the square named after the murdered leader. To these one may add the innumerable signs of commemoration such as roads, streets and institutions named after him. Of this phenomenon of reproduction, Feige wrote with a characteristic touch of irony: "The graffiti had to be placed in a frame, the slogan had to be put on a label, the candles had to have Rabin's picture, the day of remembrance had to be given the Hebrew date."[47]

In 1967, the year of the "Hebrew revolution," the sons of religious Zionism took over the reins of Israeli nationalism from its secular founders. How ironic it is that the commander-in-chief in the war fought in that year, which bought the "little Israel" to the opening-up of the ancestral areas, was murdered by a supporter of the political theology of the Greater Land of Israel! The political murder caused a division between the two commemorative sites: the grave in Jerusalem and the site of the murder in Tel Aviv. Both sites are places of pilgrimage for those who honor Rabin's memory, but the public ceremonies that take place in them are different both in essence and in character. The official ceremony takes place on the day of remembrance for Rabin next to his grave on Mount Herzl, while the ceremony in Tel Aviv is a kind of reconstruction of the gathering in the square at the end of which the prime minister was murdered. The ceremonies are also held at different times. The ceremony on Mount Herzl takes place on the Hebrew date of the murder, and the ceremony in Tel Aviv, on the secular date. The two commemorations have different narratives: the official ceremony stresses the blow to democracy and the values of citizenship, and, the other – the political significance of the event.

Apart from the commemoration of Rabin himself and his activities, the commemoration of the components of commemoration are given prominence. Instead of commemorating the things that Rabin said and did, it is the things that Clinton said about him that are commemorated. This results in a sort of commemoration at second or third hand which is not a commemoration of Rabin himself but a continual reminder of the forms of mourning in the first days after the murder. Feige said that it seems that a commemoration of the commemoration is needed in this split society in which the image of the hero is challenged and confronted. The act of commemoration requires a reminder of the first moments of commemoration which were emotional and "authentic," and around which there is a relative agreement. The "commemorative industry," which reproduces and copies and industrializes, confirms Walter Benjamin's opinion that in the modern era, the aura, the uniqueness and the authenticity of the traditional means of commemoration have disappeared. The reproduction of the rituals lost to man is made in modern times through the thing through which they were lost: namely, technology.[48] The reproduction of commemoration replaces memory itself. Feige duplicated Benjamin's insight without specifically mentioning him, and claimed that "a considerable part of the reproduction reproduces precisely the reproduction itself." The real source of the commemoration – the figure of Rabin – which does not succeed in motivating the ceremony, undergoes a processing through the rituals of mourning. The acts of the mourners are reproduced like the other elements of commemoration. The ritual of aesthetic mourning replaces the political victim.

Where there is aesthetics for aesthetics' sake, memory becomes commemoration for commemoration's sake. The aesthetic rejects the political, the form voids the content, the duplicated act replaces radical criticism. The techniques of reproduction and the media create their own community and cause a manipulation of political activity. Thus, a series of actions and results can be determined in accordance with the reactions of the consumers of commemoration, already conditioned at the time of the commemorative action. Rituals, which reproduce and industrialize memory, permit a mobilization of citizens and a "commemoration of commemoration" (which causes the political reason for the murder of Rabin – the Oslo Accords – to be forgotten), to be set in motion. The aestheticization of politics makes the citizens participate in a political game in order to remove them from politics. Benjamin's insight is not far from our considerations. Modern man, including the citizen of Israel, has brought reason, science and the media to such a high level that he experiences violence, or its representation, as an aesthetic manifestation.

The day of remembrance for Rabin has been added to the Zionist movement's and Israeli society's tradition of memorializing and commemoration, but this addition to the calendar of the Israeli "civil religion" and the rituals of the community of memory was made at a time of the uprooting of central values of Zionism. The ethos of commemoration was likewise not exempted from criticism and reflection on representations of the past. Feige pointed to two parallel and contradictory views: one, the idea that social division prevents agreement about commemoration, and the other, that it is precisely social agreement that prevents a meaningful act of commemoration. As Avishai Margalit says, "A political murder must be remembered in a political way."[49] Certain kinds of commemoration (ideological, social, ethnic) determine the boundaries of the communities of memory: who belongs to us and who shares our grief. Because the polarized Israeli society cannot have an agreed image of the murdered prime minister, it is more convenient for it to leave Rabin as an empty symbol devoid of content and to commemorate the commemoration. Anyone who wishes to honor the memory of Rabin paradoxically causes a desecration of his name, and, as Yossi Sarid said, "Yitzhak Rabin is the most alive dead person that walks among us."[50]

To remember and to forget

Apart from his researches on political radicalism, social myths and memory and commemoration in Israeli society, Feige was interested in globalization and the day after the conflict with the Palestinians, and, as he said, "a new, perhaps post-Zionist Israel, liberated from ideological fetters."[51] He showed an original approach to an examination of the boundaries of Israelism in his research with

Louis Runger on the culture of the *freier* in Israel. The study of the refusal to be a *freier* as a sociological and psychological phenomenon brought him to the conclusion that we have here authentic Israelism that derives from the discrepancy between the altruistic discourse of the 1950s, 1960s and early 1970s and the novel critical norms adopted by the new Israelis. Unlike the pioneer or the Sabra who in the past determined who belonged to the Israeli ethos, belonging today is determined by a capacity to make an intelligent use of a cultural indicator as a testimony of oneself. That is to say, the Israeli bears witness to himself as someone familiar with social norms.

Israelism has long ago discarded its collective identity, and now "Israel in the age of the *freier* is a society of people whose lives on the spot provide them with the meaning of their existence."[52] The image of the Israeli has changed from an authentic, ideal mythological figure of a pioneer with a harmonious and comprehensive world-view to a non-ideological individual, critical of heroism and sacrifice. But because sacrifice has not completely disappeared from Israeli society, there is a gray area in which questions are asked concerning the meaning of pioneering and freierdom. The discourse concerning the *freier* expresses a dialectical relationship with the myth of the Israeli rebirth, and at the same time it requires a continual confrontation with the subject of sacrifice. The concept of the *freier* is not detached from the ideals of Zionism, and conducts a reflective discussion with the image of the pioneer and his collectivist values. The *freier* is a tale that the society tells about itself, about an Israel that has not completely passed from collectivism to individualism, and the individual who refuses to be a *freier* is a by-product of the pioneer who paradoxically rises against his maker.

It is tempting to say that Feige was not a *freier*, and he refused to accept at face value the self-definition of Shalom Achshav as a movement whose sole motivation was the struggle against the annexation of the territories and the process of colonization. He proposed something else: to examine the movement as representing a class conducting a process in which the class reproduces itself in accordance with global changes.[53] The change that the movement wanted to make was described by Bruno Latour as a re-modernization of Israel with the aim of gaining the new middle class a position of leadership.[54] The process of globalization was taking place at a time when the concepts of time and space were changing because the communication technologies were penetrating the frontiers of the state. The dominance of huge trans-national companies and the world-wide distribution of labor did not exclude Israel at the beginning of the 1990s. These economic processes were accompanied by processes in the social, cultural and ideological spheres which can be described as "the privatization of Israelism." The new middle class in Israel encouraged the globalization and challenged the old middle class which was connected to the national and collectivist values and the symbolic benefits derived from them.

It was the new middle class, said Feige, that was behind Shalom Achshav, whose program refused to diverge from the agenda of the occupation. He criticized those on the left who justified a purely dovish agenda which concentrated solely on the occupation and ignored subjects such as the just distribution of wealth and social solidarity. Similarly, Feige revealed the problematic nature of the support of the members of Shalom Achshav for the process of globalization which contributed to the weakening of broad classes in the Israeli periphery and the Palestinian population. The weakening of these classes also hurt the interests of large-scale capital in that it disturbed the tranquility in which it wished to operate. Shalom Achshav's claim that advancing the cause of peace was more important than social issues was unusual in Western societies. The reason for this order of priorities was the fact that Shalom Achshav did not emerge from a protest movement against Western modernity but from a protest against that protest.

Shalom Achshav saw itself as modern and enlightened, and its rivals were regarded as not modern. Gush Emunim in particular was seen as anti-modern because of its propensity for myths from the past, national particularism and Jewish fundamentalism. Feige refused to accept this simplistic correlation and said that Gush Emunim was in a tense situation between joining globalization and rejecting it, unlike Shalom Achshav, which was not ambivalent concerning global processes. The increasing presence of the Haredim in the public sphere, the return to traditionalism and ethnic self-assertion were also seen as tendencies opposed to the forms of universal secular modernity represented by Shalom Achshav. It reacted with fear and protestation to these sociological changes which were liable to hurt the class interests of its members who saw themselves as representatives of a movement striving for a restoration of Western modernity. Its members wished to engage in a process of restoring the values of rationality, materialism, science and progress which characterized the "initial" modernism associated with the secular nationalism of the 1950s and 1960s.[55] The dark sides of modernism were excluded from the discourse of Shalom Achshav, and difficult social and economic questions were also thrust aside. Its modernistic ethos was in keeping with capitalist values.

The two examples discussed by Feige – the complex relationship to mass-demonstrations and the criticism of the use of political myths – illustrate the nature of Shalom Achshav as a modernistic movement which pursued a strategy of avoiding any hint of non-modernity. Shalom Achshav was a chorus of adherents who condemned the critics of modernity and affirmed the processes of modernization. The movement participated in the privatization of Israelism by its assertion of the values of individualism, critical thought, and a knowledgeable and educated society, which by their very nature undermine an intellectual and national collectivism. Unlike the "national camp" which the world associates with occupation and colonialism, Shalom Achshav created a mass-identity for the new middle class, and this enabled it to continue to thrive even in difficult circumstances. And, today, what will remain of the memory of Shalom Achshav?

The fickleness of memory, said Feige, will be revealed on the day after the end of the conflict between Israel and the Palestinians. Then there will be new critical thinking about it – about its causes and effects. At the end of the conflict there will be a change from a violent situation to a state of mind that will correctly assess the character of the traumas, the memories, the symbols, the rituals, the figures and the representations to which the Israelis have become accustomed. There will be a change from memory to forgetting: if the conflict depends on memory, the day after will be characterized by forgetfulness. Unlike the feeling of justice and conciliation with which conflicts based on confronting the memory of the past, such as the apartheid regime in South Africa or the decolonization in Latin America ended, the conflict in our area will not end with a sense of justice accomplished. The condition for conciliation will be disconnection from memory: each side will have to forget the hostile actions of the other. "Each side has to understand that even if the murderers of its sons are on the other side of the border, it cannot make any claims against them. It is a difficult forgetting from the emotional point of view,"[56] but it is even harder to ask the Israelis and Palestinians to forget their national narratives based on the denial of the narrative of the other. The Oslo Accords were a starting point for the possibility of forgetting. The Accords were signed at a time when there was a desire to forget the extinct memory and sacred significance of places in Judea and Samaria. Practical steps changed symbolic values, and, together with this, "forgetfulness replaced memory." But the Oslo Accords did not succeed in taking off because the two sides forgot to forget. Hanan Porat did not forget Rachel's Tomb and the Palestinians did not forget the right of return. Feige therefore once again insisted: "As I said, the day after depends above all not on the capacity to forgive but on the capacity to forget, or at least on the capacity to place memory in inverted commas."[57]

At the heart of the dispute is the unwillingness to forget. In Rabbi Zvi Yehuda Hacohen Kook's famous address on the eve of the Day of Independence in 1967, his rhetorical question is particularly striking: "Where is our Hebron – have we forgotten it?" Nothing was more important to him than the prohibition on forgetting the realms of memory in the land of Israel.[58] On the other hand, at the heart of Ben-Gurion's outlook there was the deliberate forgetfulness expressed in his answer to Geula Cohen who interviewed him on the eve of the Six-Day War: "The boundaries of your homeland are the boundaries of the State of Israel today."[59] The war suddenly removed the cobwebs of forgetfulness that had covered Jerusalem since 1948. The realignment with the biblical realms of memory "took place so quickly that it seemed that the forgetfulness that preceded it had been quite superficial."[60] Gush Emunim not only sought to return to the places of the Bible but gave the new settlements biblical names. Beyond the theoretical memory there was a political hyper-memory that gave rise to actions based on a reliance on the past.

Did this re-establishment of the biblical memory, at the center of which was the settlement enterprise aimed at connecting with the historical roots of the Jewish people, succeed in gaining a foothold among the Israelis and convincing them that it was forbidden to part from Judea and Samaria? If tens of thousands of settlers had to leave the settlements, said Feige, the trauma would not affect most Israelis, but only limited circles. The precedent of the evacuation of

Yamit left the Israelis indifferent and far from a feeling of national trauma. Although the evacuation of parts of Judea and Samaria would be far more significant, it would nevertheless be bearable and Israeli society could live with it. The memory of the evacuation would not become a motivation for return, because in many ways Israel has already forgotten the reasons for entering Judea and Samaria. As far as the Israeli public is concerned, Judea and Samaria have been lost, "but the degree to which they are forgotten depends on situations whose nature cannot be foreseen today."[61] The memory of the former settlers will coexist in the future with the process of fragmentation in which the national memory will disintegrate, and in place of it there will be the particular memories of different groups in Israeli society, each of which will nurture its own narrative.

In this scenario, religious Zionism will need to redefine its place. Many of the former settlers will see themselves as refugees, and religious Zionists will proclaim the experience of their uprooting and traumatic evacuation in the public sphere. The call for the right of return to the evacuated places will be heard in all the media and in all sites of memory, and the motivation to return to Judea and Samaria will be nurtured like the precedent of Gush Etzion. The commemoration of the commemoration of religious Zionism in the community of memory will preserve the restorative memory. The problem of the Jewish refugees will replace the problem of the Palestinian refugees in the public and international agendas, and the former settlers will reproduce the forms of commemoration used shortly before by the Palestinian refugees. The end of the conflict will find the former settlers "with many programs of memory and forgetfulness." To this change will be added many permutations expected in the post-conflict period, and here are some of them: a democratization of bereavement and its extension to other populations not previously included; a conciliation with the memory of Rabin and his expropriation from the political party to which he belonged; a raising of the status of the new historians and critical scholars because the conflict is no longer an issue; the diversion of archaeology from the investigation of the national past to the excavation of sites intended for economic development – a change that will release archaeology from the yoke of memory.

The Azrieli Towers, the beating heart of globalization in Israel, embody the future in which memory tends to be forgotten. Their geometric form is a testimony to the new Israelism, clean and direct, free from the deformity of the conflict and the distortions of the past, it is the architectural embodiment of the idea that Israel has decided to forget the conflict. The towers are symbols of a post-national age in which the mall in the center is a kind of eye of the symbolic space of the State of Israel. The globalized character of the mall represents a domestication of the Israeli political street. The towers are the temple of the new Tel Aviv. In the advertisements of the telephone company Bezek, Tel Aviv and Jerusalem have the same tariffs, but the former is represented as a capitalist in the globalization process and the latter is given the national role of commemorating an ancient king. One is detached from the place and its conflicts and the other is connected with the place through its messianic expectations. This difference expresses Israel's option in the future: to remember or to forget.

Another commercial center figures in Tamar Berger's book, *Dionysius at the Center*, which relates the history of a certain geographical area: the one now occupied by the Dizengoff Center in Tel Aviv.[62] Its past is examined from the time the land was owned by an Arab landowner from Jaffa, through the time it was the Nordia neighborhood of small Jewish businesses, to the period of the building of the mall and the tower above it. Berger in her writing gives a combination of names from different worlds which are unconnected from the point of view of the Zionist historical consciousness. It is a combination that recalls Michel Foucault in *Les Mots et les choses* (Words and Things)[63] – one that undermines the basic accepted ideas of Zionism. The space is given an Arabic name and a Hebrew, bureaucratic and literary name, a name in the present and a name in the past, a name from history and a name from memory, a private name and a collective name. This whole mixture of course contradicts the basic idea of a historical narrative. The proliferation of names of the space shows that the space has no name of its own, and, together with this, there is the question of its historical ownership and responsibility for what was done in the past. The analysis provides a basis for a fruitful discussion on the subject of the positivist historians and the critical historians and the surprising affinities between them.

The Dizengoff Center embodies the dialectic of memory and forgetfulness. Berger's book presents the stories of a small space beneath which there are archaeological strata of previous inhabitants. The building of the towers sweeps history under the carpet and causes the members of the Hinawi family and the Ashkenazi petty traders to be forgotten (they were transferred to a new neighborhood or a refugee camp). Inspired by Walter Benjamin, who asked for the fur to be brushed contrary to the direction of history,[64] Feige's project of memory illuminates great distances and likewise redeems figures which have been forgotten. The restoration of former archaeological strata is in his opinion "an interesting record of memory and forgetfulness"[65] which turns the searchlight of memory on dark areas which the national narrative has previously hidden from us.

Another small space, or, rather, reduced space – the site of "Mini-Israel" near the Latrun intersection – also serves as an occasion for a discussion on the imagined Israel.[66] The site represents an Israel that is utopian, complete, and in accordance with the precepts of beauty and order. Its beauty consists in excluding deprivation and preserving the utopian, and its success is connected with the longing for utopia. The Zionist narrative makes a critical assessment of the existing situation and demands a change in a national and modern direction. It requires a "Judaization" of the country. "Mini-Israel" does not reflect this narrative, because the latter is connected to reality and what exists and even promotes it (as in the Israel National Trail). Likewise, in more controversial matters like the occupation, the settlements and the Greater Land of Israel, the site makes the choice of disregarding them. Thus, the site is more perfect and ideal than the reality. But Feige, an artist in depicting small details within a larger picture, noticed that some of the miniature models – dolls representing Muslims praying on the Temple Mount, for example – are kept in transparent plastic boxes because the Jewish visitors damaged them again and again:

> This expression of violence, real and symbolic at the same time, shows that there are visitors who relate to the site as if it is not a model but a reality. Perhaps they express in this way a position concerning the limits of legitimate representation, and perhaps, as in the Voodoo ritual, they try to harm the thing symbolized by harming the symbol.[67]

Unlike the secular space – the Azrieli Towers, the Dizengoff Center and "Mini-Israel" – the space of Judea and Samaria is the Promised Land for the settlers – the heavenly Israel. Feige noticed that at the height of the Oslo process, Elyakim Haetzni claimed that the Rabin government, instead of evacuating the settlements – in his words, taking the fish out of the water – dried them out, took away the water and left the fish. The settlements remained where they were after Oslo, but without any water to swim in. Haetzni's image reminded Feige of another metaphor, from the historian Pierre Nora. The sea when it retreats leaves deposits behind it. The sea is the past and the deposits are remnants that attach themselves to the past but are separate from it, suspended between life and death. After the great wave of Gush Emunim and of Israel's attempt to assert its presence in Judea and Samaria has retreated, the settlements are left behind. They are no longer a pioneering enterprise intended to lead to a broader action, but they are still an integral part of the state under whose protection their members came to that place to realize their dream. Rather than realms of the biblical past after which they were named, Ofra, Shilo, Alon Moreh and Beit El are places commemorating the movement of memory that set them up. The whole process which had given them their significance had been lost.

Notes

1 Pierre Nora, "Memory: From Liberty to Tyranny," A lecture in the National Academy of the Sciences in Israel, February 16, 2016; ibid., *Realms of Memory: Rethinking the French Past*, Vol. 1–2, Colombia University Press, New York 1996.
2 Michael Walzer, *Interpretation and Social Criticism*, Harvard University Press, Cambridge MA 1987.
3 Michael Feige, *One Space, Two Places: Gush Emunim, Peace Now and the Construction of Israeli Space*, Magnes Press, Jerusalem 2003 (in Hebrew).
4 Ibid., 22–24.
5 Ibid., 18.
6 Fernand Braudel, *La Méditerranée et le monde méditerranéen à l'époque de Philippe II*, Le livre de poche, Paris 1993.
7 David Ohana. "The Myth of Nimrod: 'Canaanism' between Zionism and 'Post-Zionism'," *Modernism and Zionism*, Palgrave Macmillan, Basingstoke 2012, 122–179.
8 Feige, *One Space, Two Places*, 79.

9 Ian Lustick, *For the Land and the Lord: Jewish Fundamentalism in Israel*, Council on Foreign Relations Press, New York 1991.

10 Antonio Gramsci, *Selections from Prison Notebook*, Lawrence & Wishart, London 1971.

11 Feige, *Settling in the Hearts: Jewish Fundamentalism in the Occupied Territories*, Wayne State University Press, Detroit 2009.

12 Nehemia Stern, Review of: Michael Feige, "Settling in the Hearts: Jewish Fundamentalism in the Occupied Territories," *Review of Middle East Studies*, 45, 1 (Summer 2011), 104–105.

13 Hadas Weiss, Review of: Michael Feige, "Settling in the Hearts: Jewish Fundamentalism in the Occupied Territories," *Cultural Anthropology*, 24, 4 (November 2009), 755–757.

14 Feige, "Where is 'Here'?: Scientific Practices and Appropriating Space in the Discourse of Israeli Social Movements," in (eds.) A. Paul Hare and Gideon M. Kressel, *Israel as Center Stage: A Setting for Social and Religious Enactments*, Bergin & Garvey, Westport, CT 2001, 43–71.

15 Ibid.

16 Uri Ram, "No Border: Two Maps to the West Bank – Gush Emunim, Shalom Achsav and the Creation of the Israeli Public Sphere," *Haaretz-Books*, 9.6.2003 (in Hebrew).

17 Feige, Review of: Akiva Eldar and Idith Zertel, "Lords of the Land: The War Over Israel's Settlements in the Occupied Territories, 1967–2007," *Zmanim*, 93 (2006), 106–109 (in Hebrew).

18 Michael Feige, "The Yom Kipur War in Israeli Memory: Break and Continuiety," in (eds.) Moshe Shemesh and Ze'ev Drori, *National Trauma, Yom kippur War: After Thirty Years and Another War*, The Ben-Gurion Research Institute, Sde Boker 2008, 351–366 (in Hebrew).

19 Gideon Aran and Michael Feige, "The Movement to Stop the Withdrawal in Sinai; A Sociological Perspective," *The Journal of Applied Behavioral Science*, 23, 1 (1987), 73–88.

20 Michael Feige, "The Yamit Evacuation and Gush Emunim," *The Fourth Decade*, (eds.) Yehiam Weiz and Zvi Zameret, Yad Ben-Zvi, Jerusalem 2016, 91–105.

21 Michael Feige, "Yitzhak Rabin: His Commemoration and the Commemoration of his Commemoration," in *Memory in Controversy – Myth, Nationality and Democracy*, Research following Yitzhak Rabin's murder, (ed.) Lev Grinberg, Hamphrey Institute for Social Studies, Jerusalem 2000 (in Hebrew).

22 Michael Feige, "Rabin's Assassination and the Ethnic Margins of Religious Zionism," *Theory and Criticism*, 45 (Winter 2015), 31–56 (in Hebrew).

23 Ibid.

24 Ibid.

25 Michael Feige and Zvi Shiloni, (eds.) *Archeology and Nationalism in Israel*, Ben-Gurion Research Institute, Sde Boker 2008 (in Hebrew).

26 Shmuel Schnitzer, "With the Company against Zionism," *Ma'ariv*, 29.7.1983. The article is quoted by Feige in: Feige and Shiloni, *Archeology and Nationalism in Israel*, 5 (in Hebrew).

27 Michael Feige, "The Vision of the Broken Bones: Haredim vs. Archeologists in the City of David, 1981," in (eds.) Emmanuel Sivan and Kimmy Kaplan, *Israeli Haredim: Integration without Assimilation*, Van Leer Institute, Jerusalem 2003, 56–81 (in Hebrew).

28 Michael Feige, "Identity, Ritual and Pilgrimage: The Meetings of the Israeli Exploration Society," in (eds.) Deborah Dash Moore and S. Ilan Troen, *Divergent Jewish Cultures: Israel and America*, Yale University Press, New Haven 2001, 87–106.

29 Michael Feige, "Archaeology, Anthropology and the Development Town: Constructing the Israeli Place," *Zion*, 63:4 (1998), 441–459 (in Hebrew).

30 Michael Feige, "Archaeology's Imagined Communities: On Nationalism, Otherness and the Surface Level," *Democratic Culture*, 12 (2009), 167–206 (in Hebrew).

31 Michael Feige, "Gush Emunim and Biblical Names of Settlements," in (ed.) Dani Yaakobi, *Nation Building*, Magnes Press, Jerusalem 2000, 121–130 (in Hebrew).

32 Michael Feige and David Ohana, "Funeral at the Edge of a Cliff: Israel Bids Farewell to David Ben-Gurion," *Journal of Israeli History*, 31:2 (2012), 249–281.

33 Uri Binder, "Everything is Political," *Zman HaNegev*, 8.12.2000; Oded Bar-Meir and Gal Levinson, "We Should Look in his Way," *Kol HaNegev*, 8.12.2000.

34 In this context, an interesting observation is the growing legitimacy that Ben-Gurion wins in the Israeli right-wing camp, a legitimacy that can be found in Begin's speech at the ceremony for the foundation of the Likud in September 1973, "The pupils of Ben-Gurion and Jabotinsky."

35 Vered Vinitzky-Seroussi, "Michael's Glasses: Funerals, Memory, Commemoration and the Israeli Society," a lecture delivered at the conference of the Israeli Sociology Society, February 2014.

36 Shlomo Givon, "Menahem Begin in Sde Boker: Commemoration of Ben-Gurion," *Ma'ariv*, 17.11.1977.

37 Michael Feige and David Ohana, "Ben-Gurion's Commemorative Rituals: State Rituals at the Edge of the Desert," *Israel*, 22 (2014), 159–181 (in Hebrew).

38 Ernest Renan, Qu'est-ce qu'une nation, Conférence Faite en Sorbonne, 11.3.1882, Paris 1892.

39 Michael Feige, "Privatizing Commemoration: The Helicopter Disaster Monument and the Absent State," in (eds.) Rachel S. Harris and Ranen Omer-Sherman, *Narratives of Dissent: War in Contemporary Israeli Arts and Culture*, Wayne State University Press: Detroit 2012, 44–64 (in Hebrew).

40 Michael Feige, "Let the Dead Go: Commemoration Practices in Gush Emunim and Peace Now," in (eds.) David Ohana and Robert Wistreich: *Myth and Memory: Transfigurations of Israeli Consciousness*, Van Leer Institute, Jerusalem 1996, 304–320 (in Hebrew); ibid., "Do Not Weep Rachel: Fundamentalism, Commemoration and Gender in a West Bank Settlement," *Journal of Israeli History*, 21, 1–2 (2002), 119–138; ibid., "Rescuing the Person from the Symbol: Peace Now and the Ironies of Modern Myth," *History and Memory*, 11:1 (1999): 141–168.

41 Feige, "Yitzhak Rabin: His Commemoration and the Commemoration of his Commemoration."

42 David Ohana, "Commemorational lecture in honor of Michael Feige," Ben-Gurion University of the Negev, Israel, 12.7.2016.

43 Jonathan Frankel, "The 'Yizkor' Book of 1911: A Note on National Myths in the Second Aliya," *Religion, Ideology and Nationalism in Europe and America: Essays presented in Honor of Yehoshua Arieli*, Historical Society of Israel, Jerusalem 1986, 355–384.

44 Feige, "Let the Dead Go: Commemoration Practices in Gush Emunim and Peace Now."

45 Ibid.

46 Feige, *One Space, Two Places*, 213.

47 Feige, "Yitzhak Rabin: His Commemoration."

48 Walter Benjamin, "Theories of German Fascism," *New German Critique*, Spring (1979), 120–128; ibid., *The Work of Art in the Age of Mechanical Reproduction*, CreateSpace Independent Publishing Platform, Seattle 2010.

49 Quoted by Yeshayahu Libman in *Political Murder: The Murder of Rabin and Political Murder Throughout The Middleast*, Am Oved, Tel Aviv 1998 (in Hebrew).

50 Yossi Sarid, "Died Twice: Yossi Sarid Commemorates the Forgotten Rabin," *Ma'ariv*, 26.10.2015 (in Hebrew).

51 Luis Roniger and Michael Feige, "From Pioneer to Freier: The Changing Models of Generalized Exchange in Israel," *European Journal of Sociology* 33:2 (1992), 280–307.

52 Ibid.
53 Feige, "Peace Now and the Legitimation Crisis of 'Civil Militarism'," *Israel Studies*, 3:1 (1998): 85–111.
54 Bruno Latur, *We Have Never Been Modern*, (trans.) Catherine Porter, Cambridge MA 1993.
55 Shmuel N. Eisenstadt, *Multiple Modernities*, Routledge, London 2002.
56 Michael Feige, "The Morning After Remembers the Night Before," 521–568, in (ed.) Meron Benvenisti, *The Morning After: The Age of Peace – Not a Utopia*. Truman Institute, Magnes Press, Jerusalem 2002 (in Hebrew).
57 Ibid., 505.
58 Gideon Aran, "From Religious Zionism to Zionist Religion: The Roots of Gush Emunim," *Studies in Contemporary Jewry*, 2 (1986), 116–143.
59 *Ma'ariv*, 12.5.1967 (in Hebrew).
60 Feige, "The Morning After Remembers the Night Before."
61 Ibid.
62 Michael Feige, "The Names of the Place: New Historiography in Tamar Berger's Dionysus at the Center," *Israel Studies Review*, 19:2 (2004): 54–74.
63 Michel Foucault, *The Order of Things: An Archaeology of the Human Sciences*, Routledge, London 1994.
64 David Ohana, "Walter Benjamin, Ernst Bloch and the Fascist Myth," in David Ohana, *Homo Mythicus*, Sussex Academic Press, Eastbourne and Chicago, 2009, 95–105.
65 Feige, "The Morning After Remembers the Night Before."
66 Feige, "Mini Israel: The Israeli Place Between the Global and the Miniature," in (eds.) Julia Brauch, Anna Lipphardt and Alexandra Nocke, *Jewish Topographies: Visions of Space, Traditions of Place*, Ashgate, Aldershot, UK 2008, 327–342.
67 Ibid.

7   Settlers and the Land of the Bible

The connection between the Bible and the Land of the Bible – the realms of memory of Judea and Samaria – is the most important matter in the settlers' political theology. The attitude to the Bible is a seismograph for scrutinizing the attitude of Zionism, in general, and that of the settlers, in particular, to their ideological and political world-view. To where in the Bible are the settlers returning? To the Land of Canaan, to the land of the Patriarchs, or perhaps to the Kingdom of David? And what is the meaning of this return? It is not only the land that is basic to this question, but the relationship of the Land of Israel to the people of Israel. This *credo* is the basis of the settlers' ideal. The early leaders of the Zionist movement and the figures of the Second Aliyah turned to the Bible to establish their claims to the land. They were reluctant to base their right to the land on the divine promise.[1] Religious Zionism combined the divine promise with Zionist ideology, which is essentially secular. It was only after the Six-Day War in 1967 that the religious settling project made the biblical promise of the land the sole basis of the legitimacy, at once political and theological. *Gush Emunim* [The Bloc of the Faithful], was an Israeli Orthodox Jewish, messianic, right-wing activist movement, which fine-tuned the project and brought it to fruition was the most decisive, methodical political theology in the seventy years of the existence of the State of Israel.

For broad circles of religious Zionism, the State of Israel is a stage in the Redemption, about which it was said, in the religious kibbutz movement as well, that it is "the first manifestation of the approach of our redemption."[2] The secular political echelon in the State of Israel would be absorbed into the messianic movement as a *sine qua non*, as an essential stage that cannot be dispensed with. This attitude to the State, as a stage in the process of redemption, permeated the philosophy of history of the followers of Rabbi Abraham Isaac Hacohen Kook, his son Rabbi Tzvi Yehuda Kook, the leaders of *Gush Emunim*, and major rabbis of settler Zionism, for whom the biblical kingdom of Israel is a restorative model destined to take over from the secular political structure.

Gershom Scholem distinguished between a restorative (regenerative) messianism intended to revive a political or social model from the past, as in "renew our days as of old," and a "utopian messianism" that takes place after an apocalyptic crisis and diverges from historical time, entering a different kind of time.

The restorative utopia, in his view, is a redemption that takes place in the future but restores a historical golden age, or as he puts it, "This utopianism seizes upon all the restorative hopes turned toward the past [...]."[3] In this sense, the biblical land of secular Zionism is not the settlers' land. Native-born Israelis like Amos Kenan, Haim Guri and other secular figures longed for the biblical homeland, the land of the Bible, but did not put their yearnings to practical effect and did not participate in the settler movement.

For this reason, this chapter will not deal with secular Zionists but only with the biblical land of faith, in which the settlers attempt to create a restorative utopia.[4] I shall examine how the scholars among the settlers reconstructed the locations and names of biblical places as part of the process of the restorative vision. I shall present various positions with regard to the claim that there is a linkage between settlers and the Canaanite ideal and the contradictory assertion represented by the settlement movement thinker Yosef Ben-Shlomo that constitutes the foundation of the restorative vision: the future legitimization is bound up with the land of the Bible and not with any state entity. I shall describe how the Zionism of faith changed from a national-Zionist enterprise into a religious-messianic enterprise, a notion that puts into practice the restorative ideal, or more precisely, some models of restorative utopias prevalent among the settlers, such as the hyper-statist theocracy of Rabbi Zvi Yisrael Tau; the kabbalistic model of absolute monarchy of Rabbi Yitzchak Ginsburgh as opposed to a secular state; and the a-political model of Rabbi Menachem Froman. These models do not encompass the entire range of broad settler faith, or all the streams of settlement in the areas occupied in 1967. In this chapter, I shall mainly address the radical theological facets of the settler movement, not the proponents of Greater Israel, not the prominent settler leaders like Hanan Porat and Yoel Bin Nun, nor the pragmatic faction of *Gush Emunim* (Gershon Shefet, Meir Har-Noy, and others), on whom many studies have been conducted. Here I shall focus on the replication of settler theology from the first stage of *Gush Emunim* and the act of settlement, which in the opinion of the settlers is in accord with the continuation and completion of the Zionist project, to a more metaphysical phase, in which the centrality of the act of settlement gives way to Hassidic or kabbalistic thinking. The models which I present, make possible a fresh look at the utopian thinking and radical theology that are nourished by the settler movement and reflect a new, non-homogeneous stage. Of course, the proponents of the messianic-theological program in Judaism do not constitute the whole picture.

The broader theological perspective

Classical Catholic reading holds that the coming of Christ changed the development of sacred history and specifically the relation between God and the Israelites and their relation to the Holy Land. According to Augustine, the Christian Church, as the body of Christ, formed a new covenant that abolished the historical role of the Jews. According to Augustine's *Replacement Theology*, the Jews were kept only as witnesses and lost their unique role in sacred history. With that, their claim to the land of Israel was abolished as well.[5]

An alternative view of the role of the Jews and their relation to the land of Israel was based on the writings of Paul, and had a substantial impact on the development of the Protestant tradition:

> God hath not cast away his people which he foreknew. [...] all Israel shall be saved: as it is written, there shall come out of Sion the Deliverer, and shall turn away ungodliness from Jacob: For this is my covenant unto them, when I shall take away their sins.
>
> (*Roman* 11:2, 26–27(KJ))

The vision of the twelfth-century mystic Joachim of Fiore marked a gradual restoration of the Jews' role in the Christian eschatological scheme of the unfolding of history: "The coming third stage of history would include the return of the Jews to their land. There, they would convert to Christianity and live in brotherhood with a revitalized church."[6] John Calvin, the most influential theologian in Anglo-American Protestantism, stated that beside the Jews' historical role, they still had a central place in God's plan of salvation: "As the Jews are the first-born, what the Prophet declared must be fulfilled":[7] "God has by no means cast away the whole race of Abraham."[8] Rumors of a Jewish Messiah (Shabbatai Zevi, 1626–1676) and Jews who were selling their homes and setting out for Jerusalem, together with major theological-political events such as the execution of the English monarch Charles I, were understood as signs of the approach of the last phase of history.[9] This sensitivity to the Jews only emphasized the centrality of the Jews in the Protestant eschatological mind. By the eighteenth century, the return of Jews to the land of Israel had become part of mainstream American Protestant teachings, as was expressed by Jonathan Edwards, one of the most important American Protestant theologians:

> It is the more evident, that the Jews will return to their own land again, because they never have yet possessed one quarter of that land, which was so often promised them, from the Red Sea to the river Euphrates.[10]

With the establishment of the state of Israel in 1948, one witnessed a shift from a hypothetical idea to a theological reality. This shift involved a demand for an actual participation in the restoration of Jews and their Land. Wilbur Smith, a professor of English Bible at Fuller Theological Seminary, wrote in 1951, that the establishment of Israel was the "greatest event in Palestine certainly since the destruction of Jerusalem, infinitely more important than the Crusades."[11] John Hagee, one of the most prominent Evangelical pastors, declared that "the birth of the State of Israel confirmed the accuracy of Bible prophecy."[12] The idea that the establishment of Israel and the return of the Jews to the Land of the Bible was part of sacred history radicalized the commitment of the evangelical movement toward the Jewish people and the Land of Israel, for "I will bless those who bless you" (Gen. 12). The Six-Day War augmented the theological significance of the historical events which brought together Christianity, the teachings of Judaism, and the return to the Land of Israel and particularly to Jerusalem. A statement published in the *New York Times* by liberal Protestant theologians, led by Reinhold Niebuhr, a month after the war, affirmed:

> Judaism has at its center an indissoluble bond between the people of Israel and the land of Israel. For Christians, to acknowledge the necessity of Judaism is to acknowledge that Judaism presupposes inextricable ties with the land of Israel and the City of David [Jerusalem], without which Judaism cannot be truly itself.[13]

As we have seen in this section, classical Catholic doctrine, as is expressed for example by Augustine, rejected the future role of the Jews and with that, their claim to the land of Israel. However, an alternative eschatological view based on the writings of Paul gave the Jews and their return to Zion a central role in God's salvation plan. The establishment of the State of Israel profoundly affected evangelical Christianity and radicalized its involvement in the restoration of the Jews in the Holy Land as part of their messianic function. John S. Feinberg articulates this involvement:

> If we recognize that the modern state of Israel may well be the fulfillment of OT prophecies about the return of Israel to the land preparatory to the tribulation, we should be careful not to do anything which would contribute to her removal from the land. If God is wrapping up His program with the people of Israel at this time, and if that program demands that Israel be present in the land, who are we to try to stop the accomplishment of His purposes?[14]

Christianity, throughout its development, was confronted with the questions of the status and validity of the *Old Testament*, Israel as the elected people and their claim to the land of Israel. This confrontation shaped its identity and eschatological mission. In contrast, Islam's relationship to Judaism is much simpler and is not related to its essence. Islam regards Judaism as an obsolete religion. Jewish minorities living under the rule of Islam were treated as a second-class subjects, required to pay a special tax called the *jizya*. Consequently, the Jews' claim to the Land of Israel (also called *al-Ard al-Muqaddasa*) is invalid. Hillel Cohen summarizes this as follows: "Islam [...] which sees itself as a revealed religion which replaces Judaism – would contradict its own principles if it adhered to the doctrine of the election of the people of Israel and its right to the Land of Israel."[15] As a result of the century-old Israeli-Palestinian conflict, an interesting debate has arisen concerning the status of the Jews in Islam and the Jews' right to the land of Israel. Though some scholars claim that in ancient Islamic sources the land was promised to the Jews,[16] most scholars reject this claim.[17] However, despite this fruitful discussion which may be important for the future, it cannot be denied that such a discussion is alien to the historical tradition of Islam and their understanding of the Jews. Consequently, whereas the Christian discussion opened new perspectives in this matter, this is not the case with Islam.[18]

Name and place

Secular Zionist settlement did not locate itself in the land of the Patriarchs, but in the land of the Philistines, not in Judea and Samaria, but largely in the coastal plain. The names it chose, many of which are foreign to the place or are those that express yearning. Zionism secularized the biblical language endowing places with mythical significance. For example, Petach Tikva [Entrence of Hope], Rishon LeZion [First in Zion], did not represent a deep theological connection to the land of the Patriarchs, but rather a secular, modern national vision. This secular use of the ancient language was a major tool in shaping the national community.[19]

In this way, a two-fold dissociation was created – geographic and linguistic. In contrast to secular Zionism, the settler Zionists, reverting to the cradle of the Bible, displayed a theological return both to the place and to the ancient biblical language, even though a large proportion of the proponents of the Greater Israel movement was secular. It is not surprising that in the settlers' journal *Nekuda*, M. Simon criticizes the irony that is reflected in the secular Zionist yearnings to return to the valley and the coast and their disregard of the land of the Bible:

> For whom did our hearts yearn in the two thousand years – for Degania and Netanya, or for Beit–El and Shilo? What was the dream of the Jewish people in the darkness of its exile – Caesarea and Herzliya-Pituach or Nablus and Hebron?[20]

The return to Philistia stemmed from historical constraints, since the mountains were settled whereas the swamps and the sand-dunes remained vacant.[21] This impediment was made into a secular, technological ideal by the pioneers through redemption of the land by making the wilderness bloom and draining the swamps. Settler Zionism did not return to the wilderness but to the abandoned and destroyed historical sites. While the secular ideal of making the wilderness bloom represented hope for the future arising out of the desolate past, the settler project espoused restoration of a ruined place and an attempt to revive it.[22]

In settling the land of the Philistines, secular Zionism did not manage to find a substitute for the places of sacred history preserved in the biblical narrative. The inability to reach the regions mentioned in Genesis which were in eyeshot and accessible reinforced the sense of deprivation felt about those places, just as Moses felt when overlooking the Promised Land from Mount Nebo. In this way, Zionism preserved the unrequited yearning and desire for the Land of the Bible.[23] In America, the replication of the name of Jericho in the United States formed a link between the Jericho in that country and the biblical Jericho, but at the same time it emphasized its emptiness and distance from the original place.[24] However, the proximity yet inaccessibility of Jericho for secular Zionist settlement only reinforced its "absent presence," to use Martin Heidegger's expression.[25] A good illustration to the creativity and power of the restorative imagination can be found in the words of Ezra Stiles (1727–1795), the president of Yale College. Stiles spoke of the New Republic of the United States as "God's American Israel." However, the establishment of the new American Israel and the duplication of names did not nullify the old Israel and the old places. On the contrary, "the future prosperity and splendor of the United States [...] will be literally fulfilled; when this branch of the posterity of Abraham shall be nationally collected, and become a very distinguished and glorious people."[26]

Diaspora Jewry related to the holy places by means of language and prayer, thereby neutralizing their immediate presence. The use of the name Jerusalem, for towns, such as the Jerusalem of Lithuania (Yerushalayim de Lita) or the name of Hebron for yeshivas, created an indirect connection with the sacredness of the name. Similarly, secular Zionism maintained unrequited yearnings for places which were within reach. This inaccessibility amplified the role of the language, replacing their absence with the messianic thrust of the Hebrew language.[27] In the early days of the State, three major works were published by Orthodox intellectuals that warned of the danger of the secular yearning for the Land of the Bible, and of combining the political with the theological. The three articles were published in consecutive years: the article by the educational thinker Ernst Akiva Simon, "Are we still Jews?" (1951);[28] the article by the literary critic Baruch Kurzweil, "The essence and sources of the Young Hebrew (Canaanite) movement" (1952);[29] and the article by the philosopher and scientist Yeshayahu Leibowitz, "After Qibiya" (1953).[30] In all three, the religiously observant scholars warned against the bear hug of the new Israeli nationalism's appropriation of biblical language; they warned of the radical conclusions of the secular Israeli nationalism that verged on Canaanism, and they expressed their concern at the rise of "national messianism." These desires burst out when these places were conquered in the Six-Day War. Much has been said about the postwar euphoria, but not enough attention has been paid to the emotional facet of secular Zionism which longed to return to Jerusalem's wellspring.

The land of Israel became nearer and more accessible after 1967. While secular Zionism returned to David, Saul, and Samson employing a moderated interpretation of the literal meaning of the Bible, an interpretation whose purpose was to bolster its ideological precepts,[31] the settlers' "homecoming" to the formative locations made them move from a toned-down interpretation of the Bible to an unmediated interpretation – to a messianic reading. For them, the soil became the *ground*, an interpretative foundation anchoring their mystical messianism.[32]

Both secular Zionism and the settlement movement harked back to the biblical names, making widespread use of archaeology, through which they returned to places of origin. But their purpose was different. Secular Zionists did so for national reasons, with the aim of forging a collective identity and to justify the return to the land;[33] but the motivation among the settlers was to return to the biblical source, to the places and names in the Bible, through which they could draw nearer to the theological ideal central to their outlook. For example, the archaeologist Adam Zartal who claimed to have located an altar on Mount Ebal from the time of Joshua, reasoned that this discovery provided confirmation of the Biblical story.[34] Zartal was educated in the left-wing *Hashomer Hatzair* youth movement, so that he cannot be accused of being a settler, but the settlers adopted his research discoveries and appropriated them for their own political needs.

Access to the formative places of the Bible brought ancient history closer and made the land of the Bible accessible to the new Israelis. Bible stories were made concrete. The settlers succeeded in replacing the political-security dis-course about the territories with a theological discourse. Areas of land that only the day before had been enemy territory became holy sites. Many Israelis rushed, after 1967, to visit Rachel's tomb in Bethlehem and the Tomb of the Patriarchs in Hebron.

Using philological and archaeological tools, Yoel Elitzur, Ze'ev Erlich and other settlers embarked on a project to reconstruct and assign biblical names to the settlements in Judea and Samaria. Elitzur claimed that it is possible to identify (and cross-reference) many of the names mentioned in the Bible with the names of Israeli localities corresponding to their locations, that at times were precisely preserved and at other times underwent changes. In this way, these researchers wished to create a correlation between the ancient occurrence and the new settlements in the territory, and to prove that the latter were not a foreign element but rather a continuation of an existence that had been cut short. In the introduction to his book, Yoel Elitzur wrote:

> In the modern age, starting with the journey of Robinson and Smith in 1838, that produced their basic study, *Biblical Researchers in Palestine*, and up to the present, the point of departure of every geographical, histor-ical study of the land of Israel has been a methodical tracking of the names that were preserved by the Arabs. Based on this, the various historical sources are examined and archeological evidence is collected. The large proportion of names that have been preserved in their biblical form or close to it, have been perceived by many as a kind of "cultural miracle" that has enabled us to return after many years to the land of the Bible.[35]

In accordance with Elitzur's words, it could, for example, be said that while the changing of the name Jerusalem to Aelia Capitolina by the Roman conquerors was intended to root out the Jewish foundations of the city and invalidate the Temple, the preservation of the original names by the Arabs forms a bridge to the original places and times. The demand to return to the biblical names of the biblical places is not a simple demand but is intended to legitimize the new settlements and their residents, who, not only are not strangers to the place but are even continuing the original biblical settlement.[36] The return to the land of Genesis is not a return to a place that has been defiled by having been settled by foreigners. The act of settlement does not redeem the place from its impurity but expresses the return of members of the family to their home after many years of wandering in exile – years in which others settled in their homestead.[37]

Secular Zionism, entrenched as it is in European nationalism, distorted the place names in many cases, thereby positioning itself as a foreign intruder. In this sense, preserving the linkage to the place and the name brought the settlers closer to the Arabs than to the secular Zionists, who had come from Christian Europe. Has the Canaanite-indigenous common denominator between the Palestinians and the settlers displaced the foreign, European Crusader nationalism? Did the "Crusaders" who settled this land become "Canaanites"?[38] Secular Zionism did indeed return to the land of Israel and reconstruct biblical names, but it did so in a way that was perceived as Canaanite by many, rather than as religious. Ashkelon and Hatzor are not focuses of Jewish sacredness and are not charged with religious sentiment, but are names that belong to the biblical story divested of religious motifs. Harry Emerson Fodsdick wrote in 1927 that many American Christians, guided by their restorative imagination, perceived Zionism to be a religious movement, not understanding that the Zionist pioneers were almost entirely secular socialists: "Accustomed to think of Judaism in terms of religion, [American Christians] naturally interpret Zionism in the same terms, and picture pious colonists for the love of their God endeavoring to re-people and reclaim their Holy Land."[39] This discrepancy between the religious anticipation and the secular reality only accentuates the symbiosis of American Evangelists and the Israeli settlers after 1967, when the Biblical Lands of Judaea and Samaria were retaken.

While the place names were effectively preserved by the inhabitants of the land during Hellenistic rule and up to the Ottomans, Elitzur claims that the Zionist project gave new names to many of the localities, thereby harming the chain of transmission of biblical names. Foreign names of Zionist pioneers like Witkin, Sirkin, Warburg and Hess, in memory of whom villages were established and named in the 1930s, created an estrangement between the biblical localities and the Zionist villages. In many cases, historical names were assigned in places that were not in the correct biblical location, such as Massada, Kiryat Sefer, Yavne, Mevo Horon, and even Efrat. An emphasis on the inaccuracy reveals the radicalism (in the sense of *radix*, root) of Elitzur's claim, which strives to reconstruct the past with precision.[40]

The present-day nationalist movements, including Zionism, secularized the language that conceptualized metaphysical sanctity replacing it with modern terms that conceived the physical place as having mythical significance.[41] As the scholar of religion, Mircea Eliade, puts it, constructing the sacredness of a place gives meaning to a person in his world.[42] Sanctifying the space imparts to the chaotic reality an order and organization, thereby elevating the actual place to a transcendent dimension, a place that is more than a place. A person moves from a simple existence in a space without meaning and in time without purpose, to an existence imbued with deep significance in time and space. This mythologizing of the secular space was one of the main instruments for constructing national communities.[43]

In contrast to secular Zionism that turned the land of the Patriarchs into a "modern graveyard," as Elitzur defiantly puts it, he views the settlers as having been charged with guarding the biblical heritage.[44] In a similar vein, Ze'ev Erlich thinks that "The Land of Israel preserved place names throughout the vicissitudes of history [...] It is proper that we too be punctilious in preserving the identity of the land and the footsteps of our forefathers in it."[45]

Perhaps the greatest success that the settlers had in identifying a link between the land of the Bible and the occupied territories is to be found in the naming of Judea and Samaria, a restorative replication of the name in the Bible.[46] Since the 1970s, and especially after the Likud, the rightist party, came to power in 1977, there was an increase in the use of biblical terms for what had previously been called the West Bank.

Settlement and Canaanism

In Jewish tradition, the land belongs to God and is given to the people temporarily under the conditions of the covenant between God and Abraham, so that it could be taken away from them. The autochthonous (indigenous) myth, the linkage and the correlation between the people and the territory are not unequivocal in the national consciousness, as the case of Uganda demonstrates.[47] Canaan is indeed the Promised Land, but the territorial validation and the sovereignty is granted by the Holy One Blessed Be He. The biblical narrative is not autochthonous, because the Father of the Nation (Abraham), who was not an indigenous inhabitant, was sentenced to de-territorialization; the framer of the constitution (Moses) transmitted it in the desert, with no locality; and the first settler (Joshua) came to the land from outside. The claim is that although the Hebrews became a nation in the desert on the way to inherit and conquer the land from the indigenous inhabitants living in it, they were only recovering the land for its first, natural owners from the seven peoples who had stolen it.

A different position was expressed by David Ben-Gurion, Israel's first prime minister. His biblical-Canaanite perception, whereby he claimed that "the people of Israel or the Hebrew people was born and raised in this land, even before the days of Abraham, as one of the Canaanite people [...],"[48] was not so different from his contribution to the phrasing of the Israel's Declaration of Independence in 1948, in which he stated that "the Land of Israel was the birthplace of the Jewish people." Ben-Gurion, like the Zionist ideologist A.D. Gordon and the first chief rabbi of British Mandatory Palestine, Abraham Isaac Hacohen Kook, wanted to combine the image of the land of Jewish destiny with the image of the homeland.[49] But there was a discordance in Ben-Gurion's social thinking between the idea of destiny and the local-Canaanite conception, and his secular leanings prevented him from sanctifying the land and nurturing messianic

Canaanism – a messianism that prioritizes the Land of Israel, a task which religious Zionism took upon itself.

The scholar of Jewish thought, Aviezer Ravitzky, maintained that the Land of Israel fascinated and attracted its sons, especially in exile, and threatened them, frightening them with the metaphysical demand it contained, so that the exiles recoiled at the overwhelming sacredness of the land that was sometimes taboo, untouchable. Zionism's return to its constitutive place tried to dispel this tension, to banish the fear, and to re-establish the Jew in his Hebrew homeland.[50]

Despite the marginal importance of the Canaanite group as put forward by Yonatan Ratosh, an Israeli poet and the founder of the group, the Canaanite ideal, that emphasized the centrality of the land as its most important component, played a serious role in the Israeli discourse after the conquest of the territories in the Six-Day War. An unholy alliance was formed between Rabbi Zvi Yehuda Kook and Aharon Amir,[51] in which the head of the Mercaz Ha-Rav Yeshiva offered the Canaanite poet a financial contribution towards the re-establishment of the Canaanite group. Religious Zionism perceived the Torah, the people and the land as a holy trinity in which each of the elements are equal – a people and a land without the Torah are meaningless, just as the Torah alone is not sufficient.[52] In each era, the order of priorities of these equal elements changes. Scholars who identify *Gush Emunim* as a right-wing iteration of religious neo-Canaanism[53] point out that while religious Zionism previously emphasized Torah, people and land, in that order, *Gush Emunim* changed this order to land, people, Torah. So, *Gush Emunim*, in this era, views the land as the key to the entire structure. *Gush Emunim*'s sanctification of the place, combining political theology with the myth of settlement in the boundaries of Greater Israel, dictated its political agenda.

There are those who consider this precedence as a fetishization of the land, an act that provides justification for transgressions related to Torah commandments concerning the preservation of the integrity of the land, an attitude that might lead to the Canaanization of the settlers. Major figures in religious circles warned of messianic and Canaanite tendencies and a potentially disastrous alliance between them. The thinker and religious kibbutz member Eliezer Goldman called Gush Emunim "simplistic messianism."[54] Baruch Kurzweil, who at an early stage perceived the Canaanite tendencies of the culture of the Hebrew revival, wrote ironically after the Six-Day War that "the land-based messianism had achieved its goals."[55] In 1968, Yeshiyahu Leibowitz expressed a fear that "the State would not be Jewish, but Canaanite."[56] Likewise Gershom Scholem, who saw Gush Emunim as a modern version of the Sabbatean movement, said: "I am not interested in a State of Canaan … what the Canaanites will do, and the Arabs are not Indians."[57]

According to Boaz Evron, the Canaanites' belief that the absorption of the non-Jewish inhabitants of the occupied territories would destroy the Jewish character of the state made them support the colonization project of the Greater Land of Israel, so creating a right-wing neo-Canaanite-religious synthesis: "The religious Gush Emunim settlement was a dialectical step towards the Hebrew 'Land of Kedem (Old)' which was beyond any ethnic or religious divisions and united the entire population within the framework of a single nation, the Hebrew nation."[58] The scholar of Israeli studies, Anita Shapira, described it thus: "There are Canaanite elements in *Gush Emunim*'s ideology that are moderated, to a certain extent, by their religious connection. Like the Canaanites, they too adopted the Land of Israel as a formative factor in shaping their main identity."[59] Or, in the words of the Israeli author Haim Be'er,

> the people of *Gush Emunim* place their trust in the myth of the Land of Israel. From the trinity in which they were brought up – the Torah of Israel, the people of Israel, and the land of Israel – they select, first and foremost, the land. For them, the land, like myth for the nativists, is the expression of a reality that is more original, more elevated and more important.[60]

Amnon Rubinstein, the former Israeli minister of education, considered that just as the Canaanites in the Jewish community of the 1940s were a latter-day expression of the Hebrew education of the 1930s, which viewed the negation of the Diaspora as a supreme value, *Gush Emunim* – most of whom were the products of the state-religious education system and graduates of the Bnei Akiva religious youth movement in high-school yeshivas – are the product of the Israeli society of the 1960s."[61]

In 1975, the founding of *Gush Emunim* was announced in Kfar Etzion. Kfar Etzion was a religious kibbutz established during the British mandate in 1927, evacuated during the 1948 War of Independence, and re-established as the first settlement after the Six-Day War. According to the theology of indigenous inhabitants propounded by Hanan Porat, a resident of Kfar Etzion and one of the founders of *Gush Emunim*, the long-standing biblical time period (*la longue durée*) of the Jewish people linked up with the present settlers' Israeli time. Porat and his colleagues succeeded in instilling in the Israeli national consciousness the idea of Judea and Samaria – the ancient names of the biblical kingdoms that comprise the West Bank – as an intersection in which time and space are integrated: the biblical-historical time of the Jewish people and the holy place of present-day Mount Hebron and Gush Etzion (the area where Kfar Etzion is located).

In this way, the settlement narrative was diverted from the secular time of the War of Independence and the State of Israel to the messianic time of *Gush Emunim* ("the birth of the Messiah together with our region") and the biblical place, the birthplace of the nation and the Messiah. This development had clear political implications. As the critics of the settlers saw it, the messianism of *Gush Emunim* combined religious-messianic and secular-Canaanite principles. One example of this can be seen in the words of Haim Be'er where he describes the intensive cult worship associated with an oak tree in his classic article, "*Gush Emunim* – Canaanites who wear phylacteries."

In the wake of the Six-Day War, upon their return here, it seemed as though the tree had sunk – like love letters to the beloved one who married you – into the surrounding silence of the hills. But the tree became the center for an intensive cult worship. Experts were brought in who poured concrete into its trunk, so that it wouldn't break during one of the storms. The buildings of the regional school that was established nearby were erected lower than usual, so as not to block the view of the tree even for someone standing at the top of Mount Ora in the Jerusalem Corridor. (Would they have behaved like that, with such emotional consideration, if it were a person?) They imprinted its green silhouette on every piece of writing paper, envelope, pamphlet or book they produced. And when the time came to choose a name for the locality, a name that would give expression to the longings for the place, for the land of their forefathers, for nineteen years, they chose a very Canaanite name, the Oak of Moreh [Elon Moreh], associated with ancient times, when people vested their best feelings in trees and stones.[62]

Haim Be'er thought that *Gush Emunim* changed the order of priorities of religious Zionism. During the Canaanization process, religious Zionist youth, which had suddenly "woken up," turned to the almost pre-biblical experience of Genesis, to the Land of Israel myth, to the conquest of Canaan. Like Baruch Kurzweil, who maintained that the Canaanites of the 1940s based themselves on the myth of the Land of Israel, in Be'er's opinion the leitmotif of the settlers was the neo-Canaanite myth. Evidence of this can be gleaned from the universal names, Sa'ad [aid], Shluchot [branches], Alumim [youth], or the names of rabbis or intellectuals (Ein Hanatziv [named after Rabbi Naftali Zvi Yehuda Berlin], Tirat Zvi [named after Rabbi Zvi Hirsch Kalischer], Sde Eliyahu [named after Rabbi Eliyahu Guttmacher], Be'erot Yitzhak [named after Rabbi Yitzhak Nisanboim], Kfar Haroe [named after Rabbi Abraham Isaac Kook], Sde Yaakov [named after Yitzchak Yaacov Reines], and Beit Meir [named after Rabbi Meir Bar-Ilan] assigned to their settlements by the religious kibbutz movement. *Gush Emunim* in contrast, gave its settlements Canaanite names like Kiryat Arba, Elon Moreh, Kedumim, and Karnei Shomron. The sanctification of the oak tree is a symbol and also a symptom of the process of Canaanization of Kfar Etzion.

Does *Gush Emunim* really have a neo-Canaanite aspect that worships the soil of the land as Haim Be'er, Anita Shapira, Amnon Rubinstein, and others think? In response to these claims Yosef Ben-Shlomo answered that this is a shallow perception bordering on the marginal and does not express the core perception of *Gush Emunim*. He asks, "why is the real, physical, Land of Israel, land of our fathers, important, and why is it the essence of Zionism itself?" and answers that there is no moral sense in preferring Sheikh Munis, where Tel Aviv resides, to the stony ground of Kedumim. When we do so, he concluded, we exchange the power of right associated with values of historical justification for the right to power given by political facts. Zionism of this type, without Zion and Jerusalem, in his view, changes Zionism into colonialism because it demolishes the moral basis for the people of Israel to settle anywhere in the Land of Israel.[63]

Ben-Shlomo claimed that identifying the settlers with the Canaanites ignores the essential difference between them: "Secular neo-Canaanism refuted the unity of the Jewish people in its historic connection to the Land of Israel." The "Jewish people" were not perceived by him in demographic terms but as an idea. The Jewish people, together with the Land of Israel, are super-political, value-based foundation-stones not subject to political law. On the contrary, it is due to these foundations that the State of Israel enjoys legitimacy: "This idea, that there are super-political values to which the political law is subjugated, originates from the people of Israel." From this, he extrapolated that in any contest between the State of Israel and the Land of Israel, he chooses to side with the latter:

> The highest value in our debate is not the political entity, but rather the historical-moral reality, even if this value is not lawful in the view of the state; and therefore, the right to settle in the Land of Israel is a super-political right. In my struggle over the territory, I am not expelling Arabs. So, I repeat once more that the question is, what is the determining value, the State or the Land?[64]

What makes Ben-Shlomo's words particularly interesting is their logic, that could serve both right-wing radical settler groups which do not recognize the sovereignty of the State of Israel for religious reasons, and left-wing extremist groups which, in placing their emphasis on democratic values and human rights, are liable to negate the legitimacy of the State of Israel. Here is the rationale expressed in the following words of Ben-Shlomo, intended to justify his loyalty to the Land of Israel over and above the State of Israel:

There are religious, moral or national values that justify deposing a government in order to achieve them. During the French Revolution, freedom and equality were super-political values. In the Second World War, too, De Gaulle left France and declared, "I am France!" while the majority of the French people preferred the Vichy regime headed by Pétain.[65]

This debate between the act of settlement as a neo-Canaanite act, and those who view it as a continuation of the divine promise, leads us to examine the differentiated and contradictory meanings of a political reading of the Bible.

The rise to prominence of the Bible in religious Zionism

The Haskalah (the Jewish Enlightenment movement) returned to the Bible as part of its renewal of the Diaspora tradition. The Haskalah was supposed to replicate the link to ancient history, but this was not a classic pilgrimage but a textual journey. Zionism, as an integral part of the building of the nation, dovetailed with nineteenth century European tradition, a tradition that believed in a universal mission, as in Giuseppe Mazzini's dream of a *third Rome*, Johan Gottlieb Fichte's idea of *the first nation*, Poland as the *Christ of the nations*, and even in our own sphere, the proto-Zionist thinker Moses Hess who conceived *Jerusalem* as a national vanguard force.[66]

The Bible became the very core of Zionist ideology because it constituted a super-narrative for the development of the nation, a thread running through the narrative of the Jewish people with its historical birth and its national future. From the time of the Second *Aliyah*, a founding Zionist immigration phase between 1904–1914, the reading of the Bible was transformed from a religious text into a national one. The Torah written in the Hebrew homeland inherited the place held by the oral law in the Diaspora. Socialist values of social justice were inspired by the admonitions of the prophets. The secular society in the Land of Israel secularized the Bible and selected only those elements that suited its values and needs. The author Aharon Megged wrote:

> The Bible was studied and read in the Land of Israel not as a religious work, but as a brilliant work of literature, as a compilation replete with treasures, as an historical source, as a geographical and archeological guide, as a spring of wisdom, as a stimulus that awakens the heart to social justice. From the outset and in retrospect, it reinforced the link between the people and the land of the Patriarchs, the cradle of its civilization.[67]

Prominent proto-religious Zionist figures in Europe like Rabbi Zvi Hirsch Kalischer and Rabbi Yehuda Alkalai understood the redemption of Israel in the historical context of the European national awakening. Since the *Hibbat Zion* (Lovers of Zion) forerunners of Zionism, religious Zionism had not based itself on the Bible but on Talmudic literature. In pointing out that secular Zionism was making the wilderness bloom, Rabbi Abraham Isaac Kook was returning to the Talmud which stated that "אין לך קץ מגולה מזה": (Sanhedrin 88, 62) the time of the redemption will be revealed when the land returns to producing fruit.[68] The religious Zionists did not come to Israel in order to establish a spiritual Jerusalem (although they did talk of the Temple). They were preoccupied with the real land of Israel, and religious Zionism was an ally and partner of secular Zionism. It was run by pragmatic leaders like Rabbi Yitzhak Yaacov Reines and most of the members of the *Mizrachi*, a moderate religious Zionist organization, who, at a certain stage, accepted the Uganda Scheme – a plan in the early 1900s to give a portion of British East Africa to the Jewish people as a homeland.

Orthodox Judaism displaced the Bible and caused it to be forgotten. Instead, it focused on the Mishnah, the Talmud, Kabbalah, Halakha, and Ethics which dealt with matters of Jewish existence without sovereignty. The Zionist project, that returned to the land and established Jewish sovereignty, challenged Orthodoxy which was now faced with a dilemma which Judaism had not had to cope with for nearly 2,000 years. On the one hand, the ultra-Orthodox rejected the Zionist project due to its secularity and shut themselves up within the Jewish cannon. On the other hand, Rabbi Abraham Isaac Kook, with the intervention of his son Rabbi Zvi Yehuda Kook and his *Gush Emunim* disciples, viewed the Zionist enterprise, despite its secularity, as a dialectical expression of sacred-ness: "יסוד כסא ה' בעולם" ("the base of the throne of God on earth").[69] This belief had a fundamental structural importance for their interpretation of the history of redemption (of which Zionism was perceived as an advanced historical stage) and for their understanding of the centrality of the political dimension. For 2,000 years, the love of Zion and its yearnings had remained constant. Its renewal and the contribution of the Zionist movement that was joined to a secular political program, led to the establishment of the State of Israel. Rabbi Kook's circle interpreted the revival of Israel as a necessary part of the logic of the history of the redemption. From the point of view of religious Zionism, the establishment of the state was not only a political event but was, first and foremost, a redemptive religious one.

The rise to prominence of the Bible among the religious Zionists after the Six-Day War did not take place all at once. The yeshiva world continued to focus on Halakha and Talmud which were dominant until the end of the 1970s. Moderate Halakhic scholars like Rabbis Yehuda Amital and Aharon Lichtenstein at the Har Etzion Yeshiva, or Rabbi Haim Yaakov Goldwicht of the Kerem Yavne Yeshiva continued to place the study of Talmud, not the Bible, at the center. The beginning of the shift to the Bible after the Six-Day War did not take place in the study halls but in the pilgrimages of youth movements and individuals in the biblical areas. The Bible served as a guide and every site was identified by means of the biblical text. The text was used as a book of pilgrimage to the actual past.

Whereas the scholar Gideon Aran identified the roots of *Gush Emunim* in the *Gahelet* Group, which was active in the 1950s and drew upon the ideas of both the Rabbis Kook,[70] the scholars Avi Sagi and Dov Schwartz maintained that the influence of those rabbis on *Gush Emunim* only became crucial several years after the founding of the movement.[71] They claimed that *Gush Emunim* was first activated by two principles – rehabilitative and romantic. Religious Zionism felt humiliated and inferior in face of the heroism and pioneering of secular Zionism that led to the establishment of the State of Israel. The rehabilitative principle wanted to enable religious Zionism to stand erect and to give it a central place in the shaping of the national identity of the State,[72] while the romantic principle wanted to turn the Bible into a factor that created a bridge between the religious aspirations and the biblical sites in the West Bank. With the conquest of the territories in 1967, the radical youth of *Gush Emunim* were exposed to a new-old theological space which allowed them to free themselves from the chains of their moderate parents who had been raised in a secular statehood. The propitious time of the return to the hills of Judea and Samaria was a historic opportunity not only to return to the land of the Bible in the territorial or geographic sense, but also to return to the foundations of Jewish existence. In this sense, the direct reading of the Bible was in practical reading.

Aran noted that *Gush Emunim* did not derive its biblical orientation from a religious heritage that opposed the central role of the Bible. In his view, *Gush Emunim*'s return to the Bible was not an expression of orthodoxy, but of liberation from it, an outcome of its openness towards the modern secular milieu.[73] The demand to bring back the Bible into the center of religious life, a demand that was religiously innovative, embodied a retreat from rabbinical Judaism and, in many senses, joined up with Hebrew secularity which had previously adopted the Bible.

Gush Emunim's attraction to the good-looking folk in the Emek (valley) and the hills stemmed from the vitality and self-confidence exuded by the secular native-born Israelis and from the contempt the latter felt for their exilic parents. The inspiration for the members of *Gush Emunim* did not come from the study halls of the yeshivas but from Hebrew poems like those of the poetess Rachel, from the "religion of labor" advocated by the secular Zionist A.D. Gordon, and from the kibbutz ethos of the model society. This inspiration and proximity also explain the attraction of important entities, such as the *Kibbutz Hameuhad* [United Kibbutz Movement] to the people of *Gush Emunim*, whom they viewed as their dialectical successors.

Sagi and Schwartz maintained that *Gush Emunim* was gradually taken over by the people of Elon Moreh and the Rabbi Kook Institute, settler leaders like Hanan Porat, and later on, Yoel Bin Nun. In this way, the rehabilitative and romantic precepts were shunted aside in favor of "sacred history" (Heilsgeschichte), an organizational precept in the messianic thinking of the school of thought of Rabbi Avraham Yitzhak Kook.[74] Whereas historical thinking in the vein of Greek traditional thought focused on the past, sacred history is directed towards the future, and is aimed at reforming and completing it. The integration of the notion of a sacred history needed a text that would guide the future reform, and the followers of Kook found this in the Bible. The spirit of the Rabbi Kook Institute, characterized by a clear prophetical foundation, embodied specifically in the figure of Rabbi Kook, found that the canonical books were not suited to the power and vitality required to give expression to the notion of sacred history. Conversely, the Bible with its rich prophetic spirit and its connection to the land, offered a powerful future reading for reform and was therefore selected as their guiding text. Two ways of understanding the Bible were created: a "lower" one, which was a literary understanding of the text and its comprehension by the believer; and a "higher" one, in which the text served as a channel for divine instructions and their ramifications in contemporary reality. The Bible functioned as a prophetic text for our times.

The *Gush Emunim* avant-garde made the religious Zionists, who had previously been a fifth wheel on the secular carriage or were considered mere "kosher inspectors," into leaders of a revolutionary process. In their perception, it was secular Zionism that had restored the land to prominence and the Bible to a position of centrality in the life of the nation, but only religious Zionism had brought this move to a conclusive end. The young people of *Gush Emunim*, the revolutionary young generation of religious Zionism, derived a political-theological program from the fundamentalist union between the Bible and the land.[75]

According to the interpretive perception of *Gush Emunim* there were no separate levels of interpretation. The reading of the Bible was undertaken "barefoot": *Gush Emunim* members read the Book, looked at the stony ground around them and saw the figures of the past as having a current presence. This unmediated reading led to a new simple interpretation that was more profound. It originated in the simplified reading of the Bible but it took it to a new level: "*Gush Emunim* appropriated the attitude to the simplified reading of the Bible from the secular revolutionary version but added to it the legitimacy of an obligatory religious commandment."[76] As long as the romantic principle guided the reading of the Bible, the text revealed and actualized the biblical location. But once the sacred history theology became *Gush Emunim*'s organizing principle, the barefoot reading of the Bible changed from one that actualized the place, to one that bolstered the understanding of the Bible. The physical place became a metaphysical place; the physical place became part of the emergence of the sacred history, and in this sense was part of a holy era.

Religious Zionism, which had grown out of secular Zionism, can be characterized by two contradictory components – one national and the other subversive. This dialectical tension between the institutional law and the ideal aspect that was expressed in the movement for perpetual correction that can never be fully satisfied, produces a failure in the logic of the idea of a sacred history. The transcendent dimension of the Zionism of settlement prevents the fulfillment that can, or is likely to, lead to the end of days. For secular Zionism bringing the project to fruition leads to post-Zionism in the sense that Zionism has completed its task in the very establishment of the State, while bringing the settlement project to fruition leads to a post-Zionism at the end of days, post-days. In this way, the settler theology maintains the non-fulfillment of the project. The ultra-Orthodox (Haredim), in contrast, who reject their messianism, maintain a dialectical tension between the eternal yearnings and prolonging the end, and so are not caught up in the illusion of realization.

The Bible: privatization and restoration

For certain groups in secular Israeli society, the estrangement from the Land of the Bible produced estrangement from the Bible too – even resulting in complete alienation from the land and the text. It should be recalled that the Bible had enjoyed consensus for the Zionism project and had bound together the various ideological factions, but with the conquest of the territories during the Six-Day War, there developed an increasing estrangement among parts of the secular public towards the biblical spaces.[77] The Israelis came face to face with the Palestinians living in these territories. The conquest became a toxic element preventing the forging of an emotional connection to the homeland and the constitutive text, and they were perceived as motivations for continuous reprehensible actions. The religious politicization of the land of the Bible, which correlated with friction with the local population, steadily gnawed away at the way the Bible had been adopted earlier, when it had been a constitutive factor in constructing the foundations of the nation. This erosion in the status of the Bible was clearly reflected in the rise of the "Tel Aviv school of Israeli archeology."[78] In the view of this discipline that was rejected by the "Jerusalem school," the Bible does not faithfully reflect ancient historical reality but is a later rewriting intended largely to serve subsequent political and religious aims;

therefore the correlation between the Bible and the findings uncovered in the field should be treated critically, and greater weight should be given to archaeological discoveries. It is not surprising that the settlers' leaders, like Hanan Porat and Yoel Bin Nun, objected strongly to the Tel Aviv scholars[79] who doubted the ability of the Bible to serve as a compass, a doubt that unraveled the imaginary (hegemonic) map of Israeli national identity. If it is not clear where we come from, then we also don't know where we are going.

The Bible became a bone of contention in Israeli society, especially among the secular public (the majority of the religious public accepted the settler narrative). In this way, the Bible lost its state position and went back to being a religious text that plays no part in the lives of most secular people. The biblical text was privatized for various attitudes in diverse sectors of Israeli society. For example, in recent years "weekly readings" of the Bible became fashionable in secular circles. This selective and sectorial reading is clear evidence of the privatization of the Bible. While the reaction to the settler movement led some of the secular elite to post-Zionist or even anti-Zionist positions, the settler ideology had difficulty in maintaining homogeneity. It became segmented into various approaches, some conservative and others radical in the sense that they did not confine themselves to existing achievements and extended their horizons further and further.

Upon the death of Rabbi Zvi Yehuda Kook in 1982, Rabbi Avraham Elkana Kahana Shapira was appointed head of the Rabbi Kook Institute. Fifteen years later, Rabbi Yisrael Tau left the yeshiva together with his senior students and founded the *Har Hamor* yeshiva.[80] His resignation was related to a dispute apparently connected to the possible establishment of a teaching institute attached to the yeshiva, that would include academic studies. In practice, the cause of the dispute went much deeper, because Rabbi Tau did not accept the subordination of the yeshiva to state institutions (Ministry of Education) and particularly the possibility that it would be subject to academic supervision. The polemics changed from a didactic disagreement into a theological-political dispute.[81] Rabbi Tau, who was deeply ingrained in the Rabbi Kook Institute's mindset, feared that the academic methods which Rabbi Shapira wanted to inculcate, would promote a "Christian reading." This reading, he explained, distant as it is from the Jewish tradition, interprets the events of the Bible in a Christian light, and is therefore unable to appreciate the exalted dimension of biblical figures. While the Rabbi Kook Institute wished to incorporate a wider range in which biblical studies could coexist with openness to ideas that challenge the state, Rabbi Tau completely sanctified the national state as well as emphasizing the act of settlement.

The discussion on the Bible spread in 2001 to broad segments of religious Zionism and has reverberations in the present. The dispute touched on the question of how the Bible should be read. A tension developed between the reading by the *boundary* yeshivas (that separate between sacred and secular spheres), *Har Hamor* and its offshoots, that attempt to get to a profound, ideal, simplified reading, and the approach of the *Har Etzion* yeshivas and their subsidiaries which read the Bible as it is.

In contrast to the *boundary* yeshivas which interpret biblical figures in a non-personal way, the Har Etzion yeshiva and its subsidiaries find independent value in the human qualities of biblical figures, and accept their moral shortcomings as having educational value. Whereas the people of the Har Etzion yeshivas and its offshoots do not deny the human characteristics of biblical figures – for example the flaws in the figure of King David – defects that constitute a basis for moral discourse, the *boundary* yeshivas totally deny the possibility that David's personality could be defective, and assert that what is perceived as a fault is an expression of inadequate interpretive methods.

There is a great deal of similarity between the notion of the profound literal meaning, posited by the dogmatic interpretations of the *boundary* yeshivas – an interpretation that denies the existence of contradictions – and the Christian story of Jesus' meeting, after his resurrection, with two of his disciples at Emmaus. The disciples, who did not recognize him, thought that their teacher had died at his crucifixion. Heartbroken by the shattering of their hope for salvation, the disciples' consternation grew when they were told that his body had disappeared from its tomb. Subsequently Jesus explained the events, untangled the contradictions, thereby leading to an understanding of the Holy Scriptures themselves. The climax of this event took place as follows:

> When he was at table with them, he took the bread and blessed and broke it and gave it to them. And their eyes were opened, and they recognized him. And he vanished from their sight. They said to each other, Did not our hearts burn within us while he talked to us on the road, while he opened to us the Scriptures?[82]

Even though there is a great difference between the texts, the beliefs and the contexts, it is hard not to see the similarity to the idea of the deep literal meaning. Just as it is Jesus through whom the disciples understand the contradictions and the written words, so the Land of Israel becomes a mediator through whom the meaning of the Torah is revealed. The incarnation of the holy word within the Land of Israel reveals the deep meaning of the word of God. Just as the Jews are unable to see in Jesus anything other than worship of the flesh, and to identify as idolatry the Christian belief in Jesus as the Messiah, son of God – in other words, worship of the material – so the opponents of the settlers cannot see in the land its interpretative function and only conceive it as a fetish – a Canaanite form of worship. As opposed to the Canaanite interpretation of the act of settlement, the settlers maintain that the failure to appreciate the centrality of the land attests to a misunderstanding of the theological enterprise. Just as, for the Christians, the role of Jesus serves as a mediator for salvation, and at the same time develops an understanding of the sacred text, so the land of Israel is, for the settlers, an essential factor for achieving the messianic goal and is also an interpretive tool for attaining the deep literal meaning of the holy text. Even if the settlers completely reject that they are neo-Canaanites, it is difficult not to notice, as Yeshayahu Leibowitz said, their affinity to Christian logic whose internal reasoning mandates a holy mediator in order to achieve salvation.[83]

The polemics on the Bible in the twenty-first century take place within all shades of religious Zionism, inside and beyond the Green Line (1949 ceasefire line). Despite the fact that they did not deal directly with the question of the justification for the settler project or the significance of a political reading of the Bible, a close look at the hawkish figures in the dispute and the tensions they expressed, reveals an additional element, political in its essence. The readings of the *Har Etzion* yeshiva as a straightforward interpretation were considered by the *Har Hamor* yeshiva to be both a theological and a political threat. Rabbi Tau's method outlined for his students an unconscious interpretative logic in reading the Biblical text, and in line with this logic the theological and the political were intertwined in such a way that the political became theological. Just as King David came to be considered a theological-political epitome of perfection, so Rabbi Tau viewed the State of Israel as an entity that was entirely sacred due to its being an essential component in the history of the redemption. Conversely, the readings of the *Har Etzion* yeshiva, which accept that David's human frailties do not detract from his theological role, allow them to see in the State of Israel not only a theological entity but also a body characterized by ethical dimensions which have an independent existence. Rabbi Tau's approach grants religious validity to the actions of the State, thereby expressing a political theology which could be termed "hyper-statism."[84]

Tau's redemptive rationalization, that legitimates events that under normal circumstances would be considered as unethical, resembles dialectical historical explanations (in the manner of Hegel's "Cunning of Reason"), that were made to explain how Hitler's Genocide served the divine plan. Harry Rimmer, not to be accused of being an antisemitic, asserted:

> All that Hitler has accomplished by his European-wide persecution may be summed up in a sentence: he has accelerated the return of Israel to Palestine, thus apparently hastening his own doom! By driving the 'preserved people' back into the preserved land, Hitler, who does not believe the Bible and who sneers at the Word of God, is helping to fulfill its most outstanding prophecy!

Resuming to the earlier discussion of King David's ethical behavior, the figure of the biblical David takes off as a political theological paradigm and continues to hold a central position in the polemics of religious Zionism, and particularly that of the settlers. While the Greeks saw the king as a sovereign who organized the natural political order, for Rabbi Tau the king embodies the inwardness and wholeness of the people of Israel. "His heart is the heart of the entire congregation of Israel."[85] This reading, based on Maimonides' ideas, saw the monarchy and the figure of the king both as a political organizing factor and an internal basis for the soul of the people.[86]

Another critical approach that developed concurrently with Rabbi Tau's position on the figure of King David, is the philosophy of Rabbi Yitzchak Ginsburgh.[87]

Ginsburgh, – born into a secular family became religious and a supporter of the *Chabad* Hasidic movement – established, in 1982, the *Od Yosef Hai* yeshiva, an ultra-Orthodox yeshiva with nationalist leanings that was initially located in the Tomb of Joseph in Nablus. He became known to the general public for praising, in his book *Baruch Hagever* [Blessed is the Man], the massacre carried out by Baruch Goldstein in the Tomb of the Patriarchs in 1994 in which he killed twenty-nine Palestinians. Ginsburgh's name was also associated with the book, *Torat Hamelech* [Law of Kings] that permits the killing of non-Jews, a book written by two rabbis closely linked to him. His precepts replace the position of the Bible with Hassidic, kabbalistic and halachic principles, precepts that resound with radical groups among the settlers, especially the "hilltop youth," anarchistic and individualistic groups of teenagers that seek to undermine the settler establishment.

Rabbi Ginsburgh defined his political philosophy and his attitude to the religious Zionist tradition by means of a typology of the monarchies of Saul and David.[88] The monarchy of Saul represents a natural secular political order in which the figure of the king has a proud and emotional disposition. Conversely, the monarchy of David represents a close and tense combination of pride and humility, a combination that facilitates a correct administration of political authority. In Ginsburgh's view, the monarchy of David is likely to "propose a person of proper authority, who, on the one hand, knows how to implement his authority, but, on the other hand, does not let it go to his head, but sees himself as the servant of his people."[89]

We have here a powerful allegory of the way Ginsburgh perceives himself in relation to religious Zionist tradition. For him, the monarchy of Saul is parallel to the secular Zionist nation-state, perceived as an external monarchy that was not able to "incorporate its internal dimension."[90] The contradiction between nation and religion was replaced for him by a contradiction between pride and humility, two components in the character of monarchy. Subsequently, he created another equivalence in which the Saul-David duality is duplicated in the Aaron-Moses duality. The accepted Midrashic (hermeneutical) image of Aaron and his gentle leadership of the people represents the religious Zionist tradition, a tradition that attributed religious value to the secular Zionist enterprise. In contrast to this image, the figure of Moses is a paradigmatic case of aggressive theocracy, a position that gives the Torah a commanding presence in political life without consideration of the will of the people.[91] In this dialectical transition[92] from the period of Saul's monarchy to that of David, Ginsburgh was pressing religious Zionism to negate its obligation to the secular state and to advance towards the messianic goal.

Tau and Ginsburgh, each in his own way, present radical theocratic perceptions of the state. Their differing interpretations of the Davidic monarchy have essential consequences for the attitudes of their supporters to the State of Israel. While in the Tau model, the State of Israel is perfectly in keeping with the messianic settler project, Ginsburgh's dialectical logic mandates destroying the secular foundations of the state which are perceived as impure.

In opposition to these trends of radical theocracy propounded by Tau, Ginsburgh and others, the moderate tradition of the *Har Etzion* yeshiva in Alon Shvut stands out – a tradition initiated by its founders, the later Rabbi Yehuda Amital and Rabbi Aharon Lichtenstein. Their successor, Rabbi Yaakov Meidan, adopted a moderate settler approach. As a representative of the school of thought of the *Har Etzion* yeshiva, Meidan focuses on the *p'shat*, the literal meaning of the Bible, through rigorous study of the text and its sources, especially the *aggadot* (tales)[93] of the Sages. His commentaries are far from any Kabbalistic or symbolic interpretation. He subscribes to the "barefoot reading" and leads his followers to a situation in which they feel they are standing directly in the place of the biblical figure. Meidan represents a non-radical approach among the settlers, an approach that does not support hastening the arrival of the Messiah but focuses on preparing one for redemption: "I do not want the Temple to be built tomorrow, but in a more distant future. We are not spiritually ready."[94] The researcher, Assaf Harel, claims that the settlers of Alon Shvut deal very little with the messianic question and emphasize the idea of redemption from which they derive their Zionist activity.[95]

Rabbi Menachem Froman was another representative from *Gush Etzion*, an unusual figure in the settler landscape and the former rabbi of Tekoa. The land, he explained, does not belong to men but is the property of the Creator, and he created man out of it.[96] In God's declaration that "the Land is mine" (Leviticus, 25, 23), Froman found the legal basis for preventing man from taking control of the land and the subjugation of people to one another.[97] He viewed conquest as the principle of male control, and the land as the female principle of limitation and inclusion. He inferred from this that we must move from the male movement of conquest towards the female love of the land, "from territorial ownership to territorial affiliation."[98] This unique theological outlook brought him to conclusions that deviate from the accepted settler perceptions. Like Yosef Ben-Shlomo, but approaching the matter from a different angle, he believed that dwelling in the homeland took precedence over the political framework – in this case the Israeli one. His friend, the author A.B. Yehoshua, commented sympathetically on his doctrine, saying that "a person residing in his homeland is not in exile, even if he is not living under the sovereignty of his people."[99]

In contrast to the moderate stance of Froman and Meidan of Gush Etzion, Rabbi Dov Lior – one of the leaders of the ultra-Orthodox nationalist stream and head of the *Nir Kiryat Arba hesder* yeshiva, among whose students were prominent settler leaders, represents the nationalist approach that legitimizes violent acts within the framework of the national struggle against the Palestinians. Lior was one of those who granted his approval for the book, *Torat Hamelech*; he viewed with favor the massacre perpetrated by Baruch Goldstein, and supported, in 2015, Meir Kahane's idea of transferring Palestinians out of Judea and Samaria.[100] In his article, "The Arabs' hatred is equivalent to Nazism," he claimed that "anyone who wants to subjugate and destroy the Jewish people is subject to the judgment of Amalek [who ought to be annihilated], with all that entails."[101] Lior was one of the rabbis who called for disobeying the order to evacuate settlements during the disengagement from Gaza in 2005, saying that "any law of the state [or] the army that is opposed to the laws of the Torah must be disobeyed!"[102] Despite this, he perceived the State as an expression of sanctity for which the *Hallel* prayers of praise must be recited on Independence Day.[103]

Back to the beginning

In this short review of the streams of religious settlers, the messianic or redemptive settler ideology can be identified with God's biblical promise concerning the people and the land. This notion derives its imagery from Joshua and the Judges' conquests of the territories of the tribes of Israel and reaches completion in the restoration of the Kingdom of David and the Temple in Jerusalem. However, this promise can be interpreted not only in terms of Joshua's conquests and the Kingdom of David but in a more primordial sense in terms of the history of the Patriarchs. Abraham's departure from his birthplace and his journey to the land of Israel is not a tale of conquest or of confrontation but of wandering in the land. Instead of settling the land in a particular place, Abraham spent all his life moving about throughout the length and the breadth of the land.[104] Even though the land had been promised to Abraham, there is no evidence of hostility towards the inhabitants of the land. The Patriarchs, even if they did not integrate with these inhabitants, did not seek to evacuate them. In contrast to the patrimony of Joshua, conquered by force and with divine support, the Tomb of the Patriarchs was purchased with money. While the conquest of the tribal lands and the establishment of the kingdom define the boundaries and the model for governance of the land and the Israelite people, during the period of the Patriarchs the borders of the land and the political entity remained open and were perceived as a promise for the future.

Although previously it had been an immensely powerful tool for shaping and preserving Israeli identity, the settler movement transformed it into a political factor through which the conquered territories are understood. The restorative visions among the religious public after 1967 represented different interpretations of "sacred history," expressing a variety of theological and political desires for the future of the State of Israel, the land of Israel and the conquered territories. The Bible's past still lies ahead.

Notes

1 Anita Shapira, "The Bible and Israeli Identity," *AJS review* 28:1 (2004).
2 For the messianic basis in religious Zionism, see Dov Schwartz, *Religious-Zionism: History and Ideology*, Academic Studies Press, Boston 2009. See also David Ohana, "Nationalizing Land: Gershom Scholem's Children and the 'Canaanite Messianism'," in *Nationalizing Judaism: Zionism as a Theological Ideology*, Lexington Books, Lanham 2017, 95–130.
3 Gershom Scholem, "Toward an Understanding of the Messianic Idea in Judaism," in *The Messianic Idea in Judaism: And Other Essays on Jewish Spirituality*, New York,

Schocken Books 1971, 13; Moshe Idel, "Messianic Scholars: On Early Israeli Scholarship, Politics and Messianism," *Modern Judaism* 32:1 (2012). Ibid., *Old Worlds, New Mirrors: On Jewish Mysticism and Twentieth-Century Thought*, University of Pennsylvania Press, Philadelphia 2010. For further reading see: Kenneth Seeskin, *Jewish Messianic Thoughts in an Age of Despair*, Cambridge University Press, New York 2012. Jonathan (Ed.) Jonathan Frankel, *Jews and Messianism in the Modern Era: Metaphor and Meaning*, Oxford University Press, New York 1991. Michael L. Morgan and Steven Weitzman, (eds.) *Rethinking the Messianic Idea in Judaism*, Indiana University Press, Bloomington 2014; Randi Rashkover and Martin Kavka, (eds.) *Judaism, Liberalism, and Political Theology*, Indiana University Press, Bloomington 2013.

4 For further reading on Messianism, Redemption and Utopianism in Jewish non-Zionist context, see Pierre Bouretz, *Witnesses for the Future: Philosophy and Messianism*, Johns Hopkins University Press, Baltimore MD 2010; Zachary Braiterman, *The Shape of Revelation: Aesthetics and Modern Jewish Thought*, Stanford University Press, Stanford CA 2007; Vivian Liska, *Giorgio Agambens leerer Messianismus: Hannah Arendt, Walter Benjamin, Franz Kafka*, Schlebrügger, Wien 2008; Stéphane Mosès, *The Angel of History: Rosenzweig, Benjamin, Scholem*, Stanford University Press Stanford CA 2009; Elke Dubbels, *Figuren des Messianischen in Schriften deutsch-jüdischer Intellektueller 1900–1933*, vol. 79, Boston: De Gruyter, Berlin 2011.

5 More on the historical development of *Replacement Theology* see Ronald E Diprose, *Israel and the Church: The Origins and Effects of Replacement Theology*, InterVarsity Press, Waynesboro, GA 2004. The *Nostra Aetate* declaration from 1965 marks a new attitude of the Catholic Church toward Judaism and acknowledges the unique relation of God to the Jews:

> The Church remembers the bond that spiritually ties the people of the New Covenant to Abraham's stock [...] God holds the Jews most dear for the sake of their Fathers; He does not repent of the gifts He makes or of the calls.

However, as opposed to the Protestant reading that was examined above, that designated the Jews with an important eschatological role, the Catholic Church "remembers": The Church, therefore, cannot forget that she received the revelation of the Old Testament through the people with whom God in His inexpressible mercy concluded the Ancient Covenant." (§4) It is for this reason that the declaration carefully distinguishes between Judaism and the Jews, and the Jewish State, i.e. the State of Israel. The full declaration can be found at: www.vatican.va/archive/hist_councils/ii_vatican_council/documents/vat-ii_decl_19651028_nostra-aetate_en.html.

6 Samuel Goldman, *God's Country: Christian Zionism in America*, University of Pennsylvania Press, Philadelphia PA 2018, 23.

7 John Calvin, *Commentaries on the Epistles of Paul the Apostle*, trans. John Owen, Eerdmans, Grand Rapids MI 1947, 438.

8 Ibid., 410.

9 See Goldman, *God's Country: Christian Zionism in America*, 140–141.

10 Jonathan Edwards, "Notes on the Apocalypse," in *Works of Jonathan Edwards Online, vol. 5, Apocalyptic Writings*, New Haven, Yale University Press 1957, 133–134.

11 Wilbur M. Smith, *World Crises and the Prophetic Scriptures*, Moddy Press, Chicago IL 1951, 181.

12 John Hagee, *Final Dawn over Jerusalem*, Thomas Nelson, Nashville TN 1998 9.

13 Reinhold Niebuhr et al., "Jerusalem Should Remain Unified," *New York Times*, July 12, 1967, 12.

14 John S. Feinberg, "Why Christians Should Support Israel," *Fundamentalist Journal* 1:1 (1982).

15 Hillel Cohen, "Islamic Renovated Traditions on the Return of Israel to its Land in the Zionist-Messianic Discourse" (in Hebrew), *Jama'a* 10 (2003): 183.

16 Muhammad Al-Hussaini, "The Qur'an's Covenant with the Jewish People Claims to the Holy Land," *Middle East Quarterly* Fall (2009).

17 Robert Spencer, "The Qur'an: Israel Is Not for the Jews Claims to the Holy Land," ibid.

18 A historical episode that reflects the rights of Judaism, Christianity and Israel to Jerusalem and the Holy Land is the crusaders' encounter with Salah ad-Din. For further reading see Paul M. Cobb, *Race for Paradise: An Islamic History of the Crusades*, Oxford University Press, Oxford 2014, 33–35.

19 David Ohana, *The Origins of Israeli Mythology: Neither Canaanites nor Crusaders*, Cambridge University Press, New York 2012, 30.

20 M. Simon, "The State of Israel is estranged from the Land of Israel," *Nekuda: The Newspaper of the Settlements in Judea, Samaria and the Gaza Strip* (in Hebrew) 100 (1986).

21 Aharon Kellerman, *Society and Settlement: Jewish Land of Israel in the Twentieth Century*, State University of New York Press, Albany NY 1993, 33–62. See also Dov Weintraub, Moshe Lissak, and Y. Atzmon, *Moshava, Kibbutz, and Moshav: Patterns of Jewish Rural Settlement and Development in Palestine*, Ithaca NY, Cornell University Press 1969.

22 Boaz Neumann offers a psychoanalytical analysis of the pioneers' motivations. See: Boaz Neumann, *Land and Desire in Early Zionism*, trans. Haim Watzman, Brandeis University Press, Waltham MA 2011, 29–34, 111–115.

23 Oz Almog, *The Sabra: The Creation of the New Jew*, trans. Haim Watzman, University of California Press: Berkeley, CA 2000, 173–184. Gideon Bar, "Reconstructing the Past: The Creation of Jewish Sacred Space in the State of Israel, 1948–1967," *Israel Studies* 13:3 (2008): 1–21.

24 Yehoshua Arieli, "Interpretations of American Nationalism," in *History and Meta-History*, ed. David Ohana, Bialik Institute, Jerusalem 2003, 306–331.

25 Heidegger locates a *not-yet* which grounds the constitution of our own selves, or the Dasein, which "exists in just such a manner that its 'not-yet' belongs to it." Death. Death is not something that comes at the end of our days, death is something one lives at each moment and through which all things attain meaning:

> In death, Dasein has not been fulfilled nor has it simply disappeared; it has not become finished nor is it wholly at one's disposal as something ready-to-hand. On the contrary, just as Dasein is already its "not-yet," and is its "not-yet" constantly as long as it is, it is already its end too. The "ending" which we have in view when we speak of death, does not signify Dasein's Being-at-an-end [Zu-Ende-sein], but a Being-towards-the-end [Sein zum Ende] of this entity. Death is a way to be, which Dasein takes over as soon as it is. "As soon as man comes to life, he is at once old enough to die."

Martin Heidegger, *Being and Time*, trans. J. Macquarrie and E. Robinson, Harper & Row, New York 1962, 287 [43], 89 [45]. More on the different senses of the *not-yet* see §§46–48. See also Carol J. White, *Time and Death: Heidegger's Analysis of Finitude*, Routledge, Ashgate 2005, 67. Following the line of Martin

Heidegger's philosophy, post-modern theologians assert that the presence of God is in his absence. An interesting use of the Heideggerian absence is made by the theologian Lous Marie Chauvet to address the mystery of the Eucharist as a "presence of absence." See, Louis Marie Chauvet, *Symbol and Sacrament: A Sacramental Reinterpretation of Christian Existence*, Liturgical Press, Collegeville MN 1995, 61–63.

26 Ezra Stiles, *The United States Elevated to Glory and Honor. A Sermon Given to the Connecticut General Assembly*, Thomas & Samuel Green, New Haven CT 1783, 6.

27 On the secular theological longing for the ancient sites which was reflected in the adoption of their names, see "A confession Regarding Our Language" (Gershom Scholem to Franz Rosenweig, December 26, 1926) in William Cutter, "Ghostly Hebrew, Ghastly Speech: Scholem to Rosenzweig," 1926, *Prooftexts* 10:3, September 1990, 417–418.

28 Ernst Akiva Simon, "Are We Israelis Still Jews?," *Commentary* 15 (1953).

29 Baruch Kurzweil, "Essence and Sources of the 'Young Hebrews' ('Canaanite') Movement," in *Our New Literature: Continuation or Revolution* (in Hebrew), Schocken, Tel Aviv 1959.

30 Yeshayahu Leibowitz, "After Qibya," in *Judaism, the Jewish People, and the State of Israel* (in Hebrew), Schocken, Jerusalem 1975, 229–234. David Ohana, "Yeshayahu Leibowitz: Radical Intellectual and the Criticism of Canaanite Messianism," in *Yeshayahu Leibowitz: Between Conservatism and Radicalism – Discussions of his Doctrine* (in Hebrew), ed. Aviezer Ravitzky, Hakibbutz Hameuhad and the Van Leer Jerusalem Institute, Tel Aviv 2007, 155–177.

31 Shapira, op. cit., 10. See also Tali Tadmor Shimony, "Teaching the Bible as a Common Culture," *Jewish History*, 21:2, June 2007, 159–178.

32 *Ground* or *Grund* in Heideggerian terms is the basic interpretative principle.

33 Shapira, op. cit., 17.

34 Adam Zartal, "Go to Mound Ebal," *Ha'aretz* (in Hebrew), November 12, 1999.

35 Yoel Elitzur, *Ancient Place Names in the Land of Israel, their Preservation and Metamorphoses* (in Hebrew), Academy of the Hebrew Language: Jerusalem: Academy of the Hebrew Language, 2009, 1.

36 On the legitimizing the settlement project see Michael Feige, *Settling in the Hearts: Jewish Fundamentalism in the Occupied Territories*, Wayne University Press, Detroit 2009, 247–282.

37 On the legitimization of the return to the land by the early Zionist pioneers versus the Arabs' claim to the land, see Neumann, *Land and Desire in Early Zionism*, trans. Haim Watzman, Brandeis University Press, Waltham MA 2011, 83–89.

38 Ohana, *The Origins of Israeli Mythology: Neither Canaanites nor Crusaders*, Cambridge University Press, New York 2012.

39 Harry Emerson Fosdick, *A Pilgrimage to Palestine*, Macmillan, New York 1927, 286.

40 For further reading see Maoz Azaryahu and Arnon Golan, "(Re)naming the Landscape: The Formation of the Hebrew Map of Israel 1949–1960," *Journal of Historical Geography* 27:2 (April 2001); Saul B. Cohen and Nurit Kliot, "Place-Names in Israel's Ideological Struggle over the Administered Territories," *Annals of the Association of American Geographers* 82:4 (1992).

41 Nachman Ben-Yehuda, *Masada Myth: Collective Memory and Mythmaking in Israel*, University of Wisconsin Press, Madison WI 1996.

42 Mircea Eliade, *Images and Symbols: Studies in Religious Symbolism*, vol. 42, Princeton University Press, New Jersey 1991. Benjamin Z. Kedar and R.J. Zwi Werblowsky (eds.),

Sacred Space: Shrine, City, Land: Proceedings from the International Conference in Memory of Joshua Prawer, Palgrave, London 1998.

43 Benedict Anderson, *Imagined Communities: Reflections on the Origin and Spread of Nationalism*, Verso, London 1983.

44 But it is ironical that several outposts in Judea and Samaria have been named after victims of terrorism.

45 Ze'ev Erlich, "House for a Child and Not for the Builder," *Nekuda: The Newspaper of the Settlements in Judea, Samaria and the Gaza Strip* (in Hebrew) 3 (1980): 16.

46 In the last decades of the twentieth century, the most commonly used expression for the settlement areas was Judea, Samaria, and Gaza.

47 Moshe Greenberg, *On the Bible and Judaism: A Collection of Articles*, Am Oved, Tel Aviv 1986 (in Hebrew).

48 David Ben-Gurion, *Studies of the Bible* (in Hebrew), Am Oved, Tel Aviv 1976, 61.

49 Eliezer Schweid, *Homeland and Land of Destiny: The Land of Israel in the Jewish People's Thought* (in Hebrew), Am Oved, Tel Aviv 1979. For the attitude of the First Aliyah (immigration) to the land of Israel, see: Yaffa Berlowitz, *Inventing a Land, Inventing a Nation: Literary and Cultural Infrastructures in the Creativity of the First Aliya* (in Hebrew), Hakibbutz Hameuhad, Tel Aviv 1996.

50 See Aviezer Ravitzky, *Messianism, Zionism, and Jewish Religious Radicalism*, trans. Michael Swirsky and Jonathan Chipman, University of Chicago Press, Chicago IL 1996.

51 Author's hearing testimony.

52 Gideon Aran, "Return to the Scripture in Modern Israel," in *Les retours aux Écritures: fondamentalismes présents et passes*, ed. Évelyne Patlagean, Louvain; Peeters, Paris 1993, 111.

53 Uri Avnery, "The Canaanites and Gush Emunim," *Ha'Olam Hazeh*, September 22, 1982 (in Hebrew).

54 Eliezer Goldman, "Simplified Messianism," *Betfotzot Hagula* (in Hebrew) (1977): 79–80.

55 Baruch Kurzweil, "Israel and the Diaspora," in *Struggle over Jewish Values* (in Hebrew), Schocken, Jerusalem 1969, 255.

56 Yeshayahu Leibowitz, *Judaism, the Jewish People, and the State of Israel* (in Hebrew), Schoken, Jerusalem, 1975, 420.

57 Ehud Ben-Ezer, "Zionism – Dialectic of Continuity and Rebellion (Interview)," in *Continuity and Rebellion – Gershom Shalom in Statement and Discourse* (in Hebrew), ed. Avraham Shapira, Schocken, Tel Aviv 1994.

58 Boaz Evron, *A National Reckoning*, Dvir, Tel Aviv 1988, 364 (in Hebrew).

59 Anita Shapira, "The People as Human Beings," *Gateway Thoughts* (n.d.), 25 (in Hebrew).

60 Haim Be'er, "Gush Emunim: Canaanites who Wear Phylacteries," *Davar*, October 15, 1982 (in Hebrew).

61 Amnon Rubinstein, *From Herzl to Rabin and Onward: One Hundred Years of Zionism* (in Hebrew), Schocken: Jerusalem, 1997, 138.

62 Be'er, op. cit.

63 Yosef Ben-Shlomo, "What is the Highest Value: The Concept of the State or the Concept of the Land? – A Response to David Ohana," in *Where Do We Live?* ed. Yona Hadari, Netanya: Ahiasaf, 2007, 275–282 (in Hebrew).

64 "I have no doubt that we will return to the 47 boundaries – interview with Prof. Yosef Ben-Shlomo," *Histadrut Hamorim* (in Hebrew) 6 (July) (1998).

65 Ben-Shlomo, ibid.

66 See J.L. Talmon, *Political Messianism: The Romantic Phase*, Praeger: New York 1960. See also David Ohana's introduction to Talmon, *Mission and Testimony: Political Essays, with Epilogue by Isaiah Berlin*, Sussex Academic Press, Chicago 2015.

67 Aharon Megged, "Bible Now," *Ha'aretz*, July 25, 1986 (in Hebrew).

68 Ravitzky, *Messianism, Zionism, and Jewish Religious Radicalism*, 58.

69 Rabbi Abraham Isaac Kook with Commentary by Rav Ze'ev Soltanowitch, *Light of Israel* (in Hebrew), Har Bracha, Machon Har Bracha, 2008, f–g.

70 Gideon Aran, *Kookism: The Roots of Gush Emunim, Settler Culture, Zionist Theology, Contemporary Messianism*, Carmel: Jerusalem 2013.

71 Avi Sagi and Dov Schwartz, *Religious Zionism and the Six-Day War*, Carmel: Jerusalem 2017 (in Hebrew).

72 See Dov Schwartz, "The Conquest of the Land and the Attitude to the Nations Inhabiting it: Approaches in Religious Zionist Theory," *Kathedra* 111 (2011): 79 (in Hebrew).

73 Aran, op. cit. 117.

74 Sagi and Schwartz, op. cit.

75 This trend had already begun during the rebellion of the young people of the National Religious Party at the beginning of the 1960s, prior to the Six-Day War. See, Dov Schwartz, "From Growth to Fulfillment: The History of the Religious Zionist Movement and Its Ideas," in *Religious Zionism: The Age of Transformations, an Anthology of Research in Memory of Zvulum Hammer*, ed. Harel Y. and A. Cohen, Mossad Bialik, Jerusalem 2004, 124–134 (in Hebrew).

76 Anita Shapira, "The Bible in Israeli Experience," in *Modern Jewish Time*, ed. Yirmiyahu Yovel, Keter, Jerusalem 2007, 169.

77 See particularly, Uriel Simon, *The Status of the Bible in Israeli Society: From National Midrash to Existential Simplification*, Arana Hass, Jerusalem 1999 (in Hebrew).

78 This school became known among the general public following the publication of the article by Ze'ev Herzog, "The Bible: There Are No Findings in the Field," *Ha'aretz*, October 29, 1999 (in Hebrew). See also Israel Finkelstein, *The Beginnings of Israel: Archeology, Bible, and Historical Memory*, Tel Aviv University Press: Tel Aviv 2003 (in Hebrew). An important representative of the Jerusalem School, that opposes Finkelstein and the Tel Aviv School, is Yosef Garfinkel who claims that his studies of Khirbet Qeiyafa refutes the latter claims. See Yosef Garfinkel, Saar Ganor, and Michael Hasel, "Khirbet Qeiyafa," ed. Daniel M. Master, *The Oxford Encyclopedia of the Bible and Archaeology*, Oxford University Press, Oxford 2013.

79 Yoel Bin Nun, for example, turns the critical demands of the "Tel Aviv school" against themselves, in the sense of demanding that they live up to their own principles:

> It is our duty to determine that this situation of biblical research … [reflect] the limitations of the research itself, that has reached a dead end and has not been able to forge ahead. It is not reasonable to base oneself on the Bible wherever an archeological-historical basis has been found, while wherever nothing has been found, there is a rush on the Bible that is changed into a later legend or it is ignored completely.

Yoel Bin Nun, "'Ba El Halth': A new solution for identifying Ai," (in Hebrew) (paper presented at the Research in Judea and Samaria, 1992).

80 Udi Abramowitz, "The Political Theology of Rabbi Zvi Tau and his Circle" (in Hebrew), Ben-Gurion University, 2014.

81 Yishai Rosen Zvi, "Metaphysics in the Making: Polemics at the Rabbi Kook Institute – A Critical View," in *A Hundred Years of Religious Zionism*, ed. Avi Sagi and Dov Schwartz, Ramat Gan, Bar-Ilan University, 2003, 421–445 (in Hebrew).

82 Luke 24: 30–32.

83 Leibowitz, *Judaism, the Jewish People, and the State of Israel*, Jerusalem 1975 (in Hebrew), 475.

84 Harry Rimmer, *The Shadow of Coming Events*, Wm. Eerdmans, Grand Rapids MI 1946, 63–64.

85 Maimonides, "Laws of Kings," in *Mishneh Torah* (in Hebrew), ed. Yohai Makbili, Haifa: Yeshivat Or Veyeshua, 2006, 3, 6.

86 For a critique of the theological sources of Rabbi Tau, see: David Sorotzkin, *Orthodoxy and the Regime of Modernity: The Production of Jewish Tradition in Modern Europe*, Hakibbutz Hameuhad: Tel Aviv 2012 (in Hebrew).

87 See particularly, Yehiel Harari, *Mysticism as Messianic: Rhetoric in the Works of Rabbi Yitzchak Ginsburgh* (in Hebrew), Tel Aviv University, Tel Aviv 2005; Raphael Sagi, *Messianic Radicalism in the State of Israel: Chapters on the Messianic Amendment in the Philosophy of Rabbi Yitzchak Ginsburgh*, Gyanim, Tel Aviv 2015 (in Hebrew). See also, Gideon Aran, "The Rabbi Who Believes that Killing Non-Jews is Sanctification of God," *Ha'aretz*, March 25, 2016.

88 Yitzchak Ginsburgh, "Renewing the Internal Monarchy," *Makor Rishon*, May 8, 2015 (in Hebrew).

89 Ginsburgh, "From the Monarchy of Saul to the Monarchy of David" (in Hebrew), www.pnimi.org.il.

90 Ibid.

91 Haviva Pedaya sees relations of humility and pride among the religious Zionists as a feeling of joy, while for Chabad this is a feeling of sadness. See Haviva Pedaya, "Land, Time, and Place – Apocalypses of End and Apocalypses of Beginning," in *The Land of Israel in Twentieth Century Jewish Philosophy*, ed. Aviezer Ravitzky, Yad Ben-Zvi, Jerusalem 2005, 560–624 (in Hebrew).

92 In Hegelian dialectics, the term *aufheben* indicates negativity and preservation in the midst of elevation.

93 Non-legalistic exegetical texts in the classical rabbinic literature of Judaism, particularly as recorded in the Talmud and Midrash.

94 "About the Place," interview of Rabbi Meidan by Yoav Sorek, *Makor Rishon*, December 12, 2014 (in Hebrew).

95 Assaf Harel, "Post Gush Emunim: On Faith, Redemption and Messianism in the West Bank Settlements," *Theory and Criticism* 47 (2016): 164.

96 Menachem Froman, *The Heavens of our Land: Peace, People, Land*, Yediot Aharonot: Tel Aviv 2014, 47 (in Hebrew).

97 Ibid., 59–60.

98 Harel, op. cit., 173.

99 A.B. Yehoshua, "Afterword." In Froman, op. cit.

100 Rabbi Meir Kahane was an Israeli ultra-nationalistic politician, one of the cofounders of the *Jewish Defense League*, a member of the Knesset. He was murdered by a Palestinian in 1990.

101 "The Arabs' Hatred is Equivalent to Nazism," Channel 7 website, March 9, 2008 (in Hebrew).

102 Dov Lior, "Disobeying the Order on Secularity in the Army" (in Hebrew), www. yeshiva.org.il/ask/?cat=373.

103 Other rabbis joined in Rabbi Shapira's call, Channel 7 website, October 24, 2004.

104 Zali Gurewitz and Gideon Aran state that "the sense of place in Genesis is a constant feeling of moving to the place, within the place and outside the place." However, Abraham's move to the Promised Land is not wandering towards a place but is moving about in the land. See, Zali Gurewitz and Gideon Aran, "Israeli Anthropology," *Alpayim* 4 (1992).

Bibliography

Aharonsohn, Ran, *Rothschild and Early Jewish Colonization in Palestine*, Rowman & Littlefield, Lanham 2000.

Abramowitz, Udi, "The Political Theology of Rabbi Zvi Tau and his Circle," Diessertation submitted to the Ben-Gurion University, 2014 (in Hebrew).

Adler, Cyrus, *Solomon Schechter: A Biographical Sketch*, Andesite Press, London 2017.

Al-Hussaini, Muhammad, "The Qur'an's Covenant with the Jewish People Claims to the Holy Land," *Middle East Quarterly* Fall (2009): 9–14.

Almog, Oz, *The Sabra: The Creation of the New Jew*, trans. Haim Watzman, University of California Press: Berkeley, CA 2000.

Améry, Jean, *At The Mind's Limits: Contemplations by a Survivor on Auschwitz and its Realities*, Indiana University Press, Bloomington 1980.

Anderson, Benedict, *Imagined Communities: Reflections on the Origin and Spread of Nationalism*, Verso, London 1983.

Appelfeld, Aharon, *First Person Essays*, Jerusalem 1979 (in Hebrew).

Aran, Gideon, "From Religious Zionism to Zionist Religion: The Roots of Gush Emunim," *Studies in Contemporary Jewry*, 2 (1986): 116–143.

Aran, Gideon, "Return to the Scripture in Modern Israel," in *Les retours aux Écritures: fondamentalismes présents et passes*, ed. Évelyne Patlagean, Peeters: Paris 1993.

Aran, Gideon, *Kookism: The Roots of Gush Emunim, Settler Culture, Zionist Theology, Contemporary Messianism*, Carmel, Jerusalem 2013 (in Hebrew).

Aran, Gideon and Michael Feige, "The Movement to Stop the Withdrawal in Sinai; A Sociological Perspective," *The Journal of Applied Behavioral Science*, 23:1 (1987): 73–88.

Arel, Niza, *Without Fear or Impropriety*, Jerusalem 2006 (in Hebrew).

Arieli, Yehoshua, *Individualism and Nationalism in American Ideology*, Harvard University Press, Cambridge MA 1964.

Arieli, Yehoshua, "Interpretations of American Nationalism," in *History and Meta-History*, ed. David Ohana, Bialik Institute, Jerusalem 2003, 306–331.

Avineri, Shlomo, *Moses Hess: Prophet of Communism and Zionism*, New York University Press, New York 1987.

Avnery, Uri, "The Canaanites and Gush Emunim," *Ha'Olam Hazeh*, September 22, 1982 (in Hebrew).

Azaryahu, Maoz, *State Rituals*, Sde Boker 1995 (in Hebrew).

Azaryahu, Maoz, "Mt. Herzl: An Historical Outline of the National Cemetery in Jerusalem," *Ophacim BeGeographia*, 64–65 (2005): 369–383 (in Hebrew).

Azaryahu, Maoz and Arnon Golan, "(Re)naming the Landscape: The Formation of the Hebrew Map of Israel 1949–1960," *Journal of Historical Geography* 27:2 (April 2001): 178–195.

Baba, Homi, *The Location of Culture*, Routledge, London 1994.

Bar, Gideon, "Reconstructing the Past: The Creation of Jewish Sacred Space in the State of Israel, 1948–1967," *Israel Studies* 13:3 (2008): 1–21.

Bar-Zohar, Michael, *Ben-Gurion*, New York 1986.

Bar-Zohar, Michael, *Ben-Gurion*, Vol. 3, Tel Aviv 1987 (in Hebrew).

Be'er, Haim, "Gush Emunim: Canaanites who Wear Phylacteries", *Davar*, October 15, 1982 (in Hebrew).

Be'er, Haim, "The Father's Branch," *Literature and Life: Poetics and Ideology in the new Hebrew Literature – To Menachem Brinker in his 70's*, eds., Iris Parush, Hamutal Zamir and Hannah Suker-Schweger, Jerusalem 2011 (in Hebrew).

Ben-Ezer, Ehud, *Unease in Zion*, ed., Robert Alter, New York 1974.

Ben-Ezer, Ehud, "Zionism – Dialectic of Continuity and Rebellion (Interview)," in: ed. Avraham Shapira, *Continuity and Rebellion – Gershom Shalom in Statement and Discourse*, Schocken, Tel Aviv 1994 (in Hebrew).

Ben-Gurion, David, *Studies of the Bible*, Am Oved, Tel Aviv 1976 (in Hebrew).

Benhabib, Dolly, "Skirts Are Shorter Now: Comments on Levantine Female Identity in the Writings of Jacqueline Kahanoff," *Theory and Criticism – An Israeli Forum*, 5 (1994): 159–164 (in Hebrew).

Benjamin, Walter, "Theories of German Fascism," *New German Critique*, Spring (1979): 120–128.

Benjamin, Walter, *The Work of Art in the Age of Mechanical Reproduction*, CreateSpace Independent Publishing Platform, Seattle 2010.

Ben-Shlomo, Yosef, "What is the Highest Value: The Concept of the State or the Concept of the Land? – A Response to David Ohana," in: ed. Yona Hadari, *Where Do We Live?* Netanya 2007, 275–284 (in Hebrew).

Benvenisti, Meron, *Sacred Landscape*, University of California Press, Berkeley 2000.

Ben-Yehuda, Nachman, *Masada Myth: Collective Memory and Mythmaking in Israel*, University of Wisconsin Press, Madison WI 1996.

Berdichevsky, Micha Yosef Bin-Gorin, "Thoughts/Age and Youth," *The Collected Works of Micha Yosef Bin-Gorin*, Tel Aviv 1951 (in Hebrew).

Berdichevsky, Micha Yosef, "Towards the Question of the Past," *The Writings of Bin-Gorin*, in: Menachem Brinker, *Narrative Art and Social Thought in Y. H. Brenner's Work*, Tel Aviv 1990 (in Hebrew).

Berkowitz, Michael, "Robert S. Wistrich and European Jewish History: Straddling the Public and Scholarly Spheres," *The Journal of Modern History*, Vol. 70 (March 1998): 119–136.

Berlowitz, Yaffa, *Inventing a Land, Inventing a Nation: Literary and Cultural Infrastructures in the Creativity of the First Aliya*, Hakibbutz Hameuhad, Tel Aviv 1996 (in Hebrew).

Bet-El, Ilana, "Rituals, Education and History: The Memorial Days of the Holocaust and the National Memorial Day in Israeli Schools," in: eds., Emanuel Atkes and Rivka Paldachi, *Education and History*, Jerusalem 1998, 457–479 (in Hebrew).

Bialik, Haim Nahman, "On the Verge of the Beth Midrash," 1893, https://benyehuda.org/bialik/bia012.html, taken in 8/3/2019 (in Hebrew).

Bialik, Haim Nahman, "On the Gathering of Spirit," A lecture in the 'Am Ivrit' congress, London 1925, in: ed. Menachem Brinker, *The Hebrew Literature as a European Literature*, Carmel Publishing Press, Jerusalem 2016 (in Hebrew).

Bialik, Haim Nachman, "Metei Midbar" (The Desert Dead), *The Writings of H. N. Bialik*, Tel Aviv 1993 (in Hebrew).

Billing, Michael, *Banal Nationalism*, SAGE Publications, London 1995.

Bilu, Yoram and Eyal Ben-Ari, "Modernity and Charisma in Contemporary Israel: The Case of Baba Sali and Baba Baruch," *The Shaping of Israeli Identity*, 224–237.

Borochov, Ber, *Selected Works of Ber Borochov*, CreateSpace 2011.

Bouretz, Pierre, *Witnesses for the Future: Philosophy and Messianism*, Johns Hopkins University Press, Baltimore MD 2010.

Braiterman, Zachary, *The Shape of Revelation: Aesthetics and Modern Jewish Thought*, Stanford University Press, Stanford CA 2007.

Braudel, Fernand, *The Mediterranean and the Mediterranean World in the Age of Philip II*, University of California Press, Berkeley 1972.

Braudel, Fernand, *La Méditerranée et le monde méditerranéen à l'époque de Philippe II*, Paris 1993.

Brenner, Yosef Haim, *Writings*, vol. III, Tel Aviv 1977–1984 (in Hebrew).

Brenner, Yosef Haim, *Collected Essays*, Tel Aviv 1985 (in Hebrew).

Brinker, Menachem, "Brenner's Judaism," *Congress of the Israeli National Academy*, 8 (1985): 211–228.

Brinker, Menachem, "The Influence of Nietzsche on the Hebrew Writers of the Russian Empire," Bernice Glatzer-Rosenthal (ed.), *Nietzsche and the Soviet Culture*, Cambridge University Press, Cambridge 1994.

Brinker, Menachem, "The Jewish Studies in Israel from a 'Secular'-Liberal Perspective," in: eds., Shlomo Fuks, Israel Shpeler and Daniel Marom *Talking Vision – An Invitation to a Discussion on The Purpose of The Jewish Education*, Jerusalem 2006 (in Hebrew).

Brinker, Menachem, "Micha Yosef Berdichevsky (Bin-Gorion)," *New Jewish Time – Jewish Culture in a Secular Age: An Encyclopedic View*, vol. I, Jerusalem 2007 (in Hebrew).

Brinker, Menachem, *Israeli Thoughts*, Jerusalem 2007 (in Hebrew).

Brinker, Menachem, "Hebrew Literature and Zionist Historiography," *Zmanim: Quarterly of History*, 105 (Winter 2009): 16–23 (in Hebrew).

Brinker, Menachem, *Modern Hebrew Literature as a European Literature*, Carmel Publishing Press, Jerusalem 2016 (in Hebrew).

Brinker, Menachem, "The Hebrew Literature is Grounded within European Literature," *Haaretz – Culture and Literature*, 4/3/2016 (in Hebrew).

Brinker, Menachem, *The Hebrew Literature as a European Literature*, Jerusalem 2016 (in Hebrew).

Buber, Martin, *Between a Nation and its Country*, Tel Aviv 1944 (in Hebrew).

Martin Buber, *A Land of Two Peoples: Martin Buber on Jews and Arabs*, ed. Paul Mendes-Flohr, Chicago University Press, Chicago 2005.

Burnce, Frances, ed. and trans., *A. D. Gordon Selected Essays*, Tel Aviv 1938.

Calvin, John, *Commentaries on the Epistles of Paul the Apostle*, trans. John Owen, Eerdmans, Grand Rapids, MI 1947.

Carmi, Na'ama, "The Nationality and Entry into Israel Case Before the Supreme Court of Israel," *Israel Studies Forum*, 22:1 (Summer 2007): 26–53.

Chaubey, Ajay Kumar, ed. *V. S. Naipaul: An Anthology of 21st Century Criticism*, New Delhi 2015.

Chauvet, Louis Marie, *Symbol and Sacrament: A Sacramental Reinterpretation of Christian Existence*, Liturgical Press: Collegeville MN 1995.

Clark, Ronald W., *Einstein: The Life and Times*, Bloomsbury, New York 1971.

Cobb, Paul M., *Race for Paradise: An Islamic History of the Crusades*, Oxford University Press, Oxford 2014.

Cohen, Hillel, "Islamic Renovated Traditions on the Return of Israel to its Land in the Zionist-Messianic Discourse," *Jama'a* 10 (2003): 169–185 (in Hebrew).

Cohen, Saul B. and Nurit Kliot, "Place-Names in Israel's Ideological Struggle over the Administered Territories," *Annals of the Association of American Geographers* 82:4 (1992): 653–680.

Connerton, Paul, *How Societies Remember*, Cambridge University Press, Cambridge 1989.

Cutter, William, "Ghostly Hebrew, Ghastly Speech: Scholem to Rosenzweig," 1926, *Prooftexts* 10:3, (September 1990): 413–433.

Diprose, Ronald E., *Israel and the Church: The Origins and Effects of Replacement Theology*, InterVarsity Press: Waynesboro, GA 2004.

Don-Yechia, Eliezer, "Mamlachtiyut and Judaism in the dictum of Ben-Gurion," Zionism, 14 (1989): 51–81 (in Hebrew).

Dubbels, Elke, *Figuren des Messianischen in Schriften deutsch-jüdischer Intellektueller 1900–1933*, vol. 79, De Gruyter, Berlin and Boston 2011.

Edwards, Jonathan, *Works of Jonathan Edwards Online, vol. 5, Apocalyptic Writings*, New Haven 1957.

Eisenstadt, Shmuel N., *Israeli Society*, CRC Press, New York 1967.

Eisenstadt, Shmuel N., *Multiple Modernities*, Routledge, London 2002.

Eldar, Akiva, and Idith Zertel, Review of Michael Feige, "Lords of the Land: The War Over Israel's Settlements in the Occupied Territories, 1967–2007," *Zmanim*, 93 (2006): 106–109 (in Hebrew).

Elgenius, Gabriella, *Symbols of Nations and Nationalism: Celebrating Nationhood*, Palgrave Macmillan, Basingstoke 2011.

Eliade, Mircea, *Images and Symbols: Studies in Religious Symbolism*, vol. 42, Princeton University Press, New Jersey 1991.

Elitzur, Yoel, *Ancient Place Names in the Land of Israel, their Preservation and Metamorphoses*, Academy of the Hebrew Language, Jerusalem 2009 (in Hebrew).

Erlich, Ze'ev, "House for a Child and Not for the Builder," *Nekuda: The Newspaper of the Settlements in Judea, Samaria and the Gaza Strip* 3, 1980 (in Hebrew).

Evron, Boaz, "Clarifications for our Time – or: Perceived Difference and Real Difference," *Etgar*, 93, 1/10/1964 (in Hebrew).

Evron, Boaz, "Generals and Caves," *Haaretz*, March 26, 1961 (in Hebrew).

Evron, Boaz, "One Revolution in the Land and the Space," *Etgar*, 22, January 12, 1962 (in Hebrew).

Evron, Boaz, "The Character of Martin Buber," *Etgar*, 22, January 12, 1964 (in Hebrew).

Evron, Boaz, "Power and its Perlis," *Etgar*, 133, April 14, 1966 (in Hebrew).

Evron, Boaz, "A Hymn for Jonathan," *Yediot Aharonot*, January 30, 1981 (in Hebrew).

Evron, Boaz, "The Action – And its Academic Reflection," *Yediot Aharonot, Culture, Literature, Art*, March 2, 1984.

Evron, Boaz, *A National Reckoning*, Dvir, Tel Aviv 1988 (in Hebrew).

Evron, Boaz, *Jewish State or Israeli Nation*, Indianapolis 1995.

Evron, Boaz, "Democratic, Not Jewish [State]," *Haaretz*, September 11, 2002 (in Hebrew).

Evron, Boaz, "Political Autobiography," *Athens and Oz*, Tel Aviv 2010 (in Hebrew).

Feige, Michael, "Let the Dead Go: Commemoration Practices in Gush Emunim and Peace Now," in: eds., David Ohana and Robert Wistreich: *Myth and Memory: Transfigurations of Israeli Consciousness*, Van Leer Institute, Jerusalem 1996, 304–320 (in Hebrew).

Feige, Michael, "Archaeology, Anthropology and the Development Town: Constructing the Israeli Place," *Zion*, 63:4 (1998), 441–459 (in Hebrew).

Feige, Michael, "Peace Now and the Legitimation Crisis of 'Civil Militarism'," *Israel Studies*, 3:1 (1998): 85–111.

Feige, Michael, "Rescuing the Person from the Symbol: Peace Now and the Ironies of Modern Myth," *History and Memory*, 11:1 (1999): 141–168.

Feige, Michael, "Gush Emunim and Biblical Names of Settlements," in (ed.) Dani Yaakobi, *Nation Building*, Magnes Press, Jerusalem 2000, 121–130 (in Hebrew).

Feige, Michael, "Yitzhak Rabin: His Commemoration and The Commemoration of his Commemoration," in: ed. Lev Grinberg *Memory in Contrevercy – Myth, Nationality and Democracy*, Hamphrey Institute for Social Studies, Jerusalem 2000 (in Hebrew).

Feige, Michael, "Where is 'Here'?: Scientific Practices and Appropriating Space in the Discourse of Israeli Social Movements," in: eds., A. Paul Hare and Gideon M. Kressel, *Israel as Center Stage: A Setting for Social and Religious Enactments*, Bergin & Garvey, Westport, CT 2001.

Feige, Michael, "Identity, Ritual and Pilgrimage: The Meetings of the Israeli Exploration Society," in: eds., Deborah Dash Moore and S. Ilan Troen, *Divergent Jewish Cultures: Israel and America*, Yale University Press, New Haven 2001, 87–106.

Feige, Michael, "Do Not Weep Rachel: Fundamentalism, Commemoration and Gender in a West Bank Settlement," *Journal of Israeli History*, 21, 1–2 (2002): 119–138.

Feige, Michael, "The Morning After Remembers the Night Before," in (ed.) Meron Benvenisti, *The Morning After: The Age of Peace – Not a Utopia*. Truman Institute, Magnes Press, Jerusalem 2002, 521–568 (in Hebrew).

Feige, Michael, "The Vision of the Broken Bones: Haredim vs. Archeologists in the City of David, 1981," in eds., Emmanuel Sivan and Kimmy Kaplan, *Israeli Haredim: Integration without Assimilation*, Van Leer Institute, Jerusalem 2003, 56–81 (in Hebrew).

Feige, Michael, *One Space, Two Places: Gush Emunim, Peace Now and the Construction of Israeli Space*, Jerusalem 2003 (in Hebrew).

Feige, Michael, "The Names of the Place: New Historiography in Tamar Berger's Dionysus at the Center," *Israel Studies Review*, 19, 2 (2004): 54–74.

Feige, Michael, "Mini Israel: The Israeli Place Between the Global and the Miniature," in, eds., Julia Brauch, Anna Lipphardt and Alexandra Nocke, *Jewish Topographies: Visions of Space, Traditions of Place*, Aldershot 2008, 327–342.

Feige, Michael, "The Yom Kipur War in Israeli Memory: Break and Continuiety," in, eds., Moshe Shemesh and Ze'ev Drori, *National Trauma, Yom kippur War: After Thirty Years and Another War*, The Ben-Gurion Research Institute, Sde Boker 2008, pp. 351–366 (in Hebrew).

Feige, Michael, and Zvi Shiloni, eds., *Archeology and Nationalism in Israel*, Ben-Gurion Research Institute, Sde Boker 2008 (in Hebrew).

Feige, Michael, *Settling in the Hearts: Jewish Fundamentalism in the Occupied Territories*, Wayne State University Press, Detroit 2009.

Feige, Michael, "Archaeology's Imagined Communities: On Nationalism, Otherness and the Surface Level," *Democratic Culture*, 12 (2009): 167–206 (in Hebrew).

Feige, Michael, "Privatizing Commemoration: The Helicopter Disaster Monument and the Absent State," in, eds., Rachel S. Harris and Ranen Omer-Sherman, *Narratives of Dissent: War in Contemporary Israeli Arts and Culture*, Wayne State University Press, Detroit 2012, 44–64 (in Hebrew).

Feige, Michael, and David Ohana, "Funeral at the Edge of a Cliff: Israel Bids Farewell to David Ben-Gurion," *Journal of Israeli History*, 31:2 (2012): 249–281.

Feige, Michael, and David Ohana, "Ben-Gurion's commemorative rituals: state rituals at the edge of the desert," *Israel*, Vol. 22 (2014): 159–181 (in Hebrew).

Feige, Michael, "Rabin's Assassination and the Ethnic Margins of Religious Zionism," *Theory and Criticism*, 45 (Winter 2015): 31–56 (in Hebrew).

Feige, Michael, "The Yamit Evacuation and Gush Emunim," *The Fourth Decade*, eds., Yehiam Weiz and Zvi Zameret, Yad Ben-Zvi, Jerusalem 2016, 91–105.

Feige, Michael, *Al Da'at Hamakom, Israeli Realms of Memory*, eds., David Ohana, Sde Boker 2017 (in Hebrew).

Feinberg, John S., "Why Christians Should Support Israel," *Fundamentalist Journal* 1, 1 (1982): 10–17.

Finkelstein, Israel, *The Beginnings of Israel: Archeology, Bible, and Historical Memory*, Tel Aviv University Press: Tel Aviv 2003 (in Hebrew).

Fosdick, Harry Emerson, *A Pilgrimage to Palestine*, Macmillan: New York 1927.

Foucault, Michel, *The Order of Things: An Archaeology of the Human Sciences*, Routledge, London 1994.

Frankel, Jonathan, "The 'Yizkor' book of 1911: A Note on National Myths in the Second Aliya," *Religion, Ideology and Nationalism in Europe and America: Essays Presented in Honor of Yehoshua Arieli*, Historical Society of Israel, Jerusalem 1986, 355–384.

Frankel, Jonathan (Ed.), *Jews and Messianism in the Modern Era: Metaphor and Meaning*, Oxford University Press, New York 1991.

Freundlich, Charles H., *Peretz Smolenskin: His Life and Thought*, Bloch Publishing, New York 1965.

Friedlander, Saul, *Nazi Germany and the Jews, 1933–1945*, New York 2009.

Froman, Menachem, *The Heavens of our Land: Peace, People, Land*, Yediot Aharonot, Tel Aviv 2014 (in Hebrew).

Garfinkel, Yosef, Saar Ganor, and Michael Hasel, "Khirbet Qeiyafa," ed. Daniel M. Master, *The Oxford Encyclopedia of the Bible and Archaeology*, Oxford University Press, Oxford 2013.

Gertz, Nurit, *The Canaanite Group: Literature and Ideology*, Tel Aviv 1987 (in Hebrew).

Ginsburgh, Issac, "From the Monarchy of Saul to the Monarchy of David," www.pnimi. org.il (in Hebrew).

Ginsburgh, Issac, "Renewing the Internal Monarchy," *Makor Rishon*, May 8, 2015 (in Hebrew).

Goldman, Eliezer, "Simplified Messianism," *Betfotzot Hagola* (1977): 79–80 (in Hebrew).

Goldman, Samuel, *God's Country: Christian Zionism in America*, University of Pennsylvania Press, Philadelphia, PA 2018.

Gramsci, Antonio, *Selections from Prison Notebook*, Lawrence & Wishart, London 1971.

Greenberg, Moshe, *On the Bible and Judaism: A Collection of Articles*, Am Oved, Tel Aviv 1986 (in Hebrew).

Gurewitz, Zali and Gideon Aran, "Israeli Anthropology," *Alpayim* 4 (1992).

Guri, Haim, "Burning of Memory," *Ha'aretz – Literary Supplement*, 22.02.2017 (in Hebrew).

Hagee, John, *Final Dawn Over Jerusalem*, Thomas Nelson, Nashville TN 1998.

Handelman, Don, *Models and Mirrors: Towards an Anthropology of Public Events*, Berghahn Books, Cambridge 1990.

Harari, Yehiel, *Mysticism as Messianic: Rhetoric in the Works of Rabbi Yitzchak Ginsburgh*, Tel Aviv University, Tel Aviv 2005 (in Hebrew).

Harel, Assaf, "Post Gush Emunim: On Faith, Redemption and Messianism in the West Bank Settlements," *Theory and Criticism* 47 (2016): 159–180.

Heidegger, Martin, *Being and Time*, trans. J. Macquarrie and E. Robinson, Harper & Row, New York 1962.

Heller, Joseph, *The Stern Gang: Ideology, Politics and Terror, 1940–1949*, London 1985.

Heller, Joseph, *Lehi, Ideology and Politics, 1940–1949*, Jerusalem 1989 (in Hebrew).

Herzl, Theodor, *The Complete Diaries of Theodor Herzl*, vol. 1, ed. Raphael Patai, trans. Harry Zohn, New York 1960.

Herzog, Ze'ev, "The Bible: There Are No Findings in the Field," *Ha'aretz*, October 29, 1999 (in Hebrew).

Hobsbaum, Eric and Terrance Ranger eds., *The Invention of Tradition*, Cambridge University Press, Cambridge 1983.

Holzman, Avner, *Towards the Tear in the Heart: Micha Josef Berdichevsky – The Formative Years (1886 1902)*, Jerusalem 1995 (in Hebrew).

Holzman, Avner, "On the Way to the Transvaluation of Values: On the Place of Nietzsche's Influence in Berdichevsky's Work," in: ed., Jacob Golomb, *Nietzsche in the Hebrew Culture*, Jerusalem 2002 (in Hebrew).

Idel, Moshe, *Old Worlds, New Mirrors: On Jewish Mysticism and Twentieth-Century Thought*, University of Pennsylvania Press, Philadelphia 2010.

Idel, Moshe, "Messianic Scholars: On Early Israeli Scholarship, Politics and Messianism," *Modern Judaism* 32:1, (2012).

Jaron, Steven, "French Modernism and the Emergence of Jewish Conciseness in the Writings of Edmond Jabes," PhD. Dissertation, Columbia University, New York 1997.

Kahanoff, Jacqueline, "Ciao," Poems in the Gnazim Institute of the Writers Association in Tel Aviv.

Kahanoff, Jacqueline, "Claude Vigée: A Portrait of a Poet," *Ma'ariv* (in Hebrew).

Kahanoff, Jacqueline, *Jacob's Ladder*, London 1951.

Kahanoff, Jacqueline, "Israel's Levantinization," 1959, Kahanoff Archive, Gnazim Institute.

Kahanoff, Jacqueline, "What about Levantinization," 1959, Kahanoff Archive, Gnazim Institute, Tel Aviv.

Kahanoff, Jacqueline, *Ramat-Hadassah-Szold: Youth Aliyah Screening and Classification Centre*, Jerusalem 1960.

Kahanoff, Jacqueline, "Wake of the Waves," *Amot*, booklet 2, 1962. Translated from Hebrew in *Mongrels or Marvels*, 136–153.

Kahanoff, Jacqueline, "Charles Péguy," *Amot*, booklet 6–7, June–July, I, 1963, 44–58, II, 1963, 50–65; Reprinted in *Between Two Worlds*, 235–288 (in Hebrew).

Kahanoff, Jacqueline, *Modern African Writing*, edition and introducing by Jacqueline Kahanoff, Tel Aviv 1963 (in Hebrew).

Kahanoff, Jacqueline, ed., *La Grande Ile: Poems Malgaches*, Tel Aviv 1964 (in Hebrew).

Kahanoff, Jacqueline, "Edmond Jabès or The Book of Questions," *Davar*, 30.4.1965 (in Hebrew).

Kahanoff, Jacqueline, "Afterword – From East the Sun," 1968, Kahanoff Archive, Gnazim Institute, Tel Aviv (in Hebrew).

Kahanoff, Jacqueline, "Culture in Becoming," *Davar*, 16.4.1973 (in Hebrew).

Kahanoff, Jacqueline, *From East the Sun*, Tel Aviv 1978 (in Hebrew).

Kahanoff, Jacqueline, "Albert Memmi, or Wilding Road to Israel," *Ma'ariv*, 18.11.1996 (in Hebrew).

Kahanoff, Jacqueline, *Between Two Worlds*, ed. David Ohana, Jerusalem 2005 (in Hebrew).

Kahanoff, Jacqueline, *Mongrels or Marvels: The Levantine Writings of Jacqueline Shohet Kahanoff*, eds., Deborah A. Starr and Sasson Somekh, Stanford University Press, Stanford 2011.

Kahanoff, Jacqueline, *Jacob's Ladder*, trans. Ophira Rahat, Jerusalem 2014 (in Hebrew).

Kedar, Benjamin Z. and R.J. Zwi Werblowsky, eds., *Sacred Space: Shrine, City, Land: Proceedings from the International Conference in Memory of Joshua Prawer*, Palgrave, London 1998.

Keidar, Nir, *Mamlachtiyut: The Civil Conception of David Ben-Gurion*, Sde Boker 2009 (in Hebrew).

Kellerman, Aharon, *Society and Settlement: Jewish Land of Israel in the Twentieth Century*, State University of New York Press, Albany 1993.

Kook, Rabbi Abraham Isaac, with Commentary by Rav Ze'ev Soltanowitch, *Light of Israel*, Har Bracha: Machon Har Bracha (in Hebrew).

Koren, Yehuda, "Relevant Even Today – Albert Camus," *Yediot Aharonot* (in Hebrew).

Kurzweil, Baruch, "Essence and Sources of the 'Young Hebrews' ('Canaanite') Movement," in *Our New Literature: Continuation or Revolution*, Schoken, Tel Aviv 1959 (in Hebrew).

Kurzweil, Baruch, "The Essence and Origins of the 'Young Hebrews' Movement ('Canaanites')," *Our New Literature – Continuity or Revolution?*, Tel Aviv 1964 (in Hebrew).

Kurzweil, Baruch, "Israel and the Diaspora," in *Struggle over Jewish Values*, Schocken, Jerusalem 1969 (in Hebrew).

Laor, Dan, "Kurzweil and the Canaanites: Between Reason and Struggle," *Keshet – Literature, Theory and Criticism Commemoration of Forty Years Since the First Publication*, Tel Aviv 1998 (in Hebrew).

Latur, Bruno, *We Have Never Been Modern*, (trans.) Catherine Porter, Cambridge MA. 1993.

Lebel, Uri, *The Road to the Pantheon: Etzel, Lechi and the Limits of the Israeli Memory*, Schocken, Jerusalem 2007 (in Hebrew).

Leibowitz, Yeshayahu, "After Qibya," in *Judaism, the Jewish People, and the State of Israel*, Schocken, Jerusalem 1975 (in Hebrew).

Leibowitz, Yeshayahu, *Judaism, the Jewish People, and the State of Israel*, Schoken, Jerusalem 1975 (in Hebrew).

Libman, Yeshayahu, *Political Murder: The Murder of Rabin and Political Murder Throughout The Middleast*, Am Oved, Tel Aviv 1998 (in Hebrew).

Liebman, Charles S., and Eliezer Don-Yehia, *Civil Religion in Israel*, Berkeley 1983.

Lindbeck, George, *The Nature of Doctorine*, John Knox Press, Philadelphia 2009.

Lior, Dov, "Disobeying the Order on Secularity in the Army" (in Hebrew), www.yeshiva. org.il/ask/?cat=373.

Liska, Vivian, *Giorgio Agambens leerer Messianismus: Hannah Arendt, Walter Benjamin, Franz Kafka*, Schlebrügger, Wien 2008.

Lustick, Ian, *For the Land and the Lord: Jewish Fundamentalism in Israel*, Council on Foreign Relations Press, New York 1991.

Maimonides, *Mishneh Torah*, ed. Yohai Makbili, Haifa 2006 (in Hebrew).

Mansel, Philip, *Levant: Splendor and Catastrophe on the Mediterranean*, Yale University Press, New Haven 2012.

Megged, Aharon, "Bible Now," *Ha'aretz*, July 25, 1986 (in Hebrew).

Mendes-Flohr, Paul, *Martin Buber: A Life of Faith and Dissent*, Yale University Press, New Haven 2019.

Morgan, Michael L., and Steven Weitzman, eds., *Rethinking the Messianic Idea in Judaism*, Indiana University Press, Bloomington 2014.

Mosès, Stéphane, *The Angel of History: Rosenzweig, Benjamin, Scholem*, Stanford University Press, Stanford CA 2009.

Moshe, HaNeomi (Zinger), "Dalia Ravikobitch Poems Collection," *Ma'ariv*, 11.12.1959 (in Hebrew).

Neumann, Boaz, *Land and Desire in Early Zionism*, trans. Haim Watzman, Brandeis University Press, Waltham, MA 2011.

Neumark, David, "Die Judische Moderne," *Allgemeine Zeitung des Judentums*, Bd. 64, no. 45 (Berlin 1900): 536–538.

Niebuhr, Reinhold, et al., "Jerusalem Should Remain Unified," *New York Times* July 12, 1967.

Nietzsche, Friedrich, *Geneology of Morals*, trans. Ian Johnston, Arlington 2009.

Nir, Henry, "Like all the Gentiles? The Zionist Pioneers in Inter-cultural Context," eds., Anita Shapira, Yehuda Reinhertz and Jacob Harris, *The Age of Zionism*, Jerusalem 2000 (in Hebrew).

Nora, Pierre, *Realms of Memory: Rethinking the French Past*, Vol. 1–2, New York 1996.

Nora, Pierre, "Memory: From Liberty to Tyranny," A lecture in the National Academy of the Sciences in Israel, February 16, 2016.

Nun, Yoel Bin, " 'Ba El Halth': A New Solution for Identifying Ai," (paper presented at the Research in Judea and Samaria, 1992) (in Hebrew).

Ohana, David, "Georges Sorel and the Rise of Political Myth," *History of European Ideas*, 13:6 (1991): 733–746.

Ohana, David, "Zarathustra in Jerusalem: Nietzsche and the 'New Hebrew'," *The Shaping of Israeli Identity*, eds., Robert Wistrich and David Ohana, Frank Cass, London 1995, 38–60.

Ohana, David, *Messianism and Mamlachtiyut: Ben-Gurion and the Intellectuals – Between Political Vision and Political Theology*, Sde Boker 2003 (in Hebrew).

Ohana, David and Robert S. Wistrich, eds., *Myth and Memory*, Tel Aviv 2005 (in Hebrew).

Ohana, David, "The Mediterranean Option in Israel: An Introduction to the Thought of Jacqueline Kahanoff," *Mediterranean Historical Review*, 21:2 (2006): 239–263.

Ohana, David, "Yeshayahu Leibowitz: Radical Intellectual and the criticism of Canaanite Messianism," in *Yeshayahu Leibowitz: Between Conservatism and Radicalism – Discussions of his Doctrine*, ed. Aviezer Ravitzky, Hakibbutz Hameuhad and the Van Leer Jerusalem Institute, Tel Aviv 2007, 155–177 (in Hebrew).

Ohana, David, "J.L. Talmon, Gershom Scholem and the Price of Messianism," *History of European Ideas*, 34:2 (2008): 169–178.

Ohana, David, "Otherness, Absence and Canonization in the Discourse of Literary Historiography: The Case of Jacqueline Kahanoff," *Times of Change: Jewish Literature in the Modern Era, Essays in Honor of Dan Miron*, eds., Michal Arbell and Michael Gluzman, Sede Boker 2008, 235–257 (in Hebrew).

Ohana, David, *Homo Mythicus*, Sussex Academic Press, Eastbourne and Chicago, 2009.

Ohana, David, *Political Theologies in the Holy Land*, London 2010.

Ohana, David, *Israel and Its Mediterranean Identity*, Palgrave Macmillan, London 2011.

David Ohana, *Modernism and Zionism*, Palgrave Macmillan, New York 2012.

Ohana, David, *The Origins of Israeli Mythology: Neither Canaanites nor Crusaders*, Cambridge University Press, New York 2012.

Ohana, David, "Jacqueline Kahanoff Between Levantinism and Mediterraneanism," *New Horizons. Mediterranean Research in the 21st Century*, eds., Mihran Dabag, Dieter Haller and Nikolas Jaspert, Schoeningh Ferdinand GmbH, Bochum 2015.

Ohana, David, "Trailing Nietzsche: Gershom Scholem and the Sabbatean Dialectics," *Nietzsche*-Studien (2016): 224–246.

Ohana, David, "The Secular Perspective of Menachem Brinker," *Haaretz – Culture and Literature*, 4/3/2016 (in Hebrew).

Ohana, David, "Nationalizing Land: Gershom Scholem's Children and the 'Canaanite Messianism'," in *Nationalizing Judaism: Zionism as a Theological Ideology*, Lexington Books, Lanham 2017.

Ohana, David, "Michael Feige's Realms of Memory," Michael Feige, *Al Da'at Ha'makom: Israeli Realms of Memory*, ed., David Ohana, Sde Boker 2017 (in Hebrew).

Ohana, David, *Nationalizing Judaism: Zionism as a Theological Ideology*, Lanham 2017.

Ohana, David, *On Land of Stones: 1967 – The Place of the Israeli Place*, Tel Aviv 2017 (in Hebrew).

Ohana, David, "It Would be a Good Thing if the God of Zarathustra were the God of Israel," *Nietzsche and Jewish Political Thought*, Routledge, London 2018, 31–41.

Ohana, David, "'Civil Cannanism' in the Philosophy of Boaz Evron," in: Israel Segal, *Civil Israelism*, Jerusalem 2018, 157–194 (in Hebrew).

Ohana, David, *Nietzsche and Jewish Political Theology*, Routledge 2018.

Ohana, David, *The Intellectual Origins of Modernity*, Routledge, London 2019.

Oz, Amos, *Unto Death*, trans. Nicholas de Lange, Boston 1978.

Oz, Amos, "The Past Belongs To Us. We Don't Belong To It," *Haaretz – Culture and Literature*, 4/3/2016 (in Hebrew).

Pachter, Henry, "Masters of Cultural History, Gershom Scholem – The Myth of the Mythmaker," *Salmagundi* 40 (Winter 1978): 9–39.

Pedaya, Haviva, "Land, Time, and Place – Apocalypses of End and Apocalypses of Beginning," in: Aviezer Ravitzky ed., *The Land of Israel in Twentieth Century Jewish Philosophy*, Yad Ben-Zvi, Jerusalem 2005 (in Hebrew).

Péguy, Charles, *Eve*, Paris 1913.

Péguy, Charles, *L'Argent*, Paris 1913.

Péguy, Charles, *Notre Jeunesse*, Paris 1957.

Péguy, Charles, *The Mystery of the Charity of Joan of Arc*, trans. Jeffrey Wainwright, Manchester 1986.

Porat, Yehoshua, *The Life Story of Yonatan Ratosh*, Tel Aviv 1989 (in Hebrew).

Rappaport, Roy, *Ecology, Meaning and Religion*, North Atlantic Books, Berkeley 1979.

Rashkover, Randi and Martin Kavka, eds., *Judaism, Liberalism, and Political Theology*, Indiana University Press, Bloomington 2013.

Ratosh, Jonathan, "The Confessions of a Dumber-Than-Average Guy," *Etgar*, 97, November 26, 1964 (in Hebrew).

Ratosh, Jonathan, Letter, Liberty, September 18, 1964 (in Hebrew).

Ravikovitch, Daliah, "Accounting of Cruelty and Compassion," *Yediot Achronot*, 11.1.1963 (in Hebrew).

Ravikovitch, Daliah, Ravikovitch's letter to Kahanoff, 12.5.63, The Gnazim Institute of the Writers Association in Tel Aviv (in Hebrew).

Ravikovitch, Daliah, *All the Poems So Far*, Tel Aviv 1995 (in Hebrew).

Ravikovitch, Daliah, "Delight," *Hovering at a Low Attitude: The Collected Poetry of Daliah Ravikovitch*, trans. Chana Bloch and Chana Kronfeld, W. W. Norton, New York 2009.

Ravikovitch, Daliah, *Daliah Ravikovitch: Complete Poems*, eds., Gidon Tikotski and Uzi Shavit, Tel Aviv 2010 (in Hebrew).

Ravitsky, Aviezer, Yeshayahu Leibowitz: Between Conservatism and Radicalism-Reflections on his Philosophy, Jerusalem 1995, 219–284 (in Hebrew).

Ravitzky, Aviezer, *Messianism, Zionism, and Jewish Religious Radicalism*, trans. Michael Swirsky and Jonathan Chipman, University of Chicago Press, Chicago, IL 1996.

Renan, Ernest, *Qu'est-ce qu'une nation*, Conférence Faite en Sorbonne, 11.3.1882, Paris 1892.

Rimmer, Harry, *The Shadow of Coming Events*, Wm. Eerdmans, Grand Rapids 1946.

Roniger, Luis and Michael Feige, "From Pioneer to Freier: The Changing Models of Generalized Exchange in Israel," *Archives Europeennes De Sociologie*, 33 (1992): 280–307.

Roniger, Luis, and Michael Feige, "From Pioneer to Freier: The Changing Models of Generalized Exchange in Israel," *European Journal of Sociology* 33:2 (1992): 280–307.

Rosen Zvi, Yishai, "Metaphysics in the Making: Polemics at the Rabbi Kook Institute – A Critical View," in: Avi Sagi and Dov Schwartz eds. *A Hundred Years of Religious Zionism*, Ramat Gan, Bar-Ilan University 2003, 421–447 (in Hebrew).

Rosenberg, Shalom, "The Affinity to Erez Israel in Jewish Thought – A Struggle of Outlooks," *Katedra*, 4 (1977): 148–166 (in Hebrew).

Rosenthal, Rubik, "I Feel Estranged in My Own Homeland," *Al-HaMishmar – Hotam*, September 26, 1983 (in Hebrew).

Rotenstreich, Nathan, "Being Zionist in 1976 – An Interview with Yeshayahu Ben Porat," *The Yearbook of Journalists*, Tel Aviv 1975 (in Hebrew).

Rubin, Nisan, *New Rituals, Old Societies: Invented Rituals in Contemporary Israel*, Academic Studies Press, Boston 2009.

Rubinstein, Amnon, *From Herzl to Rabin and Onward: One Hundred Years of Zionism*, Schocken, Jerusalem 1997 (in Hebrew).

Sadan, Dov, *A Man of Many Pains, Between Verdict and Judgment*, Tel Aviv 1965 (in Hebrew).

Sagi, Avi, "Between Love and Politics of Sovereignty," *Against Others: The Ethics of Inner Regression*, Tel Aviv 2012, 107–137 (in Hebrew).

Sagi, Raphael, *Messianic Radicalism in the State of Israel: Chapters on the Messianic Amendment in the Philosophy of Rabbi Yitzchak Ginsburgh*, Gyanim, Tel Aviv 2015 (in Hebrew).

Sagi, Avi and Dov Schwartz, *Religious Zionism and the Six-Day War*, Carmel, Jerusalem 2017 (in Hebrew).

Said, Edward, *Orientalism*, Penguin Books, New York 1978.

Sand, Shlomo, "A National Reckoning," *Theory and Criticism*, special issue: 50 to 48, ed., Adi Ophir, vol. 12–13 (Winter 1999): 339–348.

Sartre, Jean-Paul, *Selected Writings*, ed. Menachem Brinker, Tel Aviv 1972 (in Hebrew).

Sartre, Jean-Paul, *Anti-Semite and Jew*, trans. George J. Becker, Preface by Michael Walzer, New York 1995.

Jean-Paul Sartre, *The Jewish Question: Anti-antisemitism and the Politics of the French Intellectual*, University of Nebraska Press, Nebraska 2009.

Scholem, Gershom, *The Messianic Idea in Judaism: And Other Essays on Jewish Spirituality*, New York 1971 (in Hebrew).

Schorske, Carl, *Fin-de-siecle Vienna – Politics and Culture*, Random House, London 1980.

Schwartz, Dov, "From Growth to Fulfillment: The History of the Religious Zionist Movement and Its Ideas," in: Harel Y. and A. Cohen eds., *Religious Zionism: The Age of Transformations, an Anthology of Research in Memory of Zvulum Hammer*, Mossad Bialik, Jerusalem 2004, 24–134 (in Hebrew).

Schwartz, Dov, *Religious-Zionism: History and Ideology*, Academic Studies Press, Boston 2009.

Schwartz, Dov, "The Conquest of the Land and the Attitude to the Nations Inhabiting It: Approaches in Religious Zionist Theory," *Kathedra* 111 (2011): 75–104 (in Hebrew).

Schweid, Eliezer, *Homeland and Land of Destiny: The Land of Israel in the Jewish People's Thought*, Am Oved, Tel Aviv 1979 (in Hebrew).

Seeskin, Kenneth, *Jewish Messianic Thoughts in an Age of Despair*, Cambridge University Press, New York 2012.

Segev, Tom, *A State at Any Cost: The Life of David Ben-Gurion*, Farrar, Strauss and Giroux, New York 2019.

Shalev, Yizhak, *The Gabriel Tirosh Affair*, Tel Aviv 1964 (in Hebrew).

Shamir, Shimon, ed., *The Jews of Egypt: A Mediterranean Society in Modern Times*, Boulder 1977 (in Hebrew).

Shapira, Anita, "The People as Human Beings," *Gateway Thoughts* (n.d.), p. 25 (in Hebrew).

Shapira, Anita, *The Bible and Israeli Identity*, Cambridge University Press, Cambridge MA 2004.

Shapira, Anita, "The Bible and Israeli Identity," *AJS Review* 28:1 (2004).

Shapira, Anita, "The Bible in Israeli Experience," in *Modern Jewish Time*, Vol. 1, ed. Yirmiyahu Yovel, Keter, Jerusalem 2007, 161–171.

Shavit, Yaakov, *The New Hebrew Nation: A Study in Israeli Heresy and Fantasy*, London 1987.

Shilon, Avi, *Ben-Gurion: An Epilogue*, Tel Aviv 2013 (in Hebrew).

Shilon, Avi, Ben-Gurion: His Later Years in the Political Wilderness, Rowman & Littlefield, Lexington 2016.

Shilon, Avi, "The Influence of the Six-Day War on the Cannanite Idea in its Varieties," *Iyunim BeTkumat Israel*, 11 (2017) (in Hebrew).

Shimony, Tali Tadmor, "Teaching the Bible as a Common Culture," *Jewish History*, 21:2 (June 2007): 159–178.

Shperber, Moshe, ed., *Secularization Process in the Jewish Culture*, Raanana 2013 (in Hebrew).

Shumsky, Dimitry, *Beyond the Nation-State*, New Haven 2018.

Smith, Anthony, *Ethno-Symbolism and Nationalism: A Cultural Approach*, Routledge, Abingdon 2009.

Simon, Ernst Akiva, "Are We Israelis Still Jews?," *Commentary* 15 (April 1953): 357–364.

Simon, M. "The State of Israel is estranged from the Land of Israel," *Nekuda: The Newspaper of the Settlements in Judea, Samaria and the Gaza Strip* (in Hebrew) 100 (1986).

Simon, Uriel, *The Status of the Bible in Israeli Society: From National Midrash to Existential Simplification*, Arana Hass, Jerusalem 1999 (in Hebrew).

Smith, Wilbur M., *World Crises and the Prophetic Scriptures*, Moddy Press, Chicago, IL 1951.

Sorotzkin, David, *Orthodoxy and the Regime of Modernity: The Production of Jewish Tradition in Modern Europe*, Hakibbutz Hameuhad, Tel Aviv 2012 (in Hebrew).

Spencer, Robert, "The Qur'an: Israel Is Not for the Jews Claims to the Holy Land," *Middle East Quarterly* Fall (2009): 3–8.

Stern, Nehemia, Review of: Michael Feige, "Settling in the Hearts: Jewish Fundamentalism in the Occupied Territories," *Review of Middle East Studies*, 45, 1 (Summer 2011): 104–105.

Stiles, Ezra, *The United States Elevated to Glory and Honor. A Sermon Given to the Connecticut General Assembly*, Thomas & Samuel Green, New Haven, CT 1783.

Syrkin, Marie, *Nachman Syrkin: Socialist Zionist*, Herzl Press, New York 1961.

Talmon, J.L., *Political Messianism: The Romantic Phase*, Praeger, New York 1960.

Talmon, J.L., *Mission and Testimony: Political Essays*, in: eds., David Ohana, with Epilogue by Isaiah Berlin, Sussex Academic Press, Chicago IL 2015.

Teveth, Shabtai, "King of the Desert," *Haaretz*, 5/12/1973 (in Hebrew).

Ticotsky, Giddon, *Dahlia Ravikovitch: In Life and Literature*, Haifa 2016 (in Hebrew).

Tikotsky, Gideon, *Daliah Ravikovitch: Life and Literature*, Haifa University Press, Haifa 2016.

Troen, S. Ilan and Rachel Fish, *Essential Israel: Essays for the 21st Century (Perspectives on Israel Studies)*, Indiana University PressIndianapolis 2017.

Turner, Frederick Jackson, *The Frontier in American History*, Toronto 1920.

Turner, Victor, "The Center Out there: Pilgrim's Goal," *History of Religion*, 12:3 (1973): 191–230.

Vigée, Claude, "The Crooked Bridge of Man to the World," *Davar* (in Hebrew).

Vigée, Claude, *Les Artistes de la faim*, Paris 1960.

Vigée, Claude, *Révolte et louanges*, Paris 1962.

Vinitzky-Seroussi, Vered, *Forget-Me-Not: Yitzhak Rabin's Assassination and the Dilemmas of Commemoration*, SUNY Press, Albany 2009.

Volkov, Shulamit, "Exploring the Other: The Enlightenment's Search for the Boundaries of Humanity," in: ed. Robert Wistrich, *Demonizing the Other – Antisemitism, Racism and Xenophobia*, Routledge, London and New York 1999, 148–167.

Walzer, Michael, *Interpretation and Social Criticism*, Harvard University Press, Cambridge MA, 1987.

Weintraub, Dov, Moshe Lissak, and Y. Atzmon, *Moshava, Kibbutz, and Moshav: Patterns of Jewish Rural Settlement and Development in Palestine*, Cornell University Press, Ithaca NY 1969.

Weiss, Hadas, Review of: Michael Feige, "Settling in the Hearts: Jewish Fundamentalism in the Occupied Territories," *Cultural Anthropology*, 24:4 (November 2009): 755–757.

White, Carol J., *Time and Death: Heidegger's Analysis of Finitude*, Routledge, Ashgate 2005.

Wistrich, Robert S., "Karl Kraus – Jewish Prophet or Renegade?," *European Judaism*, 9:2 (Summer 1975): 32–39.

Wistrich, Robert S., "Zionism, Colonialism and the Third World," *The Jewish Chronicles*, 7.1.1976.

Wistrich, Robert S., (co-ed. Walter Laqueur and George L. Mosse), *Theories of Fascism*, London 1976.

Wistrich, Robert S., "Zionism: Revolt against Historic Destiny," *The Jewish Quarterly*, 25:2 (1977): 6–12.

Wistrich, Robert S., "Zionism: Rebellion against History," *Tfuzot Hagola*, 83–84 (1978): 98–105 (in Hebrew).

Wistrich, Robert S., *Socialism and the Jews – The Dilemmas of Assimilation in Germany and Austria-Hungary*, London 1982.

Wistrich, Robert S., *Who's Who in Nazi Germany*, Routledge, London 1982.

Wistrich, Robert S., *Hitler's Apocalypse – Jews and the Nazi Legacy*, London 1985.

Wistrich, Robert S., *The Jews of Vienna in the Age of Franz Joseph*, Oxford 1989.

Wistrich, Robert S., *Between Redemption and Perdition – Modern Antisemitism Jewish Identity*, London 1990.

Wistrich, Robert S., "Zionism and Myths of Assimilation," *Midstream* (Aug–Sept 1990), 3–8.

Wistrich, Robert S. "Antisemitism and the Origins of Zionism," *Between Redemption and Perdition – Modern antisemitism Jewish Identity*, London 1990.

Wistrich, Robert S., "Max Nordau and the Dreyfus Affair," *The Journal of Israeli History*, 16:1 (1995): 1–19.

Wistrich, Robert S., *Weekend in Munich – Art, Propaganda and Terror in the Third Reich*, London 1995.

Wistrich, Robert S. and David Ohana, *The Shaping of Israeli Identity*, eds., Frank Cass, London 1995.

Wistrich, Robert S., "From Cracow to London – A Polish-Jewish Odyssey," in: ed., Slawomir Kapralski, *The Jews in Poland*, Vol. 2, *Judaica Foundation Center for Jewish Culture*, Cracow 1999, 57–73.

Wistrich, Robert S., *Demonizing the Other – Antisemitism, Racism and Xenophobia*, Routledge, London and New York 1999, 148–167.

Wistrich, Robert S., "Max Nordau – From Degeneration to 'Muscular Judaism'," *Transversal*, 2 (2004): 3–21.

Wistrich, Robert S., "The Last Testament of Sigmund Freud," *Leo Baeck Yearbook XLIX*, 2004.

Wistrich, Robert S., "Bernard Lazare, l'affaire Dreyfus et l'antisemitisme," *Cahiers Bernard Lazare* (July/August 2007): 23–26.

Wistrich, Robert S., *Laboratory for World Destruction – Germans and Jews in Central Europe*, University of Nebraska Press, Nebraska 2007.

Wistrich, Robert S., *A Lethal Obsession – Anti-semitism from Antiquity to the Global Jihad*, Random House, New York 2010.

Wistrich, Robert S., "Antisemitism and Jewish Destiny," *The Jerusalem Post*, May 20, 2015.

Wistrich, Robert S., "The European Demons: The First World War Awake from their Slumber," http://mida.org.il/2014/03/06 taken: 2017.

Yehoshua, Abraham B., "Facing the Forest" in William Cutter and David C. Jacobson (eds.), *History and Literature: New Readings of Jewish Texts in Honor of Arnold J. Band*, Providence 2002, 409–418.

Yehoshua, Abraham B., "Menachem Brinker Proves that there is a Special Meaning to Intellectuals," *Haaretz – Culture and Literature*, 4/3/2016.

Yellin-Mor, Nathan, *Fighters of Israel's Liberty, People, Ideas, Stories*, Tel Aviv 1999 (in Hebrew).

Zartal, Adam, "Go to Mound Ebal," *Ha'aretz*, November 12, 1999 (in Hebrew).

Zerubavel, Yael, "The Desert as a Mythical Landscape and as a Memorial Site in the Hebrew Culture," in: Moshe Idel and Itamar Greenold, eds., *The Myths in Judaism: History, Thought, Literature*, Jerusalem 2004, 223–236 (in Hebrew).

Zerubavel, Yael, *Desert in the Promised Land*, Stanford University Press, Stanford CA 2018.

Index

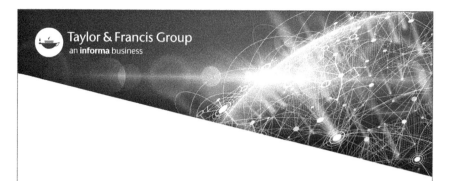